IN VITRO TOXICOLOGY:
TENTH ANNIVERSARY
SYMPOSIUM OF CAAT

ALTERNATIVE METHODS IN TOXICOLOGY
VOLUME 9

In Vitro Toxicology:
TENTH ANNIVERSARY
SYMPOSIUM OF CAAT

Editor
ALAN M. GOLDBERG

Editorial Assistant
MARILYN L. PRINCIPE

Mary Ann Liebert, Inc. publishers

ALTERNATIVE METHODS IN TOXICOLOGY SERIES

Volume 1
Product Safety Evaluation

Volume 2
Acute Toxicity Testing: Alternative Approaches

Volume 3
In Vitro Methods in Toxicology

Volume 4
A Critical Evaluation of Alternatives to Acute Ocular Irritation Testing

Volume 5
In Vitro Toxicology: Approaches to Validation

Volume 6
Progress in *In Vitro* Toxicology

Volume 7
In Vitro Toxicology: New Directions

Volume 8
In Vitro Toxicology: Mechanisms and New Technology

Volume 9
In Vitro Toxicology: Tenth Anniversary Symposium of CAAT

Copyright © 1993 by Mary Ann Liebert, Inc., Publishers, 1651 Third Avenue, New York, NY 10128

ISBN: 0-913-113-60-3

All rights reserved

No part of this book may be reproduced, stored in a retrieval system, or transmitted in any form or by any means, electronic, mechanical, photocopying, microfilming, recording, or otherwise, without written permission from the publisher.

Printed in the United States of America

Contents

Acknowledgments xiii
Contributing Authors xv

Part 1. Symposium Presentations

A. *In Vitro* Approaches to Neurotoxicity

    1. Cholinergic Cell Lines as Models for Testing Drug Efficacy and Toxicity
       J.K. Blusztajn, A. Venturini, D.A. Jackson, U. Schüler, H.J. Lee, and B.H. Wainer   3

    2. Electrophysiological Approaches to *In Vitro* Neurotoxicology
       J. van den Bercken, M. Oortgiesen, T. Leinders, and H.P.M. Vijverberg   9

    3. Development of an *In Vitro* Hippocampal Brain Slice Screen for Neurotoxicity
       S.B. Fountain and J.D. Rowan   27

    4. An *In Vitro* Model for Human Peripheral Nerve Demyelination
       J.L. Rutkowski and G.I. Tennekoon   41

B. Mechanisms of Dermatotoxicity

    1. *In Vitro* Models to Evaluate Agents that Contribute to Cutaneous Carcinogenesis
       S.H. Yuspa   49

    2. Photoimmunology
       S.E. Ullrich   55

    3. The Epidermal Response to Retinoic Acid in Cell Culture and *In Vivo*
       D.S. Rosenthal, C.E.M. Griffiths, J.J. Voorhees, and S.H. Yuspa   73

C. Development of New Biological Components for Toxicity Testing Systems

    1. Immortalization of Cells
       H.C. Isom and J-M. Hu   79

    2. Steps in Development of an *In Vitro* Nasal Toxic Response Assay: Comparison of Carboxylesterase in Human and Rat Nasal Tissue
       P.M. Mattes and W.B. Mattes   91

    3. Development of a Characterized Human Renal Proximal Tubule Cell Line
       L.C. Racusen and J.S. Rhim   101

D. Draize Eye Testing Alternatives—A Perspective
   J.P. McCulley and T.J. Stephens   107

E. A Ten-Year Progress Report of the Center

    1. Pride and Prejudice: Ten Years of CAAT—An Industry Perspective
       S.D. Gettings   121

    2. Alternatives in the 90's: What's Next?
       H. Spira   141

    3. A Ten-Year Progress Report of The Center for Alternatives to Animal Testing: A Governmental Perspective
       G.B. Guest   151

    4. A Report from the Center's Director
       A.M. Goldberg   155

F. New Technologies

    1. Flow Cytometry—High Speed Approaches to Detecting Cellular Structure, Mechanism, and Function
       L.A. Sklar   163

    2. Calcium Measurements in the Assessment of *In Vitro* Toxicity
       B.F. Trump, P.T. Jain, P.C. Phelps, S.H. Chang, and I.K. Berezesky   175

G. *In Vitro* Toxicology and Risk Assessment
   K. Krishnan, M.L. Gargas, and M.E. Andersen   185

Part 2. Poster Abstracts

A. Dermal Toxicity

    1. Inflammatory Mediators from Reconstituted Human Skin Models Treated With Formulated Cosmetic Products
       W.E. Dressler, T.J. Stephens, H. Kasbarian, and E.T. Spence   207

    2. Expression of the Antigen Presenting Cell Molecule, B7 in Normal Human Skin
       A.A. Gaspari   208

3. Use of Multiple Endpoints for Assessing Chemical Insult in an Organotypic Skin Culture
   R. Gay, M. Swiderek, A. Ernesti, D. Nelson, and A.M. Kligman — 208

4. An *In Vitro* Cytotoxicity Test on JB6 (clone 41) Mouse Epidermal Cells: A Potential Model for Prediction of *In Vivo* Toxicity
   P.T. Jain, I.K. Berezesky, and B.F. Trump — 209

5. Prediction of Eye Irritancy by a Combined Method of *In Vivo* Primary Rabbit Skin Irritation Test and *In Vitro* Cytotoxicity Test
   H. Kojima, A. Sato, S. Miyamoto, Y. Kawai, I. Ishii, and H. Konishi — 209

6. Evaluation of the Skin Irritation Potential of Petroleum Based Compounds in a Reconstituted Human Skin Model
   F.J. Koschier, R.N. Roth, T.J. Stephens, E.T. Spence, H. Kasbarian, and M.A. Duke — 210

7. Application of the Skintex™ System to the Evaluation of Cosmetic Products
   F.H. Kruszewski, M.S. Dickens, V.C. Gordon, and K.J. Renskers — 210

8. Potential Irritation by Dermatological Vehicles Assessed with *In Vivo* and *In Vitro* Tests
   S. Matsumoto, J. Cheng, R. Oda, S. Sabatine, C. Anger, O. Angelov, J. Andersen, D. Sullivan, B. Brar, G. Ewing, J. Trogden, and P. Lasker — 211

9. Interaction of Benzopsoralen with NCTC 2544, HELA, and HL60 Cells
   P.P. Parnigotto, M.T. Conconi, M. Moras, V. Bassani, and A. Chilin — 211

10. Evaluation of an *In Vitro* Photoirritation Assay
    R.J. Soto, J.S. Griesemer, V.C. Gordon, and J. Acevedo — 212

11. An *In Vitro* Skin Model for the Study of Keratinocyte Responses to Irritants
    S.R. Slivka, F. Zeigler, and R.L. Bartel — 212

12. Cytotoxicity Testing Using a Three-Dimensional *In Vitro* Model of the Human Dermis and Six Different Assay Systems
    D. Triglia, S.S. Braa, I. Kidd, and T. Donnelly — 213

13. A Three-Dimensional *In Vitro* Human Skin Model for Toxicity Testing of Topically Applied Test Materials
    D. Triglia, T. Donnelly, I. Kidd, and S.S. Braa — 213

14. Development of a Three-Dimensional *In Vitro* Oral Mucosa Model
    M.P. Zimber, L. Odioso, F. Zeigler, M. Doyle, D. Triglia, and R. Bartel — 214

B. Genotoxicity

1. Development and Application of Human Cell Lines Expressing Individual or Multiple Human Cytochrome P450s
C.L. Crespi, B.W. Penman, R. Langenbach, H.V. Gelboin, D.T. Steimel, and F.J. Gonzalez 215

2. The Assessment of a Micronuclei-Induction Assay to Evaluate the *In Vitro* Genotoxicity of Respirable Dusts
D. Nadeau and D. Lane 216

C. Hepatotoxicity

1. New Metabolite Profile of Tolbutamide in Male and Female Rats. A Study With Precision-Cut Liver Slices and Isolated Hepatocytes
P. Dogterom and G. Zbinden 217

2. *In Vitro* Culture of Fish Hepatocytes and Their Use to Assess Marine Pollution
M. Faisal and B.J. Rutan 218

3. Use of Histological and Biochemical Criteria for Assessing the Hepatocellular Alterations in Rat Liver Slices
F. Goethals, V. Allaeys, E. Caillau, P. Buc-Calderon, and M. Roberfroid 218

4. Cultured Human Hepatocytes—A Model for Drug Metabolism/Toxicity Studies
G.M. Hawksworth, L. Abernethy, S. Barnard, J.A. Coundouris, M.H. Grant, C.K. Lindsay, and V. Maitland 219

5. Liver Crude Membrane Fractions From Rat Liver Improve the Maintenance of Liver Specific Functions in Long Term, Serum Free Rat Hepatocyte Cultures
B. Saad, H. Schawalder, and P. Maier 219

6. The Enhanced Responsiveness of Hepatocytes to Growth Factors as a Result of Estrogen Treatment
N. Ni and J.D. Yager 220

7. Effect of Culture Conditions on the Maintenance of Xenobiotic Metabolism in Primary Rat Hepatocytes *In Vitro*
J. Zurlo, L.M. Arterburn, E.E. Stickler, R.M. Barry, J.M. Frazier, and J.D. Yager 220

D. Mechanisms

1. Glutathione Depletion Increases the Cytotoxic Effect of Fumonisin *In Vitro*
C. Azuka, G.D. Osweiler, D.L. Reynolds, M. Howard, and Y. Niyo 221

2. Inhibition of Protein Synthesis in Hepatocytes During Hypoxia: An Early Cytotoxic Event or an Adaptative Cellular Response?
V. Lefebvre, M. Van Steenbrugge, I. Goffin, M. Roberfroid, and P. Buc-Calderon ... 222

3. Toxicity of Formate in Dissociated Primary Neural Cultures
D.C. Dorman, B. Bolon, and K.T. Morgan ... 222

4. Mechanisms of Butylated Hydroxytoluene Hydroperoxide-Stimulated Toxicity and Changes in Gene Expression in Mouse Epidermal Cell Line PA
K.Z. Guyton, L.J. Prestigiacomo, N.E. Davidson, and T.W. Kensler ... 223

5. Regulation of Catalase Gene Expression by Copper
P.J. Lapinskas and V. Culotta ... 223

6. *In Vitro* Studies Examining the Role of Copper and Glutathione in Hydroquinone-Induced Cytotoxicity to Primary Bone Marrow Stromal Cells
Y. Li and M.A. Trush ... 224

7. Analysis of the Reactive Oxygen Species (ROS) Associated to the Respiratory Burst of Pulmonary Alveolar Macrophages (PAM) Exposed *In Vitro* to Man-Made Fibres (MMF)
D. Nadeau and D. Lane ... 224

E. Methods Development

1. Evaluation of a Group of Petrochemicals Using Clonetics' Neutral Red Bioassay to Predict Irritancy
R. Barstad, J. Janus, J. Lauten, N. Accomando, and A. Triana ... 225

2. Evaluating Teratogen Exposure Utilizing hsp 27 cDNA
N. Bournias-Vardiabasis, K. Hopkins, and B. Wang ... 226

3. A Non-Invasive Biotest for Occupational Exposure to Weak or Non-Mutagenic Toxicants
M.J.W. Chang, M.T. Chou, and R.S. Lin ... 226

4. An *In Vitro* Model for Studying Cochlear Toxicity
W.J. Clerici and L.D. Fechter ... 227

5. An *In Vitro* Assay to Evaluate Albumin Binding of Toxicants
J.M. Frazier and S. Dacosta ... 227

6. Using Real-Time/Kinetic Viability Assays to Measure Acute Toxicity *In Vitro*
J.F. Hamberger, J.S. Vaughan, and D.A. Porter ... 228

7. *In Vitro* Differentiation Using Blastocyst-Derived Euploid Embryonal Stem (E8) Cells of the Mouse: A New Approach to *In Vitro* Teratogenesis Testing
G. Klein, A. Pöting, and H. Spielmann ... 228

8. A Novel Cytotoxicity Screening Assay Using a Multi-Well Fluorescence Scanner: Correlation With LDH Release and Draize Eye Scores
   A.L. Nieminen, P. Merrick, R.A. Harper, G.J. Gores, J.M. Bond, R. Imberti, B. Herman, and J.J. Lemasters ... 229

9. An *In Vitro* Model for Investigating the Effects of Xenobiotics on the Differentiation of Monocytic Cells
   S.J. Rembish, R.W. Craig, and M.A. Trush ... 229

10. Specific Application of *In Vitro* Technologies for Product Development
    P.M. Silber and C.E. Ruegg ... 230

11. Human Bronchial Cell Culture System
    J. Stengel, J. Janus, J. Cortesi, M. Coleman, and J. Reseau ... 230

F. Neurotoxicity

1. Multicentre Initial Validation of a Tiered System for the *In Vitro* Detection of Neurotoxicity
   C.K. Atterwill ... 231

2. Cytotoxic Effects of Organophosphorus Esters and Other Neurotoxic Chemicals on Cultured Cells
   A.C. Nostrandt, T.K. Rowles, and M. Ehrich ... 232

3. Acrylamide Toxicity Studied in Culture Neuroblastoma Cells
   L. Odland, L. Romert, C. Clemedson, and E. Walum ... 232

4. Early Morphologic Changes in SH-SY5Y Neuroblastoma Cells After Exposure to a Neuropathy-Inducing Organophosphorus Compound, MIPAFOX
   D. Taylor, T.K. Rowles, A.C. Nostrandt, and M. Ehrich ... 233

5. A Multiple Cell-Culture Toxicity Test Scheme for the Identification of Neurotoxic Compounds
   E. Walum ... 233

6. An *In Vitro* Model of Drug Neurotoxicity in the Developing Nervous System
   A.D. Weissman and B.L. Crenshaw ... 234

G. Ocular Toxicity

1. Evaluation of Two *In Vitro* Methods as Predictors of Ocular Irritation of Shampoo Formulations
   L. Bernhofer, C. Juneja, and C.W. Stott ... 235

2. Surfactants Toxicity Determined *In Vitro* by Silicon Microphysiometer
   P. Catroux, A.C. Eber, P. Panfili, K.G. Dossou, A. Rougier, G. Humphries, and M. Cottin ... 236

3. Evaluation of the Eytex System for Use as a Predictor of Ocular Irritancy of Shampoos
   D. Decker and R. Harper ... 236

4. A 10-Company Collaborative Evaluation of Alternatives to the Eye Irritation Test Using Chemical Intermediates
   D.M. Galer, R. Curren, S.C. Gad, P. Gautheron, B. Leong, K. Miller, E. Sargent, P.V. Shah, J. Sina, and R.G. Sussman ... 237

5. Characterization and Evaluation of an Ordered Macromolecular Matrix to be Used to Predict *In Vivo* Ocular Irritation
   V.C. Gordon ... 237

6. Application of the Computer Automated Structure Evaluation for Toxicology (Case Tox) Methodology to the *In Vitro* Assessment of the Eye Irritation Potential of Chemicals, Chemical Mixtures, and Polymers
   G. Klopman, D. Ptchelintsev, M. Frierson, S. Pennisi, K. Renskers, and M. Dickenson ... 238

7. Use of Four *In Vitro* Assays to Evaluate the Ocular Irritation Potential of Hair Care Products
   L.K. Lake, T.J. Stephens, and E.T. Spence ... 238

8. An *In Vitro* Method to Formulate Low Adverse Effects Shampoos
   M. Marinovich, B. Viviani, and C.L. Galli ... 239

9. The Trans-Epithelial Permeability Assay as an *In Vitro* Assay for Predicting Ocular Irritation of Surfactant Formulations
   K.M. Martin and C.W. Stott ... 239

10. A Toxicity Evaluation by the Microtox Assay of Twenty Surfactant-Containing Products and Their Constituent Surfactants and Preservatives
    K.A. Miller, R.W. Stahl, F.S. Marchesani, J.W. Harbell, K.A. Wallace, F.H. Kruszewski, K.J. Renskers, and R.D. Curren ... 240

11. Cytotoxicity of Benzalkonium Chloride (BAK) is Dependent on the Alkyl Chain Length of the Homologs
    R.M. Oda, A. Hayashi, S. Hickok, and S. Matsumoto ... 240

12. Development of an *In Vitro* Assay for Ocular Irritancy Assessments of Aqueous Incompatible Substances
    R. Osborne, M.A. Perkins, D.A. Roberts, and L.H. Bruner ... 241

13. The Chicken Enucleated-Eye-Test (CEET) as an Alternative to the Draize Eye Test
    M.K. Prinsen and H.B.W.M. Koëter ... 241

14. The Computer Automated Structure Evaluation for Toxicology (Case Tox) Methodology as an *In Vitro* Assessment of the Eye Irritation Potential
   D. Ptchelintsev, M. Frierson, S. Pennisi, K. Renskers, M. Dickens, and G. Klopman   242

15. The Use of a Three-Dimensional Skin Model for Predicting Ocular Irritancy
   B. Reece and M. Rozen   242

16. Results of the German Validation Project of Alternatives to the Draize Eye Test
   H. Spielmann, M. Liebsch, I. Gerner, S. Kalweit, and T. Wirnsberger   243

17. *In Vitro* Cell Culture Investigation of Fish Eye Lens Cataract
   C.D. Williams, R.J. Huggett, and M. Faisal   243

H. Validation

1. The Use of Normal Human Keratinocytes and the Neutral Red Uptake Bioassay to Assess the First 30 MEIC Compounds
   R.D. Curren, K.A. Wallace, J. Janus, and J.W. Harbell   245

2. Preliminary Results of the MEIC Programme—A Summary
   B. Ekwall and E. Walum   246

3. IVT Databank Project Results: PC Software for Managing *In Vitro* Toxicity Testing Data
   M.R. Green and J.M. Frazier   246

4. The Problem of Collinearity and the Validation of *In Vitro* Tests
   R.L. Lipnick   247

Acknowledgments

This Symposium and the Center's programs are made possible by funding from the following:

Corporate Sponsors

3M
Alberto-Culver Company
ARCO
Avon Products, Inc.
Bernice Barbour Foundation, Inc.
Bristol-Myers Squibb Company
Charles River Laboratories, Inc.
CIBA-GEIGY Corporation
The Cosmetic, Toiletry & Fragrance Association
The Geraldine R. Dodge Foundation
Exxon Corporation
Hoffmann-La Roche Inc.
IBM Corporation
Johnson & Johnson
L'Oreal
Mary Kay Cosmetics, Inc.

Federal Sponsors

Environmental Protection Agency
Health Effects Research Laboratory, National Institutes of Health

Corporate Patrons
BP America, Inc.
The Clorox Company
E.I. du Pont de Nemours & Company
Gillette Medical Evaluation Laboratories
Glaxo Inc.
ICI Pharmaceuticals Group
Kraft General Foods, Inc.
S.C. Johnson Wax
The Procter & Gamble Company
Unilever (UK)

Corporate Benefactors
Abbott
Allied-Signal, Inc.
Amoco Foundation, Inc.
The Body Shop Inc.
Colgate-Palmolive Company
Hoechst Celanese Corporation
Kimberly-Clark Corporation
Maybelline
Merck Sharp & Dohme Research Laboratories
Neutrogena Corporation
Parfums Christian Dior
Pfizer Inc.
Rhone-Poulenc Rorer
The Upjohn Company
Wyeth-Ayerst Research

Corporate Contributors
Louis & Ann Abrons Foundation, Inc.
Allergan
Block Drug Company Inc.
Boyle-Midway Household Products, Inc.
Chanel, Inc.
Church & Dwight Co.
The Coca-Cola Company
The Dow Chemical Company
Dow Corning Corporation
Guerlain Inc.
Helene Curtis, Inc.
Hershey Foods Corporation
In Vitro Technologies, Inc.
L'Arome
L&F Products
Microbiological Associates, Inc.
Monsanto Company
Parfums Nina Ricci, U.S.A. Limited
Rickett & Colman Household Products
Society of Cosmetic Chemists
Sterling Winthrop Pharmaceuticals Research Division
Tiffany and Company

Contributing Authors

L. Abernethy
University of Aberdeen, Departments of Biomedical Sciences and Medicine & Therapeutics, Aberdeen, AB9 2ZD, United Kingdom

N. Accomando
Clonetics Corporation, 9620 Chesapeake Drive, San Diego, CA 92123-1324

J. Acevedo
In Vitro International, 16632 Milliken Avenue, Irvine, CA 92714

V. Allaeys
Université Catholique de Louvain, Unité de Biochimie Toxicologique et Cancérologique, Brussels, Belgium

Melvin E. Andersen
Duke University Medical Center, P.O. Box 3210, Durham, NC 27710

J. Andersen
Allergan, Inc., Irvine, CA 92713-9534

O. Angelov
Allergan, Inc., Irvine, CA 92713-9534

Claude Anger
Allergan, Inc., Irvine, CA 92713-9534

L.M. Arterburn
W.R. Grace & Company Research Division, Columbia, MD 21045

C.K. Atterwill
Hatfield Polytechnic, CellTox Centre, Division of Biosciences, Hatfield, Herts, AL10 9AB, United Kingdom

Charles Azuka
Veterinary Pathology and Veterinary Medical Research Institute, Iowa State University, Ames, IA 50011

S. Barnard
University of Aberdeen, Departments of Biomedical Science and Medicine & Therapeutics, Aberdeen, AB9 2ZD, United Kingdom

R.M. Barry
W.R. Grace & Company Research Division, Columbia, MD 21045

R. Barstad
Clonetics Corporation, 9620 Chesapeake Drive, San Diego, CA 92123-1324

Ronnda L. Bartel
Advanced Tissue Sciences, Inc. (formerly Marrow-Tech), 10933 North Torrey Pines Road, La Jolla, CA 92037

V. Bassani
Department of Pharmaceutical Sciences, University of Padua, 35100 Padua, Italy

I.K. Berezesky
Department of Pathology, University of Maryland School of Medicine and Maryland Institute for Emergency Medical Services Systems, Baltimore, MD 21201

Lauren Bernhofer
Johnson & Johnson Consumer Products, Inc., Skillman, NJ 08558

Jan Krzystof Blusztajn
Departments of Pathology and Psychiatry, Boston University School of Medicine, 85 East Newton Street, Boston, MA 02118

B. Bolon
C.I.I.T., Research Triangle Park, NC 27709

John M. Bond
University of North Carolina, Department of Cell Biology and Anatomy, Chapel Hill, NC 27599-7090

Nicole Bournias-Vardiabasis
California State University, San Bernardino, CA 92407

Sonia Sherard Braa
Advanced Tissue Sciences, Inc. (formerly Marrow-Tech), 10933 North Torrey Pines Road, La Jolla, CA 92037

B. Brar
Allergan, Inc., Irvine, CA 92713-9534

Leon H. Bruner
The Procter & Gamble Company, Human & Environmental Safety Division, Miami Valley Laboratories, Cincinnati, OH 45239-8707

Pedro Buc-Calderon
Université Catholique de Louvain, Unité de Biochimie Toxicologique et Cancérologique, Brussels, Belgium

E. Caillau
Université Catholique de Louvain, Unité de Biochimie Toxicologique et Cancérologique, Brussels, Belgium

Philippe Catroux
L'OREAL Basic Research Center, Aulnay sous Bois, France

Ming J.W. Chang
Chang Gung Medical College and National Taiwan University, Taiwan, Republic of China

S.H. Chang
Department of Pathology, University of Maryland School of Medicine and Maryland Institute for Emergency Medical Services Systems, Baltimore, MD 21201

J. Cheng
Allergan, Inc., Irvine, CA 92713-9534

A. Chilin
Department of Pharmaceutical Sciences, University of Padua, 35100 Padua, Italy

M.T. Chou
Chang Gung Medical College and National Taiwan University, Taiwan, Republic of China

Cecilia Clemedson
Department of Neurochemistry & Neurotoxicology, Stockholm University, S-106 91, Stockholm, Sweden

William J. Clerici
Johns Hopkins University School of Hygiene & Public Health, Division of Toxicological Sciences, Baltimore, MD 21205

M. Coleman
Clonetics Corporation, 9620 Chesapeake Drive, San Diego, CA 92123-1324

M.T. Conconi
Department of Pharmaceutical Sciences, University of Padua, 35100 Padua, Italy

J. Cortesi
Clonetics Corporation, 9620 Chesapeake Drive, San Diego, CA 92123-1324

M. Cottin
L'OREAL Basic Research Center, Aulnay sous Bois, France

J.A. Coundouris
University of Aberdeen, Departments of Biomedical Science and Medicine & Therapeutics, Aberdeen, AB9 2ZD, United Kingdom

Ruth W. Craig
Department of Physiology, Johns Hopkins School of Medicine, Baltimore, MD 21205

Benjamin L. Crenshaw
Neuroscience Branch, Addiction Research Center, National Institute for Drug Abuse, Baltimore, MD 21224

Charles L. Crespi
GENTEST Corporation, Woburn, MA 01801

Valeria L. Culotta
Johns Hopkins University School of Hygiene & Public Health, Division of Toxicological Sciences, Baltimore, MD 21205

Rodger D. Curren
Microbiological Associates, Inc., 9900 Blackwell Road, Rockville, MD 20850

Shelly Dacosta
Johns Hopkins University School of Hygiene & Public Health, Division of Toxicological Sciences, Baltimore, MD 21205

Nancy E. Davidson
Johns Hopkins Oncology Center, Baltimore, MD 21205

Denise Decker
Helene Curtis, Inc., Chicago, IL 60639

Michael S. Dickens
Avon Products, Inc., Suffern, NY 10901

Michael Dickenson
Avon Products, Inc., Suffern, NY 10901

Peter Dogterom
Institute of Toxicology, Swiss Federal Institute of Technology and University of Zürich, CH-8603 Schwerzenbach, Switzerland

Tracy Donnelly
Advanced Tissue Sciences, Inc. (formerly Marrow-Tech), 10933 North Torrey Pines Road, La Jolla, CA 92037

David C. Dorman
C.I.I.T., Research Triangle Park, NC 27709

K.G. Dossou
L'OREAL Basic Research Center, Aulnay sous Bois, France

Matthew Doyle
Procter and Gamble, Cincinnati, OH 45239

William E. Dressler
Clairol, Inc., Toxicology Department, Stamford, CT 06922

Mary Ann Duke
Thomas J. Stephens & Associates, Inc., Carrollton, TX 75006

A.C. Eber
L'OREAL Basic Research Center, Aulnay sous Bois, France

Marion Ehrich
Virginia-Maryland Regional College of Veterinary Medicine, Blacksburg, VA 24061-0442

Björn Ekwall
Department of Toxicology, University of Uppsala, Box 594, S-751 24 Uppsala, Sweden

A. Ernesti
Organogenesis, Inc., Cambridge, MA 02142

G. Ewing
Herbert Laboratories, Inc., Irvine, CA 92713-9534

Mohamed Faisal
Virginia Institute of Marine Science, College of William and Mary, Gloucester Point, VA 23062

Laurence D. Fechter
Johns Hopkins University School of Hygiene & Public Health, Division of Toxicological Sciences, Baltimore, MD 21205

Stephen B. Fountain
Department of Psychology, Kent State University, Kent, OH 44242

John M. Frazier
Johns Hopkins University School of Hygiene & Public Health, Division of Toxicological Sciences, Baltimore, MD 21205

Manton Frierson
Biofor Ltd., Waverly, PA 18471

Shayne C. Gad
Becton Dickinson and Company, Medical Affairs Technical Services, Research Triangle Park, NC 27709-2016

D.M. Galer
Warner-Lambert Company, Corporate Industrial Toxicology Research, Morris Plains, NJ 07950

Corrado L. Galli
Research Center on Cosmetic Toxicology, University of Milan, Via Balzaretti 9, 20133 Milan, Italy

Anthony A. Gaspari
Department of Dermatology, University of Rochester School of Medicine and Dentistry, Rochester, NY 14642

P. Gautheron
Merck Sharp & Dohme Chibret Research Center

Michael L. Gargas
ChemRisk, A Division of McLaren/Hart, 29225 Chagrin Boulevard, Cleveland, OH 44122

Roger Gay
Organogenesis, Inc., Cambridge, MA 02142

H.V. Gelboin
National Institutes of Health, National Cancer Institute, Bethesda, MD 20892

I. Gerner
ZEBET, Bundesgesundheltsamt, Pf. 330013, D-1000 Berlin 33, Germany

Stephen D. Gettings
The Cosmetic, Toiletry & Fragrance Association, Inc., Washington, DC 20036

Fabienne Goethals
Université Catholique de Louvain, Unité de Biochimie Toxicologique et Cancérologique, Brussels, Belgium

I. Goffin
Université Catholique de Louvain, Unité de Biochimie Toxicologique et Cancérologique, Brussels, Belgium

Alan M. Goldberg
Johns Hopkins Center for Alternatives to Animal Testing, 615 North Wolfe Street, Baltimore, MD 21205

F.J. Gonzalez
National Institutes of Health, National Cancer Institute, Bethesda, MD 20892

Virginia C. Gordon
In Vitro International, 16632 Milliken Avenue, Irvine, CA 92714

Gregory J. Gores
University of North Carolina, Department of Cell Biology and Anatomy, Chapel Hill, NC 27599-7090

M.H. Grant
University of Aberdeen, Departments of Biomedical Sciences and Medicine & Therapeutics, Aberdeen, AB9 2ZD, United Kingdom

Mildred R. Green
Technical Database Services (TDS), 10 Columbus Circle, New York, NY 10019

J.S. Griesemer
S.C. Johnson & Son, Racine, WI 53403-5011

Christopher E.M. Griffiths
Department of Dermatology, University of Michigan Medical Center, Ann Arbor, MI 48109

Gerald B. Guest
Center for Veterinary Medicine, Food & Drug Administration, Rockville, MD 20857

Kate Z. Guyton
Johns Hopkins University School of Hygiene & Public Health, Division of Toxicological Sciences, Baltimore, MD 21205

John F. Hamberger
Cell Biology Department, Bausch & Lomb, Rochester, NY 14692

John W. Harbell
Microbiological Associates, Inc., 9900 Blackwell Road, Rockville, MD 20850

Robert A. Harper
Division of Research & Development, Helene Curtis, Inc., Chicago, IL 60639

Gabrielle M. Hawksworth
University of Aberdeen, Departments of Biomedical Sciences and Medicine & Therapeutics, Aberdeen, AB9 2ZD, United Kingdom

Ava Hayashi
Allergan, Inc., Irvine, CA 92715

Brian Herman
University of North Carolina, Department of Cell Biology and Anatomy, Chapel Hill, NC 27599-7090

Shawn Hickok
Allergan, Inc., Irvine, CA 92715

K. Hopkins
California State University, San Bernardino, CA 92407

M. Howard
Veterinary Pathology and Veterinary Medical Research Institute, Iowa State University, Ames, IA 50011

Jian-Ming Hu
Department of Microbiology and Immunology, The Milton S. Hershey Medical Center, The Pennsylvania State University College of Medicine, 500 University Drive, Hershey, PA 17033

Robert J. Huggett
Virginia Institute of Marine Science, College of William and Mary, Gloucester Point, VA 23062

G. Humphries
Molecular Devices, Menlo Park, CA 94025

Roberto Imberti
University of North Carolina, Department of Cell Biology and Anatomy, Chapel Hill, NC 27599-7090

Izumi Ishii
Biochemical Research Institute, Nippon Menard Cosmetic Co., Ltd., 4-66 Asakusa, Ogaki, Gifu-ken 503, Japan

Harriet C. Isom
Department of Microbiology and Immunology, The Milton S. Hershey Medical Center, The Pennsylvania State University College of Medicine, 500 University Drive, Hershey, PA 17033

Darrell A. Jackson
Department of Pathology, Boston University School of Medicine, Boston, MA 02118

P.T. Jain
Department of Pathology, University of Maryland School of Medicine and Maryland Institute for Emergency Medical Services Systems, Baltimore, MD 21201

J. Janus
Clonetics Corporation, 9620 Chesapeake Drive, San Diego, CA 92123-1324

Chandni Juneja
Johnson & Johnson Consumer Products, Inc., Skillman, NJ 08558

S. Kalweit
ZEBET, Bundesgesundheltsamt, Pf. 330013, D-1000 Berlin 33, Germany

Hillary Kasbarian
Thomas J. Stephens & Associates, Inc., Carrollton, TX 75006

Yoshifumi Kawai
Biochemical Research Institute, Nippon Menard Cosmetic Co., Ltd., 4-66 Asakusa, Ogaki, Gifu-ken 503, Japan

Thomas W. Kensler
Johns Hopkins University School of Hygiene & Public Health, Division of Toxicological Sciences, Baltimore, MD 21205

Inger Kidd
Advanced Tissue Sciences, Inc. (formerly Marrow-Tech), 10933 North Torrey Pines Road, La Jolla, CA 92037

G. Klein
Federal Health Office, Bundesgesundheltsamt, ZEBET, Pf. 330013, D-1000 Berlin 33, Germany

A.M. Kligman
Department of Dermatology, University of Pennsylvania, Philadelphia, PA 19104

Gilles Klopman
Case Western Reserve University, Department of Chemistry, Cleveland, OH 44106

Herman B.W.M. Koëter
TNO Toxicology & Nutrition Institute, P.O. Box 360, 3700 AJ Zeist, The Netherlands

Hajime Kojima
Biochemical Research Institute, Nippon Menard Cosmetic Co., Ltd., 4-66 Asakusa, Ogaki, Gifu-ken 503, Japan

Hiroaki Konishi
Biochemical Research Institute, Nippon Menard Cosmetic Co., Ltd., 4-66 Asakusa, Ogaki, Gifu-ken 503, Japan

Francis J. Koschier
ARCO, Los Angeles, CA 90017

Kannan Krishnan
Département de Médecine du Travail et d'Hygiéne du Milieu, Faculté de Médecine, Université de Montréal, Case Postale 6128, Succursale A, Montréal, PQ, Canada H3C 3J7

Francis H. Kruszewski
Avon Products, Inc., Suffern, NY 10901

Leslie K. Lake
S.C. Johnson & Son, Inc., Racine, WI 53403-5011

Denis Lane
Université de Sherbrooke, Laboratoire de Biochimie et de Toxicologie Pulmonaires, Département de Biologie, Sherbrooke, Québec J1K 2R1, Canada

R. Langenbach
National Institutes of Health, National Institute for Environmental Health Sciences, Research Triangle Park, NC 27709

Paula J. Lapinskas
Johns Hopkins University School of Hygiene & Public Health, Division of Toxicological Sciences, Baltimore, MD 21205

P. Laskar
Herbert Laboratories, Inc., Irvine, CA 92713-9534

J. Lauten
Clonetics Corporation, 9620 Chesapeake Drive, San Diego, CA 92123-1324

Henry J. Lee
Departments of Pharmacological & Physiological Sciences, The University of Chicago, Chicago, IL 60637

V. Lefebvre
National Fund for Scientific Research, Belgium

Trese Leinders
Research Institute of Toxicology, University of Utrecht, P.O. Box 80.176, NL-3508 TD Utrecht, The Netherlands

John J. Lemasters
University of North Carolina, Department of Cell Biology and Anatomy, Chapel Hill, NC 27599-7090

B. Leong
The Upjohn Company, Kalamazoo, MI 49009

Yunbo Li
Johns Hopkins University School of Hygiene & Public Health, Division of Toxicological Sciences, Baltimore, MD 21205

M. Liebsch
ZEBET, Bundesgesundheltsamt, Pf. 330013, D-1000 Berlin 33, Germany

R.S. Lin
Chang Gung Medical College and National Taiwan University, Taiwan, Republic of China

C.K. Lindsay
University of Aberdeen, Aberdeen, AB9 2ZD, United Kingdom

Robert L. Lipnick
US Environmental Protection Agency, Office of Pollution Prevention and Toxics (TS-796), Washington, DC 20460

Peter Maier
Institute of Toxicology, Swiss Federal Institute of Technology and University of Zürich, CH-8603 Schwerzenbach, Switzerland

V. Maitland
University of Aberdeen, Aberdeen, AB9 2ZD, United Kingdom

Frank S. Marchesani
Microbiological Associates, Inc., 9900 Blackwell Road, Rockville, MD 20850

Marina Marinovich
Research Center on Cosmetic Toxicology, University of Milan, Via Balzaretti 9, 20133 Milan, Italy

Katharine M. Martin
Johnson & Johnson Consumer Products, Inc., Skillman, NJ 08558

Steven Matsumoto
Allergan, Inc., Irvine, CA 92713-9534

Pamela M. Mattes
Department of Pediatrics, University of Connecticut School of Medicine, Farmington, CT 06032

William B. Mattes
CIBA-GEIGY Corporation, Environmental Health Center, Farmington, CT 06032

James P. McCulley
Department of Ophthalmology, University of Texas Southwestern Medical School, Dallas, TX 75235

Pipsisewa Merrick
University of North Carolina, Department of Cell Biology and Anatomy, Chapel Hill, NC 27599-7090

Karen A. Miller
Microbiological Associates, Inc., 9900 Blackwell Road, Rockville, MD 20850

Satoru Miyamoto
Biochemical Research Institute, Nippon Menard Cosmetic Co., Ltd., 4-66 Asakusa, Ogaki, Gifu-ken 503, Japan

M. Moras
Department of Pharmaceutical Sciences, University of Padua, 35100 Padua, Italy

K.T. Morgan
C.I.I.T., Research Triangle Park, NC 27709

Denis Nadeau
Université de Sherbrooke, Laboratoire de Biochimie et de Toxicologie Pulmonaires, Département de Biologie, Sherbrooke, Québec J1K 2R1, Canada

D. Nelson
Organogenesis, Inc., Cambridge, MA 02142

Nan Ni
Johns Hopkins University School of Hygiene & Public Health, Division of Toxicological Sciences, Baltimore, MD 21205

Anna-Liisa Nieminen
University of North Carolina, Department of Cell Biology and Anatomy, Chapel Hill, NC 27599-7090

Y. Niyo
Veterinary Pathology and Veterinary Medical Research Institute, Iowa State University, Ames, IA 50011

Amy C. Nostrandt
Virginia-Maryland Regional College of Veterinary Medicine, Blacksburg, VA 24061-0442

Roger M. Oda
Allergan, Inc., Irvine, CA 92715

Linda Odioso
Procter and Gamble, Cincinnati, OH 45239

Lena Odland
Department of Neurochemistry & Neurotoxicology, Stockholm University, S-106 91, Stockholm, Sweden

Marga Oortgiesen
Research Institute of Toxicology, University of Utrecht, P.O. Box 80.176, NL-3508 TD Utrecht, The Netherlands

Rosemarie Osborne
The Procter & Gamble Company, Human & Environmental Safety Division, Miami Valley Laboratories, Cincinnati, OH 45239-8707

G.D. Osweiler
Veterinary Pathology and Veterinary Medical Research Institute, Iowa State University, Ames, IA 50011

P. Panfili
Molecular Devices, Menlo Park, CA 94025

Pier Paolo Parnigotto
Department of Pharmaceutical Sciences, University of Padua, 35100 Padua, Italy

B.W. Penman
GENTEST Corporation, Woburn, MA 01801

Stephen Pennisi
Avon Products, Inc., Suffern, NY 10901

Mary A. Perkins
The Procter & Gamble Company, Human & Environmental Safety Division, Miami Valley Laboratories, Cincinnati, OH 45239-8707

David A. Porter
Cell Biology Department, Bausch & Lomb, Rochester, NY 14692

P.C. Phelps
Department of Pathology, University of Maryland School of Medicine and Maryland Institute for Emergency Medical Services Systems, Baltimore, MD 21201

A. Pöting
Federal Health Office, Bundesgesundheltsamt, ZEBET, Pf. 330013, D-1000 Berlin 33, Germany

Laura J. Prestigiacomo
Johns Hopkins Oncology Center, Baltimore, MD 21205

Menk K. Prinsen
TNO Toxicology & Nutrition Institute, P.O. Box 360, 3700 AJ Zeist, The Netherlands

Dmitri Ptchelintsev
Case Western Reserve University, Cleveland, OH 44106

Lorraine C. Racusen
Department of Pathology, The Johns Hopkins University School of Medicine, 720 Rutland Avenue, Baltimore, MD 21205

Barry T. Reece
Mary Kay Cosmetics, Inc., 1330 Regal Row, Dallas, TX 75247

Stephen J. Rembish
Johns Hopkins University School of Hygiene & Public Health, Division of Toxicological Sciences, Baltimore, MD 21205

Kevin J. Renskers
Avon Products, Inc., Suffern, NY 10901

J. Reseau
Clonetics Corporation, 9620 Chesapeake Drive, San Diego, CA 92123-1324

D.L. Reynolds
Veterinary Pathology and Veterinary Medical Research Institute, Iowa State University, Ames, IA 50011

Johng S. Rhim
Laboratory of Cellular and Molecular Biology, National Cancer Institute, Bethesda, MD 20894

Marcel Roberfroid
Université Catholique de Louvain, Unité de Biochimie Toxicologique et Cancérologique, Brussels, Belgium

Deirdre A. Roberts
The Procter & Gamble Company, Human & Environmental Safety Division, Miami Valley Laboratories, Cincinnati, OH 45239-8707

Lennart Romert
Department of Genetic and Cellular Toxicology, Stockholm University, S-106 91, Stockholm, Sweden

Randy N. Roth
ARCO, Los Angeles, CA 90017

Dean S. Rosenthal
Department of Biochemistry and Molecular Biology, Georgetown University School of Medicine, Silver Spring, MD 20906

André Rougier
L'OREAL Basic Research Center, Aulnay sous Bois, France

Teresa K. Rowles
Department of Animal Science, University of Tennessee, Knoxville, TN 37901

James D. Rowan
Department of Psychology, Kent State University, Kent, OH 44242

Michael Rozen
Mary Kay Cosmetics, Inc., 1330 Regal Row, Dallas, TX 75247

Charles E. Ruegg
In Vitro Technologies, Inc., 5202 Westland Boulevard, Baltimore, MD 21227

B.J. Rutan
Virginia Institute of Marine Science, College of William and Mary, Gloucester Point, VA 23062

J. Lynn Rutkowski
Division of Pediatric Neurology, The University of Michigan, Ann Arbor, MI 48019

Bashar Saad
Institute of Toxicology, Swiss Federal Institute of Technology and University of Zürich, CH-8603 Schwerzenbach, Switzerland

S. Sabatine
Allergan, Inc., Irvine, CA 92713-9534

E. Sargent
Merck & Co., USA

Atsushi Sato
Biochemical Research Institute, Nippon Menard Cosmetic Co., Ltd., 4-66 Asakusa, Ogaki, Gifu-ken 503, Japan

Hanspeter Schawalder
Institute of Toxicology, Swiss Federal Institute of Technology and University of Zürich, CH-8603 Schwerzenbach, Switzerland

Ulrike Schüler
Department of Pathology, Boston University School of Medicine, Boston, MA 02118

P.V. Shah
Hoffmann-La Roche, Inc., Nutley, NJ 07110

Paul M. Silber
In Vitro Technologies, Inc., 5202 Westland Boulevard, Baltimore, MD 21227

J. Sina
Merck Sharp & Dohme, Rahway, NJ

Larry A. Sklar
National Flow Cytometry Resource, Los Alamos National Laboratory, Los Alamos, NM 87544

Sandra R. Slivka
Advanced Tissue Sciences, Inc. (formerly Marrow-Tech), 10933 North Torrey Pines Road, La Jolla, CA 92037

Richard J. Soto
S.C. Johnson & Son, Inc., Racine, WI 53403-5011

E. Tiffany Spence
Thomas J. Stephens & Associates, Inc., Carrollton, TX 75006

Horst Spielmann
Federal Health Office, Bundesgesundheltsamt, ZEBET, Pf. 330013, D-1000 Berlin 33, Germany

Henry Spira
Animal Rights Coalitions, P.O. Box 214, Planetarium Station, New York, NY 10024

Richard W. Stahl
Microbiological Associates, Inc., 9900 Blackwell Road, Rockville, MD 20850

D.T. Steimel
GENTEST Corporation, Woburn, MA 01801

J. Stengel
Clonetics Corporation, 9620 Chesapeake Drive, San Diego, CA 92123-1324

Thomas J. Stephens
Thomas J. Stephens & Associates, Inc., Carrollton, TX 75006

Elizabeth E. Stickler
Johns Hopkins University School of Hygiene & Public Health, Division of Toxicological Sciences, Baltimore, MD 21205

Charles W. Stott
Johnson & Johnson Consumer Products, Inc., Skillman, NJ 08558

D. Sullivan
Allergan, Inc., Irvine, CA 92713-9534

R.G. Sussman
Warner-Lambert Company, Corporate Industrial Toxicology Research, Morris Plains, NJ 07950

M. Swiderek
Organogenesis, Inc., Cambridge, MA 02142

Delana Taylor
Virginia-Maryland Regional College of Veterinary Medicine, Blacksburg, VA 24061-0442

Gihan I. Tennekoon
Division of Pediatric Neurology, The University of Michigan, Ann Arbor, MI 48109-0570

A. Triana
Clonetics Corporation, 9620 Chesapeake Drive, San Diego, CA 92123-1324

Dennis Triglia
Advanced Tissue Sciences, Inc. (formerly Marrow-Tech), 10933 North Torrey Pines Road, La Jolla, CA 92037

J. Trogden
Herbert Laboratories, Inc., Irvine, CA 92713-9534

Benjamin F. Trump
Department of Pathology, University of Maryland School of Medicine and Maryland Institute for Emergency Medical Services Systems, Baltimore, MD 21201

Michael A. Trush
Johns Hopkins University School of Hygiene & Public Health, Division of Toxicological Sciences, Baltimore, MD 21205

Steven E. Ullrich
University of Texas M.D. Anderson Cancer Center, Department of Immunology, 1515 Holcombe Boulevard, Houston, TX 77030

Joep van den Bercken
Research Institute of Toxicology, University of Utrecht, P.O. Box 80.176, NL-3508 TD Utrecht, The Netherlands

M. Van Steenbrugge
Université Catholique de Louvain, Unité de Biochimie Toxicologique et Cancérologique, Brussels, Belgium

Jeanette Schepper Vaughan
Cell Biology Department, Bausch & Lomb, Rochester, NY 14692

Amy Venturini
Department of Pathology, Boston University School of Medicine, Boston, MA 02118

Henk P.M. Vijverberg
Research Institute of Toxicology, University of Utrecht, P.O. Box 80.176, NL-3508 TD Utrecht, The Netherlands

Barbara Viviani
Research Center on Cosmetic Toxicology, University of Milan, Via Balzaretti 9, 20133 Milan, Italy

John J. Voorhees
Department of Dermatology, University of Michigan Medical Center, Ann Arbor, MI 48109

Bruce H. Wainer
Departments of Pharmacological & Physiological Sciences and Department of Pathology, The University of Chicago, Chicago, IL 60637

Kathleen A. Wallace
Microbiological Associates, Inc., 9900 Blackwell Road, Rockville, MD 20850

Erik Walum
Department of Neurochemistry & Neurotoxicology, Stockholm University, S-106 91, Stockholm, Sweden

Boris Wang
Prenatal Diagnosis Center, Beverly Hills, CA 90213

Arthur D. Weissman
Neuroscience Branch, Addiction Research Center, National Institute for Drug Abuse, Baltimore, MD 21224

Christopher D. Williams
Virginia Institute of Marine Science, College of William and Mary, Gloucester Point, VA 23062

T. Wirnsberger
ZEBET, Bundesgesundheltsamt, Pf. 330013, D-1000 Berlin 33, Germany

James D. Yager
Johns Hopkins University School of Hygiene & Public Health, Division of Toxicological Sciences, Baltimore, MD 21205

Stuart H. Yuspa
Laboratory of Cellular Carcinogenesis and Tumor Promotion, National Cancer Institute, Bethesda, MD 20892

Gerhard Zbinden
Institute of Toxicology, Swiss Federal Institute of Technology and University of Zürich, CH-8603 Schwerzenbach, Switzerland

Frank Zeigler
Advanced Tissue Sciences, Inc. (formerly Marrow-Tech), 10933 North Torrey Pines Road, La Jolla, CA 92037

Michael P. Zimber
Advanced Tissue Sciences, Inc. (formerly Marrow-Tech), 10933 North Torrey Pines Road, La Jolla, CA 92037

Joanne Zurlo
Johns Hopkins University School of Hygiene & Public Health, Division of Toxicological Sciences, Baltimore, MD 21205

Part 1
Symposium Presentations

A. *In Vitro* Approaches to Neurotoxicity

A1

Cholinergic Cell Lines as Models for Testing Drug Efficacy and Toxicity

JAN KRZYSZTOF BLUSZTAJN,[1,2] AMY VENTURINI,[1]
DARRELL A. JACKSON,[1] ULRIKE SCHÜLER,[1] HENRY J. LEE,[3]
and BRUCE H. WAINER[3,4]

*Departments of [1]Pathology & [2]Psychiatry, Boston University School of Medicine,
Boston, MA 02118*

*Departments of [3]Pharmacological & Physiological Sciences, and [4]Pathology,
The University of Chicago, Chicago, IL 60637*

INTRODUCTION

Degeneration and/or malfunction of cholinergic neurons underlies the pathophysiology of Motor Neuron Disorders, Familial Dysautonomias, Alzheimer's Disease, Tardive Dyskinesia and Huntington's Chorea. Crucial to the development of experimental approaches to study these diseases, and to design treatment strategies, is the establishment of a homogeneous cell preparation which expresses all aspects of the cholinergic phenotype. Such cell preparations will not only provide alternatives to research on experimental animals but also will be models for investigating how cholinergic neurons might behave in a defined environment. Cholinergic cell lines offer such a model system because they are homogeneous, and permit easy analysis of a large variety of treatments in a well controlled environment. We have developed cell lines derived from fusion of the murine neuroblastoma cells, N18TG2 (which lack cholinergic markers), with postnatal day 21 mouse brain septal neurons (1). Here we summarize some features of one such cell line, SN56.B5.G4, and show that these properties are similar to those characteristic of septal neurons (2). The cholinergic properties of SN56.B5.G4 cells are strikingly sensitive to pharmacological agents and thus we expect that they will become a useful model for testing effects of drugs, both beneficial and toxic, on cholinergic neurons.

MATERIALS AND METHODS

Cell culture.

The SN56.B5.G4 cells were created by fusing N18TG2 mouse neuroblastoma cells with murine (strain C57BL/6) neurons from postnatal day 21 septa (1,3). We grow the cells at 37 °C in an atmosphere of 95% air, 5% CO_2 in Dulbecco's Modified Eagle's Medium (DMEM) containing 10% fetal bovine serum (FBS), and 50 µg/ml gentamicine.

ACh accumulation.

To measure [^{14}C]ACh accumulation, the cells were incubated at 37 °C in a physiological salt solution (containing in mM: NaCl, 135; KCl, 5; $CaCl_2$, 1; $MgCl_2$, 0.75; glucose, 5; eserine, 0.015; HEPES, 10; pH 7.4) in the presence of [^{14}C]choline. The [^{14}C]ACh synthesized by the cells was extracted, purified by HPLC (4,5) and its radioactivity was determined.

ACh and choline acetyltransferase activity measurements.

ACh was determined by HPLC with an enzymatic reactor containing acetylcholinesterase and choline oxidase and an electrochemical detector using a commercial kit (Bioanalytical Systems Inc., West Lafayette, IN) based on the method of Potter et al. (6). Choline acetyltransferase (CAT) activity was determined in cell homogenates by the method of Fonnum (7).

ACh release.

To measure [^{14}C]ACh release the cells were incubated for 180 min. at 37 °C in L-15 medium containing 10 μM [^{14}C]choline and 15 μM eserine. The cells were washed with L-15 medium (as above) and then incubated for an additional 30 min. in a physiological salt solution (composition as above) and either 5 mM (control) or 40 mM potassium chloride (the concentration of sodium chloride was reduced to 100 mM). The media were collected and [^{14}C]ACh released from the cells was purified by HPLC (4,5) and its radioactivity determined.

RESULTS

SN56.B5.G4 cells extend neurites.

SN56.B5.G4 cells grown in basal medium extended few neurites. Since the analogs of the second messenger, cyclic AMP (cAMP), have been shown to cause neurite outgrowth in several murine neuroblastoma cell lines (8), rat pheochromocytoma cells (PC12)(9), and the neuroblastoma x glioma hybrid cells (NG108-15)(10), we added 1 mM $N^6,O^{2'}$-dibutyryl-adenosine-3'-5'-cyclic monophosphate (dbcAMP), a cell permeant analog of cAMP, or 10 μM forskolin, an activator of adenylyl cyclase, to the medium. Cells treated with these drugs divided slowly and developed a network of neurites. Since the dbcAMP molecule can be hydrolyzed liberating free butyric acid, we tested the effect of 2 mM butyrate in our cultures. Butyrate-treated cells were rounder than controls and few neurites were observed.

SN56.B5.G4 cells synthesize ACh from choline taken up by a sodium-dependent high-affinity transport.

In the initial step of ACh synthesis in nerve endings, choline is taken up from the extracellular space by a sodium-dependent high-affinity uptake system (SDHACU)(11). We determined the apparent affinity for choline of the ACh synthetic process by incubating the cells for 10 min. in a medium of varying [^{14}C]choline concentration and measuring [^{14}C]ACh accumulation. [^{14}C]ACh accumulation was saturable with choline and exhibited an apparent K_m of 4.6 μM, i.e. in the range characteristic of SDHACU. The uptake was sodium dependent; when the cells were incubated in medium in which sodium was replaced by lithium, accumulation of [^{14}C]ACh from 1 μM [^{14}C]choline was diminished to 29% of control. Others obtained similar results using primary cultures of rat septum (12,13). These data indicate that SN56.B5.G4 cells express SDHACU and that their ACh is synthesized from choline taken up by this system.

SN56.B5.G4 cells release ACh upon depolarization.

Non-differentiated SN56.B5.G4 cells prelabeled with 10 μM [^{14}C]choline and then incubated for an additional 30 min. in a physiological salt solution containing potassium at basal (5 mM) or depolarizing (40 mM) concentrations released little [^{14}C]ACh. However, when the SN56.B5.G4 cells were grown in the presence of 1 mM dbcAMP, 10 μM forskolin, or 2 mM butyrate for 48 hours, ACh release was reliably observed and this release was enhanced by depolarization. The spontaneous and the depolarization-evoked ACh release occurred both in neurite-free (butyrate-treated) and neurite-bearing (dbcAMP-, or forskolin-treated) cells. These data demonstrate that differentiated SN56.B5.G4 cells are capable of depolarization-evoked ACh. It would be important to determine what components of the ACh releasing mechanism are missing in undifferentiated cells.

ACh synthesis in SN56.B5.G4 cells is enhanced by retinoic acid and forskolin in an additive manner.

In cells treated with 1 mM dbcAMP or with 10 μM forskolin for two days, the activity of CAT and ACh content were 2-3-fold higher relative to controls. CAT activity and ACh content were also elevated up to four-fold in cells treated with 1 μM of all trans retinoic acid (RA) for two days. These effects were time- and dose-dependent. The EC_{50} values for dbcAMP, forskolin and RA were 1.3 mM, 0.7 μM, and 10 nM, respectively. The effects of RA and forskolin were additive resulting in a five-fold increase in ACh content in cells treated with 1 μM RA and 10 μM forskolin for two days, relative to controls.

DISCUSSION

The SN56.B5.G4 cells have been selected from other septal lines based on CAT activity. However in order to serve as a useful model of brain cholinergic neurons it was important to establish whether these cells exhibit other features of the cholinergic phenotype. The ACh content of these cells is similar to NS20 neuroblastoma cells (2 nmol/mg protein)(14), but lower than that of the human neuroblastoma LA-N-2 cells (up to 25 nmol/mg protein)(5). By comparison ACh content of rat striatum is 0.3 nmol/mg protein (15) and that of purely cholinergic synaptosomes from *Torpedo* electric organ is 130 nmol/mg protein (16). In addition to CAT activity, SN56.B5.G4 cells express SDHACU, a property which sets them apart from a variety of CAT-containing cell lines including NS20 neuroblastoma cells (17), NG108-15 neuroblastoma x glioma cells (18), PC12 pheochromocytoma cells (19), and LA-N-2 neuroblastoma cells (5), all of which synthesize ACh from choline taken up by the low-affinity transporter. Hence the SN56.B5.G4 cells resemble septal neurons, which are capable of expressing SDHACU in primary cultures (12).

SN56.B5.G4 cells grown in basal medium failed to release ACh reliably. However, differentiated cells released ACh and this release was almost doubled by depolarization. The permissive effect of dbcAMP, butyrate, and forskolin on ACh release in these cells may be due to either differentiation of the excitable properties of cell membranes, including expression of specific ion channels, or differentiation of ACh release mechanisms such as vesicular storage of ACh, or to synthesis of proteins involved in vesicular release.

Treatment of SN56.B5.G4 cells with dbcAMP stimulated CAT activity and ACh synthesis. This effect was maximal after two days of treatment suggesting that it was mediated by changes in CAT gene expression, translation, or CAT protein turnover or that ChAT was activated by a factor (perhaps an enzyme which modifies CAT), whose expression required two days to develop fully. If the effects of dbcAMP were due to the cAMP moiety of this molecule, then cells treated with forskolin, which activates the adenylyl cyclase and increases the intracellular cAMP concentration, should respond similarly. Consistent with this prediction the forskolin-treated (10 μM; 2 days) cells developed neurites and had CAT activity similar to that of dbcAMP-treated cells. The molecule of dbcAMP permeates into cells due to its butyrate moieties. Hydrolysis of dbcAMP yields free butyrate which has been shown to stimulate CAT activity in neuroblastoma cells (8,20,21). In SN56.B5.G4 cells butyrate caused elevations in CAT activity and stimulated ACh synthesis. The latter effect may be due to the conversion of butyrate to acetylCoA necessary for ACh synthesis (22).

The enhancement of ACh synthesis by agents which increase intracellular cAMP levels and by RA in SN56.B5.G4 cells suggests that ACh synthesis *in vivo* may be regulated by 1) activation of receptors for neurotransmitters, hormones, or growth factors which activate adenylyl cyclase, and 2) activation of the retinoid receptors. The data also indicate that RA and elevated intracellular cAMP levels stimulate ACh production by two different mechanisms.

Taken together, the data presented above show that SN56.B5.G4 cells are characterized by ACh synthesis and storage, SDHACU, and depolarization-evoked ACh release. These are properties characteristic of the cholinergic phenotype (23). The cholinergic features of these cells can be enhanced by pharmacologic agents. It will be important to determine whether physiologically relevant agents alter those properties as well. The list of such molecules includes: nerve growth factor (24), basic fibroblast growth factor (25), ciliary neurotrophic factor (26), CAT development factor (27), cholinergic differentiation factor (28) or leukemia inhibitory factor (29), membrane-derived factor (30), and target-derived neuronal cholinergic differentiation factor (31). It is worth noting that granulocyte-macrophage colony-stimulating factor (32) and interleukin 3 (33) have been reported to stimulate CAT activity in septal neurons as well as in one of our cell lines (SN6.10.2.2) derived from embryonic septum, indicating that these cells will be useful as models to study the molecular mechanisms of action of these and other growth- and differentiating factors on the cholinergic phenotype.

CONCLUSIONS.

Despite the fact that cholinergic function has been studied for well over half a century, to this day there is no experimental system which allows one to investigate the mechanisms of ACh synthesis and release under long term *in vitro* conditions. Our knowledge of these mechanisms derives from work on intact animals or from *in vitro* studies using freshly-obtained preparations. Animals are necessary for both of these approaches. Recently several laboratories (21,34-36), including ours (1,2,3,5), described studies on cholinergic cell lines in long term culture. The initial data, some of which are summarized in this article, are promising and they warrant further investigation of these models.

ACKNOWLEDGMENTS

Supported by: NSF BNS8808942; NS25787; MH46095; and Center for Alternatives to Animal Testing grants.

REFERENCES

1. LEE, H.J., HAMMOND, D.N., LARGE, T.H. and WAINER, B.H., (1990), Immortalized young adult neurons from the septal region: Generation and characterization. Dev.Brain Res. 52:219-228.

2. BLUSZTAJN, J.K., VENTURINI, A., JACKSON, D.A., LEE, H.J. and WAINER, B.H., (1992), Acetylcholine synthesis and release is enhanced by dibutyryl cyclic AMP in a neuronal cell line derived from mouse septum. J.Neurosci. 12:793-799.

3. HAMMOND, D.N., LEE, H.J., TONSGARD, J.H. and WAINER, B.H., (1990), Development and characterization of clonal cell lines derived from septal cholinergic neurons. Brain Res. 512:190-200.

4. LISCOVITCH, M., FREESE, A., BLUSZTAJN, J.K. and WURTMAN, R.J., (1985), High-performance liquid chromatography of water-soluble choline metabolites. Anal.Biochem. 151:182-187.

5. RICHARDSON, U.I., LISCOVITCH, M. and BLUSZTAJN, J.K., (1989), Acetylcholine synthesis and secretion by LA-N-2 human neuroblastoma cells. Brain Res. 476:323-331.

6. POTTER, P.E., MEEK, J.L. and NEFF, N.H., (1983), Acetylcholine and choline in neuronal t issue measured by HPLC with electrochemical detection. J.Neurochem. 41:188-194.

7. FONNUM, F., (1975), A rapid radiochemical method for the determination of choline acetyltransferase. J.Neurochem. 24:407-409.

8. PRASAD, K.N. and KUMAR, S. (1974), Cyclic AMP and the differentiation of neuroblastoma cells in culture, Control of Proliferation in Animal Cells, B. Clarkson and R. Baserga (Ed.) Cold Spring Harbor Laboratory, 581-594.

9. GREEN, L.A. and TISCHLER, A.S., (1976), Establishment of noradrenergic clonal line of rat adrenal pheochromocytoma cells which respond to NGF. Proc.Natl.Acad.Sci.USA 73:2424-2428.

10. DANIELS, M.P. and HAMPRECHT, B., (1974), The ultrastructure of neuroblastoma glioma somatic cell hybrids. Expression of neuronal characteristics stimulated by dibutyryl adenosine 3',5' cyclic monophosphate. J.Cell Biol. 63:691-699.

11. SUSZKIW, J.B. and PILAR, G., (1976), Selective localization of a high affinity choline uptake system and its role in ACh formation in cholinergic nerve terminals. J.Neurochem. 26:1133-1138.

12. KELLER, F., RIMVALL, K. and WASER, P.G., (1987), Choline and acetylcholine metabolism in slice cultures of the newborn rat septum. Brain Res. 405:305-312.

13. BOSTWICK, J.R., LANDERS, D.W., CRAWFORD, G., LAU, K. and APPEL, S.H., (1989), Purification and characterization of a central cholinergic enhancing factor from rat brain: Its identity as phosphoethanolamine. J.Neurochem. 53:448-458.

14. KATO, A.C., LEFRESNE, P., BERWALD-NETTER, Y., BOJOUAN, J.C., GLOWINSKI, J. and GROSS, F., (1977), Choline stimulates the synthesis of acetylcholine from acatate and the accumulation of acetate in a cholinergic neuroblastoma clone. Biochem.Biophys.Res.Commun. 78:350-356.

15. COHEN, E.L. and WURTMAN, R.J., (1976), Brain acetylcholine: control by dietary choline. Science 191:561-562.

16. MOREL, N., ISRAEL, M., MANARANCHE, R. and MASTOUR-FRACHON, P., (1977), Isolation of pure cholinergic nerve endings from *Torpedo* electric organ. J.Cell Biol. 75:43-55.

17. LANKS, K., SOMERS, L., PAPIRMEISTER, B. and YAMAMURA, H., (1974), Choline transport by neuroblastoma cells in tissue culture. Nature 252:476-478.

18. McGEE, R.,JR., (1980), Choline uptake by the neuroblastoma x glioma hybrid, NG108-15. J.Neurochem. 35:829-837.

19. MELEGA, W.P. and HOWARD, B.D., (1981), Choline and acetylcholine metabolism in PC12 secretory cells. Biochemistry 20:4477-4483.

20. SZUTOWICZ, A., MORRISON, M.R. and SRERE, P.A., (1983), The enzymes of acetyl-CoA metabolism in differentiating cholinergic (S-20) and noncholinergic (NIE-115) neuroblastoma cells. J.Neurochem. 40:1664-1670.

21. CASPER, D. and DAVIES, P., (1989), Stimulation of choline acetyltransferase activity by retinoic acid and sodium butyrate in a cultured human neuroblastoma. Brain Res. 478:74-84.

22. BIELARCZYK, H. and SZUTOWICZ, A., (1989), Evidence for the regulatory function of synaptoplasmic acetyl-CoA in acetylcholine synthesis in nerve endings. Biochem.J. 262:377-380.

23. BLUSZTAJN, J.K. and WURTMAN, R.J., (1983), Choline and cholinergic neurons. Science 221:614-620.

24. HEFTI, F., HARTIKKA, J., ECKENSTEIN, F., GNAHN, H., HEUMANN, R. and SCHWAB, M.E., (1985), Nerve growth factor increases choline acetyltransferase but not survival or fiber outgrowth of cultured fetal septal cholinergic neurons. Neuroscience 14:55-68.

25. VACA, K., STEWART, S.S. and APPEL, S.H., (1989), Identification of basic fibroblast growth factor as a cholinergic growth factor from human muscle. J.Neurosci.Res. 23:55-63.

26. SAADAT, S., SENDTNER, M. and ROHRER, H., (1989), Ciliary neurotrophic factor induces cholinergic differentiation of rat sympathetic neurons in culture. J.Cell Biol. 108:1807-1816.

27. McMANAMAN, J.L., CRAWFORD, F.G., STEWART, S.S. and APPEL, S.H., (1988), Purification of a skeletal muscle polypeptide which stimulates choline acetyltransferase activity in cultured spinal cord neurons. J.Biol.Chem. 263:5890-5897.

28. FUKADA, K., (1985), Purification and partial characterization of a cholinergic neuronal differentiation factor. Proc.Natl.Acad.Sci.USA 82:8795-8799.

29. YAMAMORI, T., FUKADA, K., AEBERSOLD, R., KORSCHING, S., FANN, M.-J. and PATTERSON, P.H., (1989), The cholinergic neuronal differentiation factor from heart cells is identical to leukemia inhibitory factor. Science 246:1412-1416.

30. ADLER, J.E., SCHLEIFER, L.S. and BLACK, I.B., (1989), Partial purification and characterization of a membrane-derived factor regulating neurotransmitter phenotypic expression. Proc.Natl.Acad.Sci.USA 86:1080-1083.

31. RAO, M.S. and LANDIS, S.C., (1990), Characterization of a target-derived neuronal cholinergic differentiation factor. Neuron 5:899-910.

32. KAMEGAI, M., KONISHI, Y. and TABIRA, T., (1990), Trophic effect of granulocyte-macrophage colony-stimulating factor on central cholinergic neurons in vitro. Brain Res. 532:323-325.

33. KAMEGAI, M., NIIJIMA, K., KUNISHITA, T., NISHIZAWA, M., OGAWA, M., ARAKI, M., UEKI, A., KONISHI, Y. and TABIRA, T., (1990), Interleukin 3 as a trophic factor for central cholinergic neurons in vitro and in vivo. Neuron 4:429-436.

34. CASHMAN, N.R., BOULET, S. and ANTEL, J., (1987), Clonal cell lines from neuroblastoma-spinal cord cell hydridization. Soc.Neurosci.Abstr. 420.7.

35. CASPER, D. and DAVIES, P., (1989), Mechanism of activation of choline acetyltransferase in a human neuroblastoma cell line. Brain Res. 478:85-94.

36. CASPER, D. and DAVIES, P., (1988), Regulation of choline acetyltransferase activity by cell density in a cultured human neuroblastoma cell line. Dev.Neurosci. 10:245-255.

A2

Electrophysiological Approaches to *In Vitro* Neurotoxicology

JOEP van den BERCKEN, MARGA OORTGIESEN,
TRESE LEINDERS, and HENK P.M. VIJVERBERG

Research Institute of Toxicology
University of Utrecht
P.O. Box 80.176
NL 3508 TD Utrecht, The Netherlands

ABSTRACT

Cultured cells are widely used for the electrophysiological investigation of properties of excitable and unexcitable membranes. From this approach cell lines are now available, which express a variety of receptors and ion channels. The detailed characterization of basic physiological and pharmacological properties of the receptors and ion channels of cultured cell lines creates valuable models for *in vitro* neurotoxicological research. Mouse neuroblastoma N1E-115 cells have been studied extensively and constitute a suitable model for *in vitro* neurotoxicological studies. The mode of action of selective compounds at the target site may be further defined down to the level of single ion channels, as demonstrated for the pyrethroid insecticides. The diversity of the model enables to compare the differential sensitivity of various potential target sites to non-selective neurotoxicants. The latter is illustrated by recent results on the effects of Pb^{2+} on voltage-dependent and receptor-operated ion channels in N1E-115 cells.

INTRODUCTION

For many years excised nerve and muscle preparations of experimental animals have been the only choice for vertebrate electrophysiology and hence for electrophysiological studies in the field of *in vitro* neurotoxicology. In particular preparations of the frog, i.e., excised myelinated nerves and single myelinated nerve fibers, ganglia, nerve-muscle preparations, the isolated spinal cord and even the brain have been used to study the effects of neurotoxic compounds. Although the toxicological gap between frog

---

¶This manuscript was unfinished at the sudden death of Joep van den Bercken on February 20, 1992. The co-authors are indebted to his ever stimulating support and appraisal of their scientific and personal endeavors, and are honored to dedicate this chapter to his memory.

and mammals, including man, is almost insurmountable from a more general viewpoint, electrophysiological studies in frog nerve preparations have contributed greatly to our present understanding of the functioning of the nervous system and of the mode of action of many neurotoxicants. In some cases results obtained in frog preparations in vitro allowed the interpretation of effects of neurotoxicants on intact animals and even to extrapolate this interpretation to the human situation.

The utility of in vitro results may be illustrated by the example of pyrethroid insecticides. At an early stage of pyrethroid development it was shown that the cutaneous touch receptor in an isolated piece of frog skin is rather sensitive to the action of these insecticides.[2] After exposure of the outside of the skin to the pyrethroid allethrin, a small mechanical stimulus, which normally produces only one nerve impulse, caused a train of impulses in the afferent nerve fiber (Fig. 1). Further investigations showed that repetitive firing in sensory nerves was the most important effect of low concentrations of pyrethroids on various parts of the peripheral nervous system. The pyrethroid-induced repetitive nerve activity was studied in detail in the lateral-line sense organ of the clawed frog, providing valuable information on the structure-activity relationship of these insecticides.[53] Cyano pyrethroids, like cypermethrin, deltamethrin and fenpropathrin, produced much more intense repetitive firing than the non-cyano pyrethroids, like allethrin, bioresmethrin, cismethrin and permethrin. In the mean time widespread practical application of these insecticides revealed that occupational exposure, in particular to cyano pyrethroids, frequently caused transient local burning or tingling sensations and also itching and numbness (paresthesia) mainly of the facial

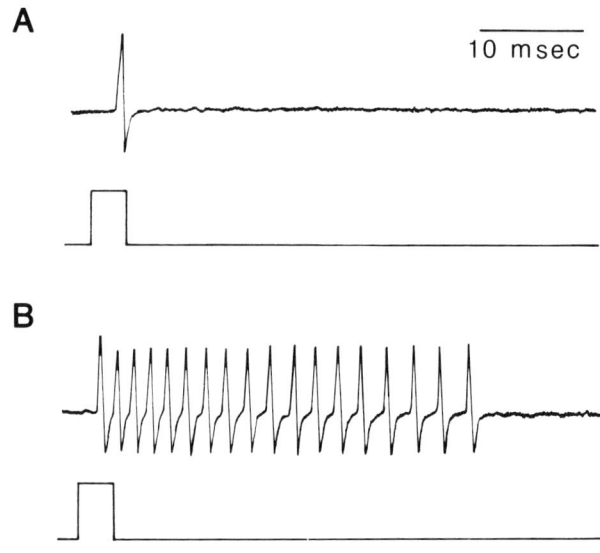

FIGURE 1. Repetitive nerve impulses induced by a pyrethroid insecticide in the peripheral sensory nervous system of the frog Xenopus laevis.
(A) Nerve impulse evoked in a single sensory nerve fibre by a brief mechanical stimulus (lower trace) in the control situation. (B) Instead of a single nerve impulse a train of repetitive nerve impulses is evoked by the same stimulus after 30 min of in vitro exposure of the skin to 10 µM of the pyrethroid allethrin. (after ref. 2: Akkermans et al., 1975)

skin.[9,13] It is now generally accepted that these skin sensations are caused by repetitive firing of sensory nerve endings in the skin, as was first observed in the frog.[17,51]

In the past decade improvements in the field of (neuronal) cell culture methods and revolutionary changes in electrophysiological techniques have advanced research into the mode of action of neurotoxicants to the molecular level. The effects of neurotoxicants on voltage-dependent and receptor-operated processes involved in the excitation of mammalian neurones can now be investigated in great detail under strictly controlled experimental conditions.

Results of recent electrophysiological investigations of effects of pyrethroid insecticides and lead, which are described below, illustrate that the *in vitro* approach contributes significantly to the understanding of the mode of action of selective and non-selective neurotoxic compounds.

NEURONAL CULTURES - NEUROBLASTOMA N1E-115 CELLS

Techniques have been developed to dissociate neuronal tissues mechanically and enzymatically to obtain neuronal cultures, which can also be used for neurotoxicological investigations. Dissociated cells, primary cultures and tissue explant cultures may be obtained from animal species ranging from insects to mammals. These cultures generally contain mixed cell populations, including diverse types of neurones and various glial cells. The finite lifetime and changes of cell properties in the course of culture are disadvantages of these *in vitro* systems. The procedures to isolate neurones need to be repeated over and over again and require experimental animals.

For a number of reasons clonal cell lines are well-suited for electrophysiological studies. With the proper management of stock cultures in liquid nitrogen, clonal cell lines can be maintained almost indefinitely with fairly consistent phenotypes and can be obtained in any quantity. Differentiation can be induced readily by changes in culture conditions. Most importantly, the cultures contain a homogeneous cell population. Cell density can be kept low and culture conditions can be adapted to restrict the outgrowth of neurites without loss of functional characteristics. These latter features are important for electrical control of the membrane potential in voltage clamp experiments. In this connection it is noteworthy that, at least in N1E-115 cells, there is little correlation between morphological differentiation, i.e., cell enlargement and outgrowth of neurites, and electrophysiological differentiation, i.e., electrical and chemical excitability.[11] Small and apparently undifferentiated neuroblastoma cells without neurites may show action potentials similar to those observed in mature neurones and may even be spontaneously active.

The neuroblastoma clone N1E-115, which is derived from the C-1300 neuroblastoma tumor of the mouse, has been used in electrophysiological investigation from a very early stage of cell culture. The C-1300 tumor originates from a part of the neural crest, which normally develops into sympathetic ganglia. Therefore, N1E-115 cells can be expected to have sympathetic properties. A detailed account of the characteristics of the C-1300 mouse neuroblastoma cells and their electrophysiology up to 1980 can be found elsewhere.[3,11,48] Four distinct types of ion currents were initially identified in these cells; two inward currents carried by voltage-dependent Na^+ and Ca^{2+} channels and two outward currents carried by voltage-dependent and by Ca^{2+}-activated K^+ channels.[23,24,25] Physiological and pharmacological properties of specific ion channels involved have been characterized in detail by electrophysiological as well as by ion flux and radioligand binding studies and are essentially similar to those of other mammalian nerve cells. Since the past decade N1E-115 cells, as well as a variety of other neuronal cell lines are being used in laboratories all over the world. N1E-115 cells contain voltage-dependent Na^+ channels and multiple subtypes of voltage-dependent K^+ and Ca^{2+} channels, Ca^{2+}-activated K^+ channels and cation channels. In addition, they contain a variety of receptors for neurotransmitters, some of which are coupled to receptor-operated ion channels. These include nicotinic and muscarinic acetylcholine (ACh) receptor-operated ion channels and serotonin ($5-HT_3$) receptor-operated ion channels. A range of receptors for other neuromodulatory substances has been demonstrated by radioligand binding and second messenger studies (for review see: ref. 50).

The availability of N1E-115 cells and other clonal cell lines, together with the development of sophisticated electrophysiological techniques, i.c. the patch clamp technique, to study the functional properties of ion channels down to the level of the individual channel molecule, have started a new era in the field of *in vitro* neurotoxicology. On the one hand the action of neurotoxicants can be studied in great detail, while on the other hand their effects on a variety of ion channels can be studied in the same cell type under the same experimental conditions.

PATCH CLAMP TECHNIQUE

The voltage clamp technique is a most powerful method to study the electrical properties of cell membranes and to investigate effects of neurotoxicants on excitable membranes. With this technique it is possible to control the voltage across the cell membrane and to simultaneously measure the ionic currents through the membrane. With the advancement of neuronal cell culture the voltage clamp technique has been adapted to record membrane currents in small isolated neurons and extended to record the miniature signals generated by the opening and closing of individual ion channels by means of the single channel patch clamp technique (Fig. 2).[8]

In the whole-cell configuration the cell is gently sucked to the opening of a glass pipette with a (sub)micrometer tip opening. The pipette tightly seals to the cell and the remaining leakage between glass and membrane, that has an electrical resistance in the order of GigaΩ, becomes negligible. Access to the cell interior is obtained by rupturing the patch of membrane inside the pipette by additional suction or by applying a current pulse. This results not only in a reduction of the access resistance to the cell required for voltage clamp, but also in a rapid exchange of diffusible components between the pipette solution and the cytoplasm. Under these conditions the ionic composition of the intra- and extracellular solutions can be manipulated and drugs and poisons can be applied to either side of the membrane. By replacing permeable ions with impermeable ones and by adding selective ion channel blockers to the experimental solutions, currents through a specific type of ion channel can be measured without interference of other signals. For single channel recording the pipette is pulled away from the cell, resulting in the isolation of a patch of membrane that is attached to the pipette tip and contains few or only one single ion channel. Depending on experimental manipulations 'inside-out' or 'outside-out' membrane patches can be obtained (see Fig. 2).

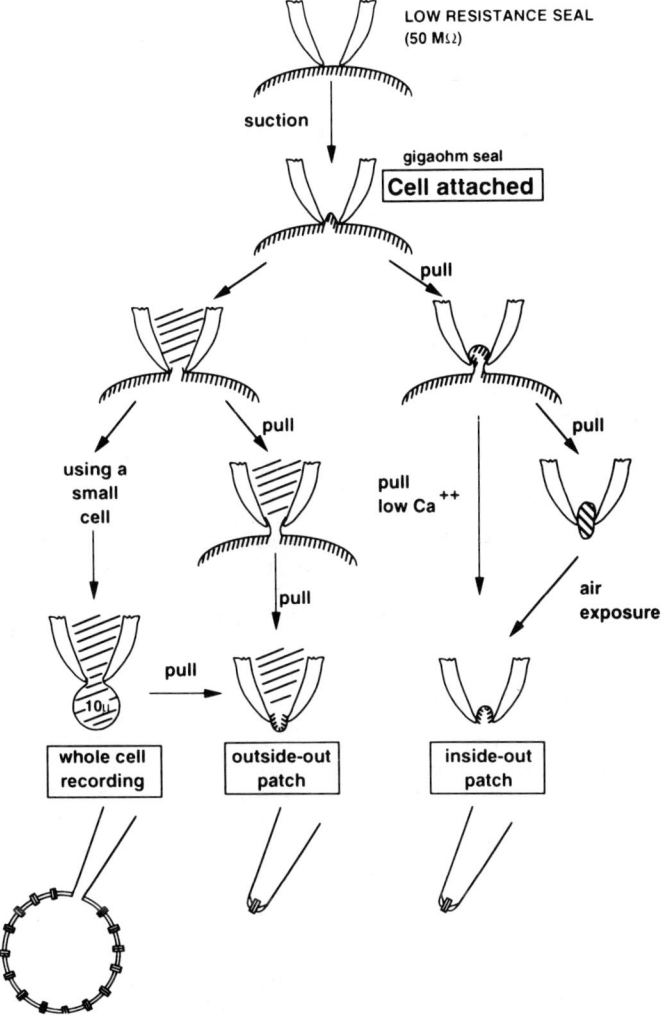

FIGURE 2. Patch pipette configurations for whole-cell voltage clamp and for single channel patch clamp of outside-out and inside-out membrane patches. (modified after ref. 8: Hamill et al., 1981).

ACTION OF PYRETHROIDS

The pyrethroids constitute a major class of synthetic and highly active insecticides with a fairly selective neurotoxic mechanism of action. They produce pronounced excitatory effects in insects as well as in mammals, including man, whenever they reach the nervous system in sufficient concentration. As mentioned above, the principal effect of pyrethroids is to induce repetitive activity in sense organs and in other parts of both the peripheral and the central nervous system. In addition, they may cause excessive neurotransmitter release due to depolarization of presynaptic nerve endings and, eventually, nerve conduction block.[51]

Voltage-dependent sodium channels. In recent years it has become evident that all insecticidally active pyrethroids share the same mechanism of action on voltage-dependent Na^+ channels in the nerve membrane. In frog myelinated nerve fibers pyrethroids induce a prolonged inward Na^+ tail current, that follows the Na^+ current evoked by a step depolarization of the membrane.[52] A similar prolonged Na^+ tail current is observed in squid giant axons and other invertebrate nerve fibers after treatment with pyrethroids.[27] The prolongation of the Na^+ current varies greatly with pyrethroid structure. Cyano substituted pyrethroids prolong the Na^+ current to a much greater extent than non-cyano pyrethroids. The time course of decay of the Na^+ tail current in frog myelinated nerve fibers correlates well with the intensity of repetitive activity in the lateral-line sense organ of Xenopus. Dependent on its size and time course the prolonged Na^+ current causes a depolarizing afterpotential, all or not associated with repetitive activity, or more permanent membrane depolarization, which may lead to excessive neurotransmitter release and to complete block of membrane excitability. In N1E-115 cells exposed to pyrethroids the Na^+ current is prolonged both during depolarization and after repolarization (Fig. 3). In addition, pyrethroids also induce an increase in the peak amplitude of the inward Na^+ current in N1E-115 cells.[44]

On the basis of macroscopic whole-cell current recordings it was hypothesized that pyrethroids selectively affect the kinetic properties of the Na^+ channels and that they keep these channels open for a much longer time than is normal. Single channel patch clamp experiments in 'outside-out' patches of N1E-115 cells have in fact confirmed that the open time of individual Na^+ channels is greatly prolonged by pyrethroids (Fig. 4).[6,55,57] Similar results were obtained in dissociated frog spinal ganglion cells.[56]

Other ion channels. It has been reported that high concentrations of pyrethroids have a suppressive effect on Na^+ as well as K^+ channels in invertebrate nerve preparations.[12,32,33,54]. However, lower concentrations of pyrethroids, which significantly affect Na^+ channels, do not affect voltage-dependent K^+ channels.[45] It has also been reported that the pyrethroid tetramethrin partially blocks one

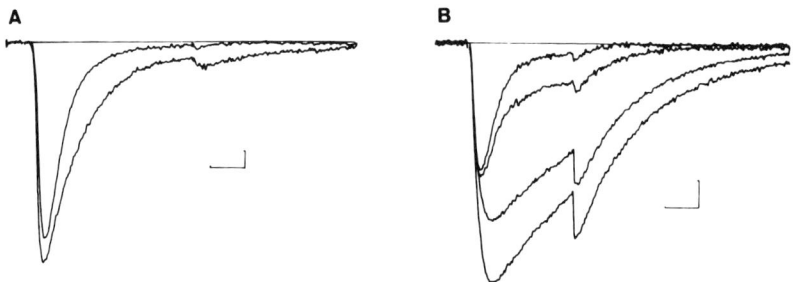

FIGURE 3. Effect of pyrethroid insecticides on Na^+ current evoked by a membrane depolarization to -5 mV in internally perfused, voltage clamped N1E-115 cells.
(A) Na^+ currents evoked by 10 ms step depolarizations of the whole cell membrane before and 20 min after external application of 100 μM phenothrin (Holding potential -95 mV; Calibrations: vertical 2 nA, horizontal 2 ms). (B) Four superimposed Na^+ current traces evoked by 15 ms step depolarizations to -5 mV before and 1.5 min, 4.5 min and 30 min after external application of 1 μM fenfluthrin (Calibrations vertical 2 nA, horizontal 5 ms). The pyrethroids prolong Na^+ currents, enhance peak amplitudes and induce prolonged Na^+ tail currents after termination of membrane depolarization. (after ref. 44: Ruigt et al., 1987)

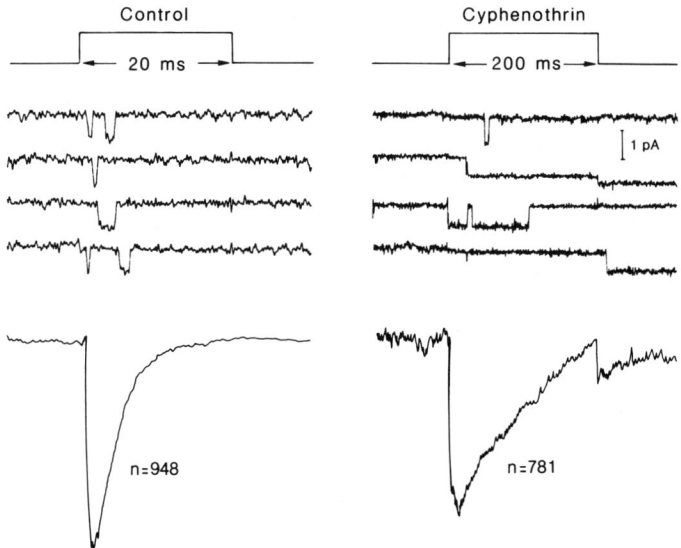

FIGURE 4. Opening and closing of individual Na^+ channels in excised patches of the membrane of cultured mouse neuroblastoma cells. Downward deflections of the current traces are discrete openings of individual ion channels.
In the presence of 10 μM of the cyano pyrethroid (1R),cis-cyphenothrin the open time of Na^+ channels is greatly prolonged and channel openings are also observed after termination of membrane depolarization. Summation of large numbers (n) of single channel records results in a rapid, transient Na^+ current in the control situation and a prolonged Na^+ current followed by a Na^+ tail current in the presence of the pyrethroid. (adapted from ref. 55: de Weille, 1986)

type of Ca^{2+} channel in N1E-115 cells.[27] This result has not been confirmed with other pyrethroids.[43]

Several studies have suggested that pyrethroids, in addition to affecting Na^+ channels, also affect ion channels that are coupled to neurotransmitter receptors. High concentrations of cyano pyrethroids cause a stereoselective partial inhibition of radioligand binding to the GABA receptor-ion channel complex.[14] From effects of pyrethroids on the properties of the ACh receptor-ion channel complex it has been suggested that these compounds delay the closing or desensitization of the ion channels coupled to the nicotinic ACh receptor.[46] Recent studies in voltage clamped N1E-115 cells have shown that relatively high concentrations of pyrethroids reduce the amplitude of the ACh response. Similar effects were observed on the 5-HT-induced response, which is mediated by an independent population of serotonin (5-HT_3) receptor-operated channels. These effects appeared to be nonspecific, as they were also produced by insecticidally inactive isomers.[36] An inhibition of nicotinic ACh receptor- and serotonin 5-HT_3 receptor-mediated responses would cause inhibitory effects rather than the excitatory symptoms observed with pyrethroids.

Although the molecular aspects of pyrethroid action are not yet understood, it can be concluded that these insecticides primarily interact with voltage-dependent Na^+ channels in the nerve membrane in a highly selective manner, keeping these channels open for a much longer time than is normal.

EFFECTS OF LEAD

Although a great deal is known about the effects of lead on the nervous system, the mechanism of lead neurotoxicity at the cellular and molecular level is still poorly understood.[47] It appears that lead acts rather nonselectively, producing dysfunction at any site to which it gains access in sufficient amounts.

Particular attention has been paid to potential effects of inorganic lead (Pb^{2+}) on synaptic transmission, both pre- and post-synaptically. Electrophysiological experiments on frog and rat nerve-muscle preparations have shown that Pb^{2+} first blocks evoked neurotransmitter release and subsequently enhances spontaneous release.[4,19,40] Similar results have been obtained in rat cortical synaptosomes.[22,49] To explain these apparently contradictory effects, it has been proposed that Pb^{2+} first blocks inward Ca^{2+} current in the presynaptic terminal, which is a prerequisite for neurotransmitter release, and subsequently penetrates into the cell and interferes with intracellular Ca^{2+} homeostasis by competing with Ca^{2+} for intracellular binding sites.[19] In addition, it has been reported that high concentrations of Pb^{2+} reduce ACh-induced depolarizations in frog muscle[19], while in the mouse hemidiaphragm 1 µM Pb^{2+} causes a transient decrease of the ACh response.[34] Comparative effects of Pb^{2+} on the various types of voltage-dependent and receptor-operated ion channels have been investigated in N1E-115 cells.

Voltage-dependent ion channels. Effects of Pb^{2+} on voltage-dependent Na^+ and Ca^{2+} channels have been studied in whole-cell voltage clamped N1E-115 cells. External application of Pb^{2+} (in the form of $PbNO_3$) at concentrations ranging from 10 - 100 µM does not affect voltage-dependent Na^+ current. Amplitude and time course of the inward Na^+ current evoked by step depolarization remain essentially unaffected. Currents through voltage-dependent Ca^{2+} channels are amplified by using external solution containing 50 mM Ba^{2+}. In addition, Ba^{2+} entry through open Ca^{2+} channels does not lead to the activation of Ca^{2+}-dependent K^+ current. Under these conditions membrane step depolarizations evoke fast transient and non-inactivating inward Ba^{2+} current components, that are carried by two distinct types of voltage-dependent Ca^{2+} channels. During superfusion with Pb^{2+} the amplitude of both Ba^{2+} current components is reversibly blocked in a concentration-dependent manner with an IC50 of 4.8 ± 0.8 µM Pb^{2+} and complete block of the Ba^{2+} current is achieved with 100 µM Pb^{2+} (Fig. 5). Effects of Pb^{2+} on whole-cell Ca^{2+} currents have been confirmed by a detailed investigation of N1E-115 cells[5] and similar results have been obtained in human neuroblastoma cells[42] and in rat dorsal root ganglion cells.[7] The IC50 obtained from N1E-115 cells is in the same order of magnitude as the value of 1 µM reported for Ca^{2+} influx inhibition by Pb^{2+} in rat synaptosomes[22,49], and as the value of 1 µM of the dissociation constant of Pb^{2+} from presynaptic Ca^{2+} binding sites in frog endplate.[19] Thus the present experiments corroborate the hypothesis that presynaptic Ca^{2+} channels are the target site for block of neurotransmitter release by micromolar Pb^{2+} concentrations.

Ca^{2+}-activated K^+ channels. N1E-115 cells contain two types of Ca^{2+}-activated K^+ channels (CaK channels). Low conductance (SK) channels with a single channel conductance of 5.4 pS in a physiological K^+ gradient are blocked by nanomolar concentrations of the bee venom peptide apamin and large conductance (BK) channels with a

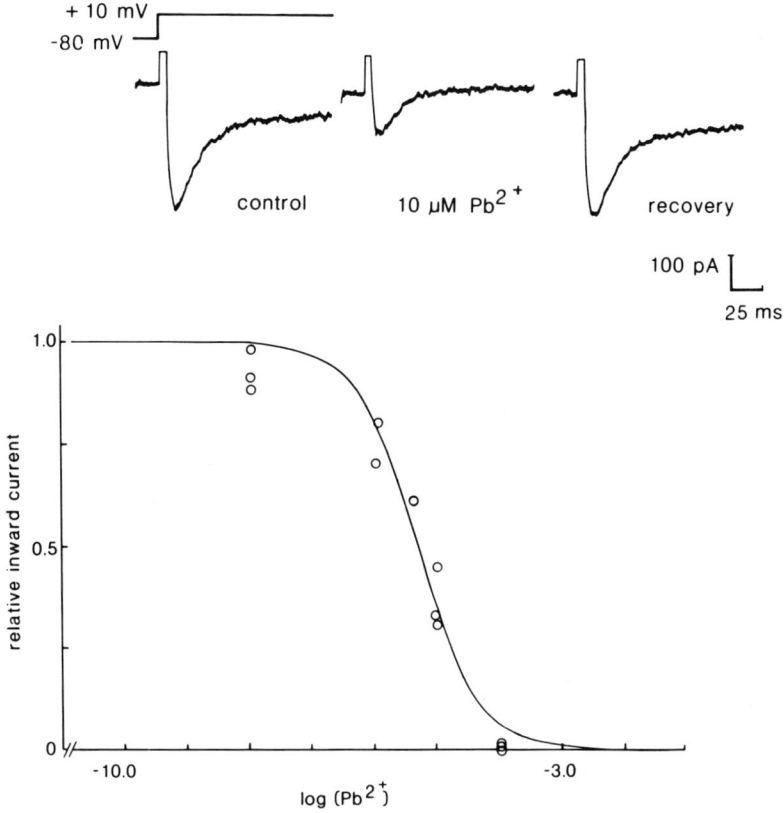

FIGURE 5. Pb^{2+} blocks voltage-dependent Ca^{2+} channels in N1E-115 cells. The upper panel shows Ba^{2+} currents evoked by step depolarizations to +10 mV in control external solution, after 5 min of superfusion with 10 μM Pb^{2+} and recovery after 5 min of washing with control external solution. The peak amplitude of the transient component of inward Ba^{2+} current was reduced to 34% of the control value by 10 μM Pb^{2+}. Holding potential is -80 mV. The lower panel shows the concentration dependence of the blocking effect of Pb^{2+}. Ordinate represents the peak amplitude of the transient inward current normalized to control value. The IC50 value and the slope factor estimated from the concentration-effect curve of block of the transient component of the Ba^{2+} current by Pb^{2+} are 4.8 ± 0.8 μM and -0.88 ± 0.14, respectively. (after ref. 35: Oortgiesen et al., 1990)

single channel conductance of 98 pS are insensitive to apamin.[15,41] BK channels play a role in the repolarization phase of the action potential[1], while SK channels are involved in the afterhyperpolarization following the action potential.[10]

Single channel patch clamp experiments on 'inside-out' patches of N1E-115 cells have revealed that Pb^{2+}, applied to the inside of the membrane, is able to activate CaK channels in the absence of Ca^{2+} (Fig. 6).[16] Pb^{2+} is more potent than Ca^{2+} in activating both types of CaK channel. At a concentration of 1 μM Pb^{2+} the open probability of the SK channel is maximally enhanced, whereas the BK channel open probability in the presence of 1 μM Pb^{2+} is only 10% of the maximum attainable with Ca^{2+}.

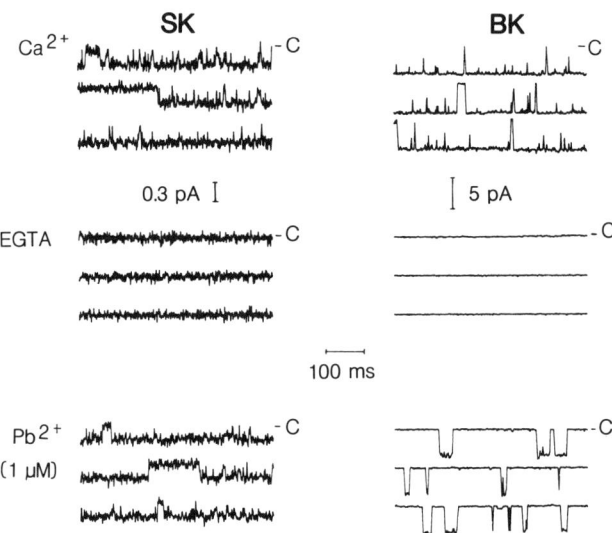

FIGURE 6. Effects of Pb^{2+} on Ca^{2+}-activated K^+ channels.
Maximum open probability of single SK (left) and BK (right) channels in two inside-out excised patches by superfusion with 14.4 and 115.2 μM buffered free Ca^{2+}, respectively. Subsequent superfusion with Ca^{2+}-free EGTA-containing solution abolished single channel activity. In the same membrane patches superfusion with 1 μM buffered free Pb^{2+} induced full activation of the SK and partial (10% of maximum open probability) activation of the BK channel. Membrane potential was held at 0 mV. (after ref. 16, Leinders et al., 1992)

Receptor-operated channels. Superfusion of voltage clamped N1E-115 cells with serotonin (5-HT) or acetylcholine (ACh) results in transient inward currents. The 5-HT-induced inward current is mediated by 5-HT$_3$ receptors. Pharmacological and physiological properties of the 5-HT$_3$ receptor-operated ion currents in N1E-115 cells have been described in detail.[29,30,31] Recently, it has been demonstrated that the 5-HT$_3$ receptor-operated ion channel protein is a member of the class of directly ligand gated ion channels and resembles the α-subunit of nicotinic receptors from *Torpedo californica*.[20] The ACh-induced inward current in N1E-115 differs from that in the end-plate by its insensitivity to block by α-bungarotoxin (α-BuTX) and its sensitivity to block by kappa-BuTX.[38] The sensitivity to kappa-BuTX is a pharmacological property of neuronal type nicotinic ACh receptors. The availability of agonists and antagonists selective to ACh and 5-HT receptors in N1E-115 cells and the heterologous desensitization of ACh and 5-HT receptor-mediated inward currents demonstrate the presence of two distinct and independent populations of ACh and 5-HT receptor-operated ion channels. The resemblance between the two may be exemplified by the fact that both ACh and 5-HT$_3$ receptor-operated ion currents in N1E-115 are blocked by the arrow poison d-tubocurarine, with IC50 values of 0.5 μM and 0.8 nM, respectively.[38,39] It is remarkable that the potency of d-tubocurarine to block 5-HT-induced ion current is much higher than that to block ACh-induced ion current.

Application of Pb^{2+} at concentrations ranging from 10 nM to 100 μM causes a reduction of the 5-HT-induced inward current, without affecting its time course. This blocking effect of Pb^{2+} is almost completely reversed by washing with external solution for 4 - 8 min. The estimated value of the IC50 of the concentration-effect curve of block by Pb^{2+} is 49 ± 18 μM.[35]

The peak amplitude of the ACh-induced inward current is 32% reduced by superfusion with 10 nM Pb^{2+} within 7 min, while the time course of the ACh response remains unaffected at this very low concentration of Pb^{2+}. At 3 μM Pb^{2+} the amplitude of the ACh-induced inward current reaches only 10% of the control value. However, after higher concentrations of Pb^{2+} the blocking effect is reversed and after superfusion with 100 μM Pb^{2+} the peak amplitude of the ACh response amounts to almost 70% of the control value. In addition, the decay of the remaining ACh-induced inward current is markedly delayed by high concentrations of Pb^{2+}. Fig. 7 shows the concentration dependence of the effect of Pb^{2+} on the inward current induced by 1 mM ACh in N1E-115 cells. The data can be fitted by the sum of a descending and an ascending concentration-effect curve with an IC50 value of 19 ± 6.3 nM and an EC50 of 21 ± 5.5 μM, respectively. The reversal of block of the ACh-induced current suggest a dual effect of Pb^{2+} on neuronal nicotinic ACh receptor-activated channels.[35]

In frog end-plate 10 mM Ni^{2+} also causes a dual effect on ACh receptor-operated ion channels; a reduction of single channel conductance and a simultaneous prolongation of channel open time.[18] Recently, Ca^{2+} has been shown to reduce single channel conductance and to increase opening frequency of ACh receptor-operated ion channels in rat central neurones.[26] Effects of Pb^{2+} on single cholinergic ion channels in N1E-115 cells remain to be investigated.

In addition to the effects described above, superfusion of N1E-115 cells with high concentrations of Pb^{2+} (> 10 μM) induce a slow, non-inactivating inward current, which is not mediated by a known type of receptor-operated or voltage-dependent ion channel. A similar current is induced by superfusion with Cd^{2+} and Al^{3+}. These currents appear mediated by a novel type of metal ion-activated (MIA) channel, which has no known physiological function at present.[37]

The results, which are summarized in Table I, show that neuronal type nicotinic ACh receptors are the most sensitive to Pb^{2+} and are selectively blocked by nanomolar concentrations of Pb^{2+}. The same low concentrations of Pb^{2+} neither affect $5-HT_3$ receptor-activated channels, nor voltage-dependent Na^+ and Ca^{2+} channels, or big Ca^{2+}-activated K^+ channels. Small Ca^{2+}-activated K^+ channels may constitute another sensitive target of Pb^{2+} after entering the cytoplasmic compartment of neurones.

Table I also demonstrates that at various fixed concentrations Pb^{2+} selectively modifies subtypes of channels of the various classes investigated. In the micromolar range external Pb^{2+} blocks voltage-dependent Ca^{2+} channels selectively as compared to Na^+ channels and internal Pb^{2+} selectively activates Ca^{2+}-dependent SK channels as compared to BK channels. The differential effects on neuronal type nicotinic ACh receptor-operated ion channels and $5-HT_3$ receptor-operated channels also suggests selective and distinct interactions of Pb^{2+} with subtypes of directly ligand gated ion channels. Although picomolar concentrations of intracellular Pb^{2+} have been reported to activate protein kinase C[21], neuronal type ACh receptors are among the most sensitive targets of Pb^{2+} known. Therefore, these effects should be considered in the interpretation of cognitive deficits resulting from low level lead exposure.[28]

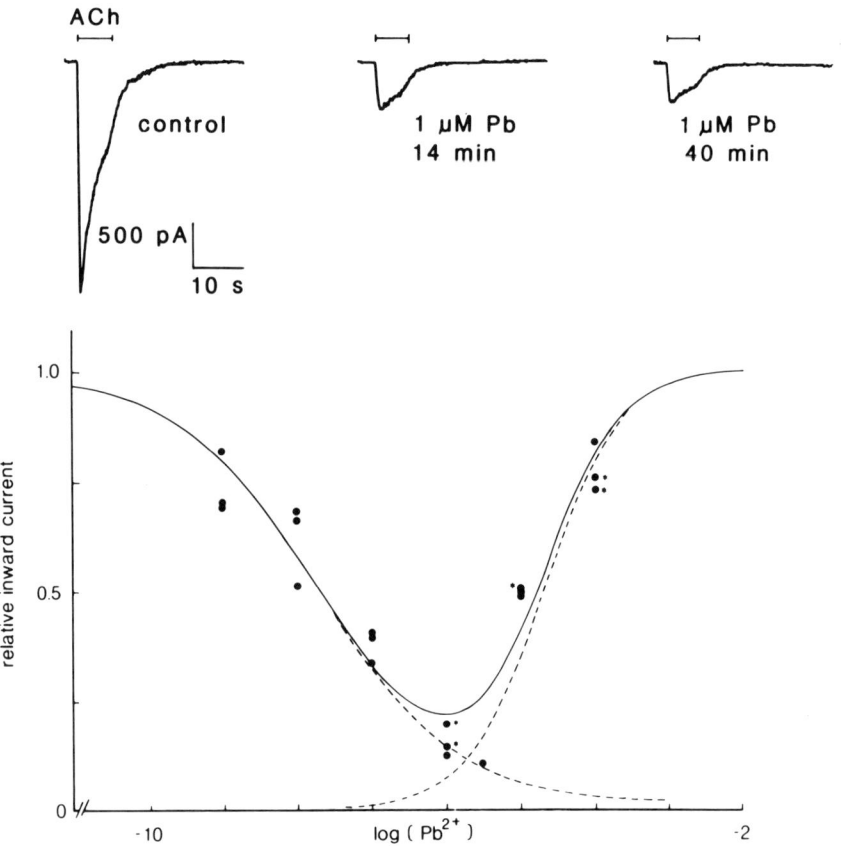

FIGURE 7. Effects of Pb^{2+} on nicotinic ACh-induced ion current. Upper panel left trace shows an inward current induced by 1 mM ACh in control external solution. During superfusion with 1 µM Pb^{2+} the peak amplitude of the ACh-induced inward current was reduced to a steady level which amounts 18% of the control value. Note that 1 µM Pb^{2+} also delays the time course of decay of the ACh-induced inward current. Membrane potential was held at -80 mV. Superfusion periods are indicated by bars. Lower panel shows the concentration dependence of Pb^{2+} effects on the nicotinic ACh-induced ion current. Ordinate represents the inward current peak amplitude normalized to control value. The data were fitted by the sum of two sigmoidal concentration-effect curves. The estimated parameters of the fitted curve (solid line) are: IC50 = 19 ± 6.3 nM; EC50 = 21 ± 5.5 µM and the slope factors are -0.45 ± 0.08 and 0.84 ± 0.15, respectively. The discontinuous lines represent the concentration-effect curve for the blocking effect of Pb^{2+} and for the reversal of block, according to the fitted parameters. (after ref. 35: Oortgiesen et al., 1990)

CONCLUDING REMARKS

N1E-115 neuroblastoma cells are highly suited for detailed electrophysiological investigations into the mechanisms of action of neurotoxicants on various types of nerve membrane ion channels. These cells contain a variety of voltage-dependent, Ca^{2+}-activated

TABLE I. Effects of Pb^{2+} on subtypes of voltage-dependent, Ca^{2+}-activated and receptor-operated ion channels in N1E-115 cells.

Channel type and effect	EC50 of Pb^{2+}
voltage-dependent	
Ca^{2+} channel block	5 µM
Na^+ channel block	>100 µM
Ca^{2+}-activated	
SK channel opening	< 1 µM
BK channel opening	>1 <90 µM
receptor-operated	
n-ACh channel block	20 nM
- reversal of block	20 µM
$5\text{-}HT_3$ channel block	50 µM

and receptor-operated channels. The investigation of structure-related effects of selective agents at the target site provides information on their intrinsic potencies and such knowledge may assist in the interpretation of effects in intact animals. The diversity of ion channels in these cells can be exploited to investigate effects of non-selective neurotoxicants over a wide concentration range and on a variety of potential targets. The example of Pb^{2+} demonstrates that this is not only confirmatory but also leads to surprising results as the finding that postsynaptic neuronal type nicotinic ACh receptors constitute a highly sensitive target for Pb^{2+} and the discovery of ion channels that are yet to be supplied with a counterpart *in vivo*. Since it is highly unlikely that a single cell type can ever be regarded as a universal model of the mammalian neuron, additional models with complementary properties, including human cell lines, are required to extend *in vitro* neurotoxicological research. Investigation of basic physiological, biochemical and pharmacological properties of distinct cell types is time consuming, but seems to be essential to adequately define and select complementary models.

Acknowledgment. The research has been financially supported by the University of Utrecht, the Netherlands Organization for Scientific Research and by Shell Internationale Research Mij. B.V.

REFERENCES

1. ADAMS, P.R., CONSTANTI, A., BROWN, D.A. and CLARK, R.B. (1982), Intracellular Ca^{2+} activates a fast voltage sensitive K^+ current in vertebrate sympathetic neurones. Nature 296:746.

2. AKKERMANS, L.M.A., van den BERCKEN, J. and VERSLUIJS-HELDER, M. (1975), Comparative effects of DDT, allethrin, dieldrin and aldrin-transdiol on sense organs of *Xenopus laevis*. Pestic. Biochem. Physiol. 5:451.

3. AMANO, T., RICHELSON, E. and NIRENBERG, P.G. (1972), Neurotransmitter synthesis by neuroblastoma clones. Proc. Natl. Acad. Sci. USA 6:258.

4. ATCHISON, W.D., NARAHASHI, T. (1984), Mechanism of action of lead on neuromuscular junctions. Neurotoxicology 5:267.

5. AUDESIRK, G. and AUDESIRK, T. (1991) Effects of inorganic lead on voltage-sensitive calcium channels in N1E-115 neuroblastoma cells. Neurotoxicology 12:519.

6. CHINN, K. and NARAHASHI, T. (1986), Stabilization of sodium channel states by deltamethrin in mouse neuroblastoma cells. J. Physiol. 380:191.

7. EVANS, M.L., BÜSSELBERG, D. and CARPENTER, D.O. (1991), Pb^{2+} blocks calcium currents of cultured dorsal root ganglion cells. Neurosci. Lett. 129:103.

8. HAMILL, O.P., MARTY, A., NEHER, E., SAKMANN, B. and SIGWORTH, F.J. (1981), Improved patch-clamp techniques for high-resolution current recording from cells and cell-free membrane patches. Pflügers Arch. 391:85.

9. HE, F., SUN, H., HAN, K., WU, Y., YAO, P., WANG, S. and LIU, L. (1988), Effects of pyrethroid insecticides on subjects engaged in packaging pyrethroids. Brit. J. Ind. Med. 45:548.

10. HUGUES, M., ROMEY, G., DUVAL, D., VINCENT, J.P. and LAZDUNSKI, M. (1982), Apamin as a selective blocker of the calcium-dependent potassium channel in neuroblastoma cells: Voltage-clamp and biochemical characterization of the toxin receptor. Proc. Natl. Acad. Sci. USA 79:1308.

11. KIMHI, Y. (1981), Nerve cells in clonal systems, *Excitable Cells in Tissue Culture*, P.G. Nelson and M. Lieberman (Eds.) Plenum Press, New York, 173-245.

12. KISS, T. (1988), Effect of deltamethrin on transient outward currents in identified snail neurones. Comp. Biochem. Physiol. C 91: 337.

13. KOLMODIN-HEDMAN, B., SWENSSON, A. and ÅKERBLOM, M. (1982), Occupational exposure to some synthetic pyrethroids (permethrin and fenvalerate). Arch. Toxicol. 50:27.

14. LAWRENCE, L.J. and CASIDA, J.E. (1983), Stereospecific action of pyrethroid insecticides on the gamma-aminobutyric acid receptor-ionophore complex. Science 221: 1399.

15. LEINDERS, T. and VIJVERBERG, H.P.M. (1992), Ca^{2+} dependence of small Ca^{2+}-activated K^+ channels in cultured N1E-115 mouse neuroblastoma cells. Submitted for publication.

16. LEINDERS, T., van KLEEF, R.G.D.M. and VIJVERBERG, H.P.M. (1992), Divalent cations activate SK and BK channels in mouse

neuroblastoma cells: selective activation of SK channels by cadmium. Submitted for publication.

17. LEQUESNE, P.M., MAXWELL, I.C. and BUTTERWORTH, S.T.G. (1980), Transient facial sensory symptoms following exposure to synthetic pyrethroids: a clinical and electrophysiological assessment. Neurotoxicology 2:1.

18. MAGLEBY, K.L. and WEINSTOCK, M.M. (1980), Nickel and calcium ions modify the characteristics of the acetylcholine receptor-channel complex at the frog neuromuscular junction. J. Physiol. 299:203.

19. MANALIS, R.S., COOPER, G.P. and POMEROY, S.L. (1984), Effects of lead on neuromuscular transmission in the frog. Brain Res. 294:95.

20. MARICQ, A.V., PETERSON A.S., BRAKE, A.J., MYERS, R.M. and JULIUS, D. (1991), Primary structure and functional expression of the 5-HT_3 receptor, a serotonin-gated ion channel. Science 254:432.

21. MARKOVAC, J. and GOLDSTEIN, G.W. (1988), Picomolar concentrations of lead stimulate brain protein kinase C. Nature 334:71.

22. MINNEMA, D.J., MICHAELSON, I.A. and COOPER, G.P. (1988), Calcium efflux and neurotransmitter release from rat hippocampal synaptosomes exposed to lead. Toxicol. Appl. Pharmacol. 92:351.

23. MOOLENAAR, W.H. and SPECTOR, I. (1978), Ionic currents in cultured mouse neuroblastoma cells under voltage-clamp conditions. J. Physiol. 278:265.

24. MOOLENAAR, W.H. and SPECTOR, I. (1979), The calcium action potential and a prolonged calcium dependent afterhyperpolarization in mouse neuroblastoma cells. J. Physiol. 292:297.

25. MOOLENAAR, W.H. and SPECTOR, I. (1979), The calcium current and the activation of a slow potassium conductance in voltage-clamped mouse neuroblastoma cells. J. Physiol. 292:307.

26. MULLE, C., LÉNA, C. and CHANGEUX, J.P. (1992), Potentiation of nicotinic receptor response by external calcium in rat central neurones. Neuron, in press.

27. NARAHASHI, T. (1986), Mechanisms of actions of pyrethroids on sodium and calcium channel gating, <u>Neuropharmacology and Pesticide Action</u>, M.G. Ford, G.G. Lunt, R.C. Reay and P.N.R. Usherwood (Eds.) Ellis Horwood Ltd., Chichester, England, 36-60.

28. NEEDLEMAN, H.L. and BELLINGER, D. (1991), The health effects of low level exposure to lead. Annu. Rev. Publ. Health 12:111.

29. NEIJT, H.C., te DUITS, I.J., and VIJVERBERG, H.P.M. (1988), Pharmacological characterization of serotonin 5-HT_3 receptor-mediated electrical response in cultured mouse neuroblastoma cells. Neuropharmacol. 27:301.

30. NEIJT, H.C., KARPF, A., SCHOEFFTER, P., ENGEL, G. and HOYER, D. (1988), Characterization of 5-HT_3 recognition sites in membran-

es of NG108-15 neuroblastoma-glioma cells by radioligand binding. Naunyn-Schmiedeb. Arch. Pharmacol. 337:493.

31. NEIJT, H.C., PLOMP, J.J. and VIJVERBERG, H.P.M. (1989), Kinetics of the membrane current mediated by serotonin 5-HT_3 receptors in cultured mouse neuroblastoma cells. J.Physiol. 411:257.

32. NISHIMURA, K., OMATSU, M., MURAYAMA, K., KITASATO, H. and FUJITA, T. (1989), Neurophysiological effects of the pyrethroid insecticides bioresmethrin and kadethrin on crayfish giant axons. Comp. Biochem. Physiol. C 93:149.

33. OMATSU, M., MURAYAMA, K., KITASATO, H., NISHIMURA, K. and FUJITA, T. (1988), Effect of substituted benzyl chrysanthemates on sodium and potassium currents in the crayfish giant axon. Pestic. Biochem. Physiol. 30:125.

34. OORTGIESEN, M., LEWIS, B.K., BIERKAMPER, G.G. and VIJVERBERG, H.P.M. (1990), Are postsynaptic nicotinic end-plate receptors involved in lead toxicity? Neurotoxicology 11:87.

35. OORTGIESEN, M., van KLEEF, R.G.D.M., BAJNATH, R.B. and VIJVERBERG, H.P.M. (1990), Nanomolar concentrations of lead selectively block neuronal nicotinic acetylcholine responses in mouse neuroblastoma cells. Toxicol. Appl. Pharmacol. 103:165.

36. OORTGIESEN, M., van KLEEF, R.G.D.M. and VIJVERBERG, H.P.M. (1989), Effects of pyrethroids on neurotransmitter-operated ion channels in cultured mouse neuroblastoma cells. Pestic. Biochem. Physiol. 34:164.

37. OORTGIESEN, M., van KLEEF, R.G.D.M. and VIJVERBERG, H.P.M. (1990), Novel type of ion channel activated by Pb^{2+}, Cd^{2+} and Al^{3+} in cultured mouse neuroblastoma cells. J. Membr. Biol. 113:261.

38. OORTGIESEN, M. and VIJVERBERG, H.P.M. (1989), Properties of neuronal type acetylcholine receptors in voltage clamped mouse neuroblastoma cells. Neurosci. 31:169.

39. PETERS, J.A., MALONE, H.M. and LAMBERT, J.J. (1990), Antagonism of 5-HT_3 receptor mediated currents in murine N1E-115 neuroblastoma cells by (+)-tubocurarine. Neurosci. Lett. 110:107.

40. PICKETT, J.B. and BORNSTEIN, J.C. (1984), Some effects of lead at mammalian neuromuscular junction. Am. J. Physiol. C 246:271.

41. QUANDT, F.N. (1988), Three kinetically distinct potassium channels in mouse neuroblastoma cells. J. Physiol. 395:401.

42. REUVENY, E. and NARAHASHI, T. (1991), Potent blocking action of lead on voltage-activated calcium channels in human neuroblastoma cells SH-SY5Y. Brain Res. 545:312.

43. RUIGT, G.S.F. (1984), An electrophysiological investigation into the mode of action of pyrethroid insecticides, Ph.D. thesis, University of Utrecht.

44. RUIGT, G.S.F., NEIJT, H.C., van der ZALM, J.M. and van den BERCKEN, J. (1987), Increase of sodium current after pyrethroid insecticides in mouse neuroblastoma cells. Brain Res. 437:309.

45. SALGADO, V.L., HERMAN, M.D. and NARAHASHI, T. (1989), Interactions of the pyrethroid fenvalerate with nerve membrane sodium channels: temperature dependence and mechanism of depolarization. Neurotoxicology 10:1.

46. SHERBY, S.M., ELDEFRAWI, A.T., DESHPANDE, S.S., ALBUQUERQUE, E.X. and ELDEFRAWI, M.E. (1988), Effects of pyrethroids on nicotinic acetylcholine receptor binding and function. Pestic. Biochem. Physiol. 26:107.

47. SILBERGELD, E.K. (1985), Neurotoxicology of lead, Drug and Chemical Toxicology, Vol. 3, Neurotoxicology, K. Blum and L. Manzo (Eds.) Marcel Dekker Inc., New York, 299-322.

48. SPECTOR, I. (1981), Electrophysiology of clonal nerve cell lines, Excitable Cells in Tissue Culture, P.G. Nelson and M. Lieberman (Eds.) Plenum Press, New York, 247-277.

49. SUSZKIW, J., TOTH, G., MURAWSKY, M. and COOPER, G.P. (1984), Effects of Pb^{2+} and Cd^{2+} on acetylcholine release and Ca^{2+} movements in synaptosomes and subcellular fractions from rat brain and *Torpedo* electric organ. Brain Res. 323:31.

50. VIJVERBERG, H.P.M. (1992), Ion channels in cultured mouse neuroblastoma cells. Submitted for publication.

51. VIJVERBERG, H.P.M. and van den BERCKEN, J. (1990), Neurotoxicological effects and the mode of action of pyrethroid insecticides. CRC Crit. Rev. Toxicol. 21:105.

52. VIJVERBERG, H.P.M., RUIGT, G.S.F. and van den BERCKEN, J. (1982), Structure-related effects of pyrethroid insecticides on the lateral-line sense organ and on peripheral nerves of the clawed frog, *Xenopus laevis*. Pestic. Biochem. Physiol. 18:315.

53. VIJVERBERG, H.P.M., van der ZALM, J.M. and van den BERCKEN, J. (1982), Similar mode of action of pyrethroids and DDT on sodium channel gating in myelinated nerves. Nature 295:601.

54. WANG, C.M., NARAHASHI, T. and SCUKA, M. (1972), Mechanism of negative temperature coefficient of nerve blocking action of allethrin. J. Pharmacol. Exp. Ther. 182: 442.

55. de WEILLE, J.R. (1986), The modification of nerve membrane sodium channels by pyrethroids. Ph.D. thesis, University of Utrecht.

56. de WEILLE, J.R. and LEINDERS, T. (1989), The action of pyrethroids on sodium channels in myelinated nerve fibres and spinal ganglion cells of the frog. Brain Res. 482:324.

57. YAMAMOTO, D., QUANDT, F.N. and NARAHASHI, T. (1983), Modification of single sodium channels by the insecticide tetramethrin. Brain Res. 274:344.

A3

Development of an *In Vitro* Hippocampal Brain Slice Screen for Neurotoxicity

STEPHEN B. FOUNTAIN and JAMES D. ROWAN

Department of Psychology
Kent State University
Kent, OH 44242

ABSTRACT

The hippocampal brain slice preparation has a number of features that make it attractive as a screening method. Chief among these is that it provides a model of CNS complexity in an *in vitro* preparation that is easily manipulated experimentally. To begin to validate the hippocampal slice approach to screening for neurotoxicity, we have tested a number of chemicals of known *in vivo* neurotoxic potential. We report results of experiments designed to use the hippocampal slice preparation to assess the neurotoxic potential of acrylamide and related compounds, lead compounds, and methylmercury. In the course of conducting these experiments, we also examined the suitability of methods that might prove effective in obtaining dose-response information using within-slice measurements to speed assessment and to reduce animal use. The results continue to favor the view that an *in vitro* hippocampal slice screen may prove to be a valid method of neurotoxicity screening.

INTRODUCTION

In recent years, explant methods for maintaining CNS tissue *in vitro* have become well-developed and are finding wide use in the fields of neurobiology, pharmacology, and, more recently, toxicology. The first demonstration of a method for maintaining physiologically viable slices of mammalian CNS tissue was described by Yamamoto and McIlwain (28). Since then, these methods have been used for analyzing the physiology of CNS tissue (7,23), for studying the mechanisms of synaptic plasticity thought to underlie learning and memory (8,15), and for analyzing the impact of drugs and toxic chemicals on neural circuits, single cells and synapses, and even specific receptors and ion channels (1,2,4,6,9,10,11,13,14,19,20,21,27). The hippocampal formation, a limbic system structure, is particularly well suited for use in brain-slice methods because of its lamellar structure. When cut in thin sections in the appropriate plane, the classic trisynaptic circuit of the hippocampus is preserved for study in each slice. This circuit can be studied using standard electrophysiological methods, and the results from *in vitro* brain slice studies generally parallel the results from comparable *in vivo* studies (24). Several investigators have suggested that the brain slice preparation could profitably be used as a screen for neurotoxicity (10,12,17,22).

The present chapter has two goals. First, we provide an update of our continuing efforts to assess the utility of the hippocampal slice preparation as a screen for neurotoxicity [cf. (12)]. We report experiments using the hippocampal slice preparation as a means of assessing the neurotoxicity of acrylamide and related compounds, lead acetate compared to triethyllead, and methylmercury. These studies were designed to determine whether the hippocampal slice could detect the neurotoxicity of these agents and, in addition, provide information regarding the relative neurotoxicity of related compounds. Second, we discuss in greater detail the rationale behind the hippocampal slice screen concept. In particular, we distinguish between two separate phases of neurotoxicity assessment that we believe to be required when using a screening method like that proposed. As we have suggested before (10,12), the screening phase should be distinguished from an analytical phase designed to determine mechanism of action. We argue that this two-phase screening approach can yield more efficient screening.

THE HIPPOCAMPAL SLICE PREPARATION

Our methods for preparing and studying the hippocampal slice *in vitro* are comparable to well-established methods that are widely used. Transverse hippocampal slices 400-450 μm thick are obtained from the middle third of the hippocampal formation of male Long-Evans hooded rats 60-90 days of age using our standard methods (10,12,18,24). Slices are placed on nylon netting stretched over the depression of a glass depression microscope slide. The depression slide is placed on a Plexiglas stage that is located in a chamber (see Figure 1) providing a humid atmosphere of adequate oxygen content (95% O_2/5% CO_2). Slices are maintained using a perfusion procedure wherein a constant flow (approximately 0.7-1.0 ml/min) of oxygenated artificial cerebrospinal fluid (aCSF: 124 mM NaCl, 3.3 mM KCl, 1.25 mM NaH_2PO_4, 1.2 mM $MgSO_4$, 2.4 mM $CaCl_2$, 25 mM $NaHCO_3$, and 10 mM glucose) flows under the nylon netting and through the pool formed by the depression below the hippocampal slices and is drawn off via a perfusion pump. Slices are allowed to equilibrate for one hour prior to study.

A concentric microbipolar stimulating electrode (approximately 50-100 μm in diameter) is positioned in the Schaffer collaterals of stratum radiatum. A glass micropipette (5-20 μm tip diameter) filled with 2 M NaCl (2-4 MΩ resistance) is used to record extracellularly from the CA1 pyramidal cell body layer of the hippocampus (see Figure 2 for approximate electrode placements). Stimulus pulses used to produce evoked potentials in CA1 range from 0-10 V with a duration of 0.1 msec. Monosynaptically driven field potentials are amplified, filtered (1 Hz-3 kHz), then digitized (10 kHz sampling rate), analyzed, and displayed on a CRT using an XT-compatible microcomputer equipped with an analog-to-digital converter (IBM Data Acquisition and Control Adaptor) and a software system developed by the first author (using Borland TurboC). At the end of each day's testing session, the waveform data are recorded on floppy disks for later analysis. The relative magnitude of the field potential population spike and EPSP are the primary measures of hippocampal excitability. Secondary measures can include spike latency, spike width at half amplitude, and area under the spike and EPSP. All measures are performed by the computer system.

Prior to exposing the slice to agents, a 15-min preexposure baseline is obtained by recording evoked responses at 1-min intervals using a stimulus intensity sufficient to produce a 1-3 mV population spike (designated the "standard stimulus"). Stability of the evoked response is deemed acceptable if the amplitude of the population spike varies less than 15% over 15 min; slices that fail to meet this criterion are rejected from the experiment. The status of local inhibitory systems is

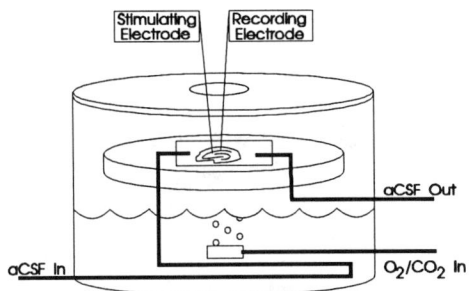

Figure 1. The chamber used for maintaining hippocampal slices *in vitro*. Slices rested on a nylon net at the interface of a pool of perfusing medium containing the agent of interest.

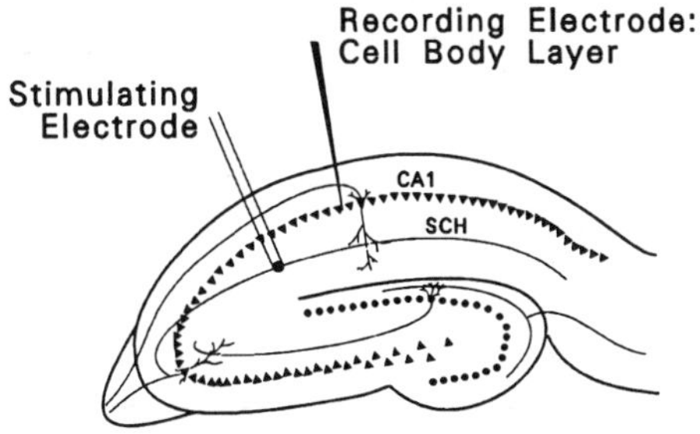

Figure 2. Stimulating and recording electrodes are positioned in the Schaffer collaterals (SCH) and pyramidal cell body layer of area CA1, respectively, of the hippocampal slice.

assessed on each trial by administering paired-pulse "conditioning/test" (C/T) stimulation with an interpulse delay of 25 msec. Slices that fail to demonstrate at least 75% inhibition of the population spike evoked by the test stimulus, i.e., the second stimulus of the pair, are likewise rejected from the experiment.

If the foregoing baseline criteria are met, the experiment proper begins. Prior to agent exposure, an input/output (I/O) profile is obtained; the I/O profile consists of CA1 responses recorded for increasing stimulus intensities in the range producing 0-5 mV population spike field potentials. Samples for the I/O profile are obtained at 60-sec intervals. Next, 2 baseline evoked waveforms are obtained at 5-min intervals prior to the onset of agent exposure using the standard stimulus. Agent exposure is then accomplished by switching from normal to agent-bearing medium reservoirs using an in-line switch; agent exposure is maintained throughout the remainder of the experiment. Changes in excitability due to agent exposure are monitored by recording field potentials elicited by paired-pulses of the standard stimulus at 5-min intervals following the onset of exposure. Monitoring is terminated after 120 min and a final I/O profile is obtained. For the I/O profile, stimulus intensities are increased where necessary until the original population spike is obtained. However, stimulus intensities are typically not increased beyond twice that of the standard stimulus.

Developing an Efficient Method for Obtaining Initial Dose-Response Information

Any practical assay must efficiently assess the neurotoxicity of agents whose biological properties are unknown. We wish to develop procedures for rapidly determining the appropriate dose range for initially studying an agent of unknown properties. We are currently evaluating the utility of the "cumulative dose response function" (cDRF), a procedure in which the dose of an agent is incremented periodically within the same preparation. This procedure can potentially provide initial dose-response information quickly using a minimum number of slices.

Our cDRF procedure monitors brain slice excitability beginning with a low dose of an agent, and successively higher doses are introduced every 30 min. The resulting cDRF may not necessarily produce the dose response function which would be obtained from independent samples (due to the cumulative effects of the preceding weaker doses), but it may suffice to identify an approximation of between-samples effects.

To determine the feasibility of this approach, the first neurotoxin to be tested in this way should have a known dose response function determined with separate slices. We recently collected cDRF data for acrylamide after collecting dose-response data using the standard between-slice protocol. We also tested lead acetate and triethyllead with the cDRF procedure because their relative neurotoxicity *in vivo* is known and because we have worked with heavy metals before. Most recently, we used the cDRF procedure to determine whether the hippocampal slice preparation would detect neurotoxic effects of methylmercury. The results of these studies will be reported below.

Hypothetically, if the cDRF data were to indicate that an agent has no effect at doses likely to be encountered in the environment, it may be possible to consider terminating the assessment at this point. Using this type of technique might speed assessment. On the other hand, this technique might entail greater risk of Type II errors, especially if other measures are not included, for example, measures of the status of processes involved in neuronal plasticity.

FURTHER VALIDATION OF THE HIPPOCAMPAL SLICE SCREEN CONCEPT

The value of the hippocampal slice preparation as a screen for neurotoxicity must ultimately be determined empirically by evaluating its ability to detect the neurotoxicity of some chemicals while rejecting other agents as relatively non-neurotoxic. We have continued the process of validating the hippocampal slice screen concept by using our standard protocol to assess the neurotoxicity of a variety of agents representative (to the extent possible) of several classes of chemicals or of classes of agents having common sequelae. The chemicals listed in Table 1 have been identified as appropriate for validating the method.

These chemicals were chosen for validating the hippocampal slice screen for several reasons. Much is already known about the relative neurotoxicity of these agents. Some of the chemicals, such as parathion/paraoxon and methylmercury, were chosen to answer specific questions concerning the performance of the screen in detecting the neurotoxicity of agents requiring biotransformation to express their neurotoxicity and chronic neurotoxicants, respectively. Most of the other chemicals were chosen as representatives of classes of chemicals or neurotoxic mechanisms. Several other considerations contributed to the latter choices. We sought to choose chemicals targeted by the EPA Superfund and/or United Auto Workers neurotoxic chemicals lists. More importantly, most of the listed agents were drawn from a list of known neurotoxins and negative controls currently being used for validating the Functional Observational Battery (FOB), the behavioral test battery being evaluated and standardized by a number of laboratories under the auspices of the U.S. EPA and the World Health Organization. This will allow direct comparison of slice results to effects observed using a standardized behavioral test battery. Most of the chemicals selected have also been targeted by the World Health Organization in a proposed project designed to develop and validate neurotoxicological assessment procedures using *in vitro* methodologies.

Acrylamide and Related Compounds

Our beginning work with acrylamide (ACR) sought to obtain initial information concerning dose-effect relationships in the hippocampal brain slice preparation. Using standard procedures, we exposed hippocampal slices to either 0, 1, 3, 5, 7, or 15 mM ACR in the aCSF medium. As described above, slices were monitored through a 2-hr postexposure period. In previous studies, we have used single-pulse stimulation of s. radiatum to evoke responses in hippocampal CA1. When the slice is stimulated every 5 min using this method, it is possible to monitor changes in pyramidal cell excitatory circuitry. Paired-pulse stimulation, where 2 stimuli are presented with a

Table I. Chemicals identified as appropriate for screen validation.

trimethyltin	neurotoxic organometal
triethyltin	neurotoxic organometal
lead acetate	inorganic heavy metal, less neurotoxic
triethyllead	neurotoxic organometal
methylmercury	neurotoxic organometal
acrylamide	ester of acrylic acid, produces central peripheral axonopathy
N,N'-methylene-bis-acrylamide	non-neurotoxic analogue of acrylamide
methacrylamide	related, moderately neurotoxic agent
p,p'-DDT	organochlorine insecticide
gamma-lindane	organochlorine insecticide
deltamethrin	type II pyrethroid insecticide
parathion	organophosphate insecticide, non-neurotoxic precursor
paraoxon	neurotoxic metabolite of parathion
toluene	organic solvent, aromatic hydrocarbon
trichloroethylene	organic solvent, halogenated hydrocarbon
benzene	organic solvent, aromatic hydrocarbon
arsenic trioxide	negative control
sodium salicylate	negative control

short inter-stimulus interval (e.g., 25 msec used here), has been used before and after monitoring to assess the status of inhibitory circuitry. One new aspect of our current procedure is that we now present paired-pulse stimuli on every "trial" so that we can observe changes in the status of local inhibitory circuitry throughout the monitoring period. Using the foregoing methods, we found that 1, 3, and 5 mM ACR produced little change in excitatory systems (as measured by changes in evoked population spike amplitude), though both 3 and 5 mM ACR produced an increase in excitability near the end of the 2-hr exposure (see Figure 3). In contrast, 7 and 15 mM ACR suppressed excitability, with the suppression appearing earlier for 15 mM compared to 7 mM ACR (see Figure 3). Although not apparent from Figure 3, it should be noted that in some slices 7 and 15 mM ACR produced an initial suppression, but the response recovered back to baseline levels by the end of the experiment. EPSP data appear to parallel the population spike results. No effects on inhibitory systems were observed at any dose.

In two additional studies, we compared the effects of N,N'-methylene-bis-acrylamide (MBA) and methacrylamide (MTA) to the effects of ACR to determine whether the hippocampal slice preparation could assess the relative neurotoxicity of the three agents *in vitro*. The relative *in vivo* neurotoxicity of these agents is MBA < MTA < ACR. Hippocampal slices were exposed to 15 mM ACR, MBA, or MTA and monitored for 2 hr. As shown in Figure 4, 15 mM ACR (data reproduced from Figure 3) produced suppression of excitability, MBA produced a slight increase in excitability, whereas MTA produced a larger increase in excitability. A further comparison of

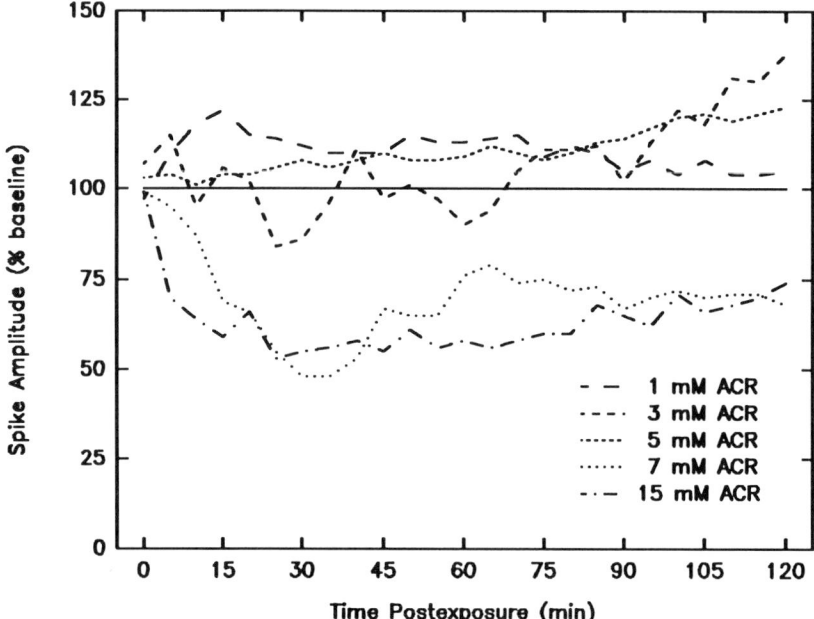

Figure 3. Timecourse of changes in population spike amplitude (as percent of baseline) for 120 min following 1, 3, 5, 7, or 15 mM acrylamide (ACR).

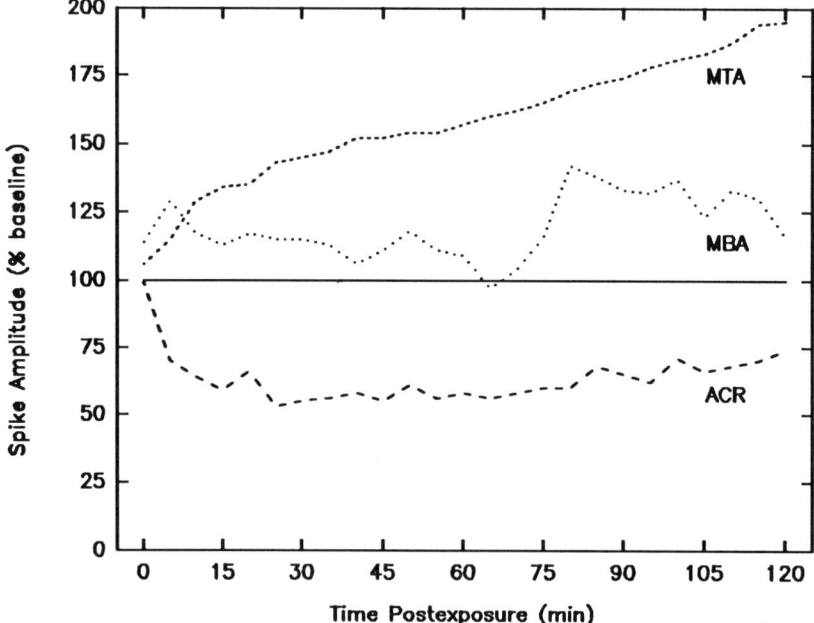

Figure 4. Timecourse of changes in population spike amplitude (as percent of baseline) for 120 min following 15 mM ACR, 15 mM MBA, or 15 mM MTA.

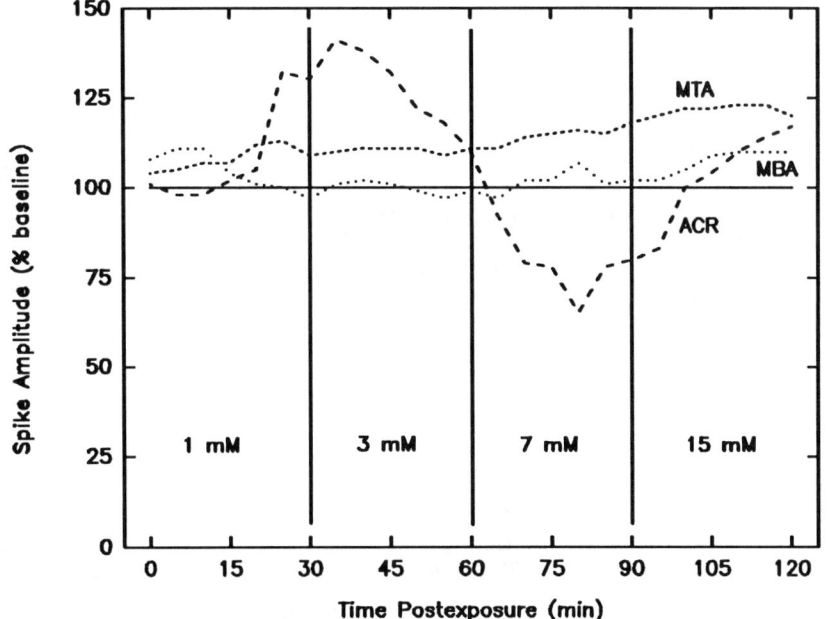

Figure 5. Timecourse of changes in population spike amplitude following ACR, MBA, or MTA exposure in the cDRF procedure. Exposures were 1, 3, 7, and 15 mM concentrations in successive 30-min periods.

these three chemicals was performed in the next experiment using the cDRF procedure we are evaluating. In this experiment, hippocampal slices were exposed for 2 hr as before, but the dose was increased every 30 min. In this case, slices were exposed to 1, 3, 7, and 15 mM concentrations of either ACR, MBA, or MTA. The results, shown in Figure 5, are generally consistent with the between-slice results of Figures 3 and 4. ACR produced an increase in excitability at lower doses (1 and 3 mM) and suppression at the 7 mM concentration. (One surprise was recovery of the response observed after the initial suppression caused by 7 mM ACR that continued through the 15 mM exposure period, but a comparable recovery was also observed in some slices of Figure 3 when exposed to 7 and 15 mM ACR.) MBA produced little change from baseline. Finally, MTA produced a step-wise increase in excitability corresponding to increasing doses.

If one were to speculate on the neurotoxic potential of these chemicals based on these data, ACR would be judged to be more neurotoxic than MBA. MTA's facilitatory effects are reminiscent of those of lower doses of ACR, and thus it might be concluded that MTA should be viewed as having more neurotoxic potential than MBA but less than ACR. This ordering of the agents' neurotoxicity, MBA < MTA < ACR, parallels the known neurotoxicity of these agents *in vivo*. This is particularly surprising (and encouraging, from our perspective) given that other *in vitro* screening methods (using protein content, LDH activity, and cumulative glucose consumption) have found MBA to be more neurotoxic than both ACR and MTA (16) despite its low *in vivo* neurotoxicity. Although the authors of the latter study urge caution in relying on *in vitro* methods for neurotoxicity assessment because of MBA's unexpected neurotoxicity in their *in vitro* studies, we can be encouraged because our initial work with acute exposure of these agents in the hippocampal slice produced results that parallel those obtained *in vivo*.

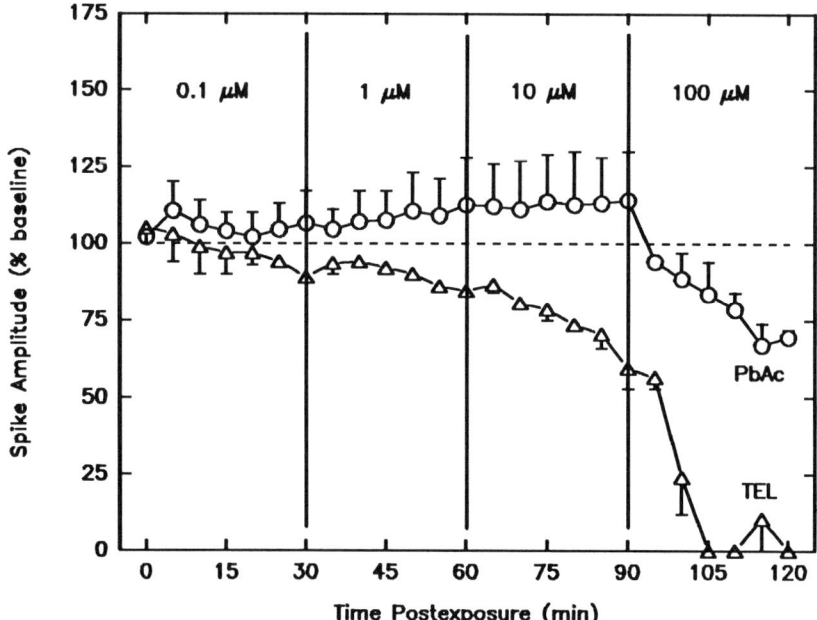

Figure 6. Timecourse of changes in population spike amplitude following PbAc or TEL exposure in the cDRF procedure. Exposures were 0.1, 1, 10, and 100 μM concentrations in successive 30-min periods.

Lead Acetate and Triethyllead

Our second objective was to determine whether the hippocampal slice preparation could provide information concerning the relative neurotoxicity of heavy metal compounds that would parallel the relative neurotoxicity established using *in vivo* methods. In our work comparing lead acetate (PbAC) and triethyllead (TEL) chloride, we have gathered some provocative initial data. Hippocampal slices were exposed to 0.1, 1, 10, and 100 μM PbAc or TEL under the cDRF protocol. Exposures were in successive 30-min periods. As shown in Figure 6, PbAc produced a slight increase in excitability until the 100 μM exposure began, then an abrupt suppression of excitability to approximately 70% of baseline was observed. In contrast, TEL appeared considerably more toxic than PbAc; initial indications of suppression of excitability appeared with doses as low as 1 μM and profound suppression was observed at the 100 μM level. These results are consistent with the known *in vivo* neurotoxicity of PbAc and TEL, where TEL is considered to be much more neurotoxic than PbAc.

Methylmercury

In our most recent work, we have sought to determine whether the cDRF procedure can be used to assess the neurotoxicity of methylmercury. Hippocampal slices were exposed to 0.1, 1, 10, and 100 μM methylmercury chloride under the cDRF protocol. As before, exposures were in successive 30-min periods. As shown in Figure 7, methylmercury produced a slight increase in excitability at the 1 μM exposure, but this was followed by profound suppression of excitability at the 100 μM level of exposure. Interestingly, methylmercury appears to have suppressed inhibitory

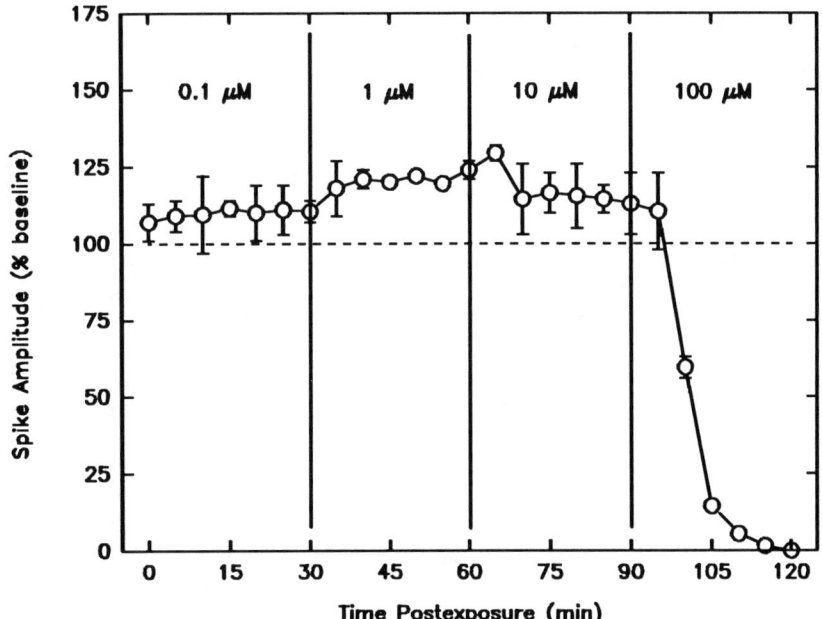

Figure 7. Timecourse of changes in population spike amplitude following methylmercury exposure in the cDRF procedure. Exposures were 0.1, 1, 10, and 100 μM concentrations in successive 30-min periods.

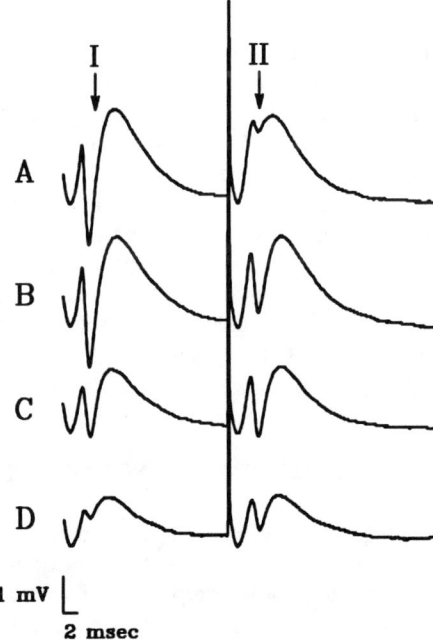

Figure 8. Waveforms recorded before and at 5, 10, and 15 min following onset of exposure to 100 μM methylmercury (Waveforms A-D, respectively). Waveforms exhibit responses to paired stimulus pulses separated by 25 msec.

systems before any effects on excitatory systems were observed. Selected waveforms recorded from the CA1 area of a representative hippocampal slice exposed to methylmercury are shown in Figure 8. Waveform A illustrates a fairly normal response recorded for paired-pulse stimulation (25-msec inter-stimulus-interval) recorded at the time of onset of 100 μM methylmercury. A negative-going population spike is observed following the first stimulus (at position I), but the population spike observed following the second stimulus (at position II) is suppressed as the result of local inhibitory processes, including recurrent and feedforward systems (3,5). Waveform A is comparable to those recorded during the preexposure baseline period of the experiment. Waveform B was recorded 5 min after the onset of 100 μM methylmercury. At this point, no change was observed in the amplitude of the population spike in position I (representing no change in pyramidal cell excitability), but the population spike in position II was considerably larger than before (representing a loss of local inhibitory processes). By 10 min of 100 μM methylmercury exposure (Waveform C), both population spikes changed compared to baseline. The amplitude of the population spike in position I was smaller than at baseline (viz., approximately 60% of baseline), indicating that pyramidal cell excitability was suppressed. The amplitude of the population spike in position II remained larger than that in position I, indicating suppression of local inhibitory properties. Both systems continued to be suppressed further, as observed in Waveform D which was recorded 15 min after the onset of 100 μM methylmercury exposure. Methylmercury, then, suppressed local inhibitory systems prior to suppressing excitatory systems in hippocampal area CA1.

Comparisons to Other Agents

The results of the foregoing experiments should be compared to the results we have obtained in other studies for the purpose of determining whether the hippocampal slice preparation is producing data on relative neurotoxicity that make sense in light of the putative neurotoxicity of the various agents. In past studies, for example, we have determined that hippocampal excitatory or inhibitory systems are rapidly suppressed by trimethyltin and triethyltin at 1-10 μM (10,11,27). By comparison, comparable response suppression was observed in the cDRF procedure for 10 μM triethyllead, 100 μM lead acetate, and 100 μM methylmercury. These results are consistent with the known neurotoxicity of heavy metals. Acrylamide, by comparison, produced comparable suppression at approximately 7-15 mM, and the related compounds MBA and MTA that are less toxic *in vivo* were found to be less toxic *in vitro* using the hippocampal slice preparation as a screen. Finally, our earlier study with aspartame (9), the non-nutritive (and putatively non-neurotoxic) sweetener, produced no suppression of response at any dose studied (0.01-10 mM). Although these comparisons should be made with caution because the data were collected with methods that differed somewhat between studies, these results are generally consistent with the putative relative neurotoxicity of these heavy metals, acrylamide, and aspartame. Such results clearly would have flagged all of the heavy metal agents and acrylamide to be passed on to an analytical phase for further assessment.

THE PROBLEM OF CNS TOXICITY

You will have noticed that until now mechanism of action has hardly been mentioned for the agents studied in the foregoing experiments. There is good reason for approaching these studies and the results in this manner. The strategy of the proposed hippocampal slice screen for neurotoxicity is to use a battery of tests to assess agent-induced electrophysiological changes in the status of a model neural system (namely, the hippocampal slice preparation) following exposure to chemical agents. We have argued in the past that this model system has as its primary conceptual advantage the fact that the *in vitro* hippocampal slice reflects the complexity of the *in vivo* nervous system (12). The hippocampal slice screen concept, then, is founded on the idea that chemical neurotoxicity, whatever its relative specificity within the CNS, should be expressed as some measurable perturbation of function within a system as complex as the hippocampal slice. Whether this assumption will ultimately be found to be proper is a matter of empirical test.

One approach to assessment is to distinguish between a screening phase and an analytical phase of assessment (12). In the screening phase, one would use relatively few tests that are broadly sensitive to a potentially large number of causative factors. The screening phase would be designed to determine that some agents require closer scrutiny because of their potential neurotoxicity. In the analytical phase, determining the mechanism of action of the agent's effects in the screening phase would be the paramount goal. This is the general approach that has met with considerable success in behavioral screening, and this is the approach that we have adopted for our proposed *in vitro* screening method. One prerequisite for this strategy to succeed, however, is to assemble a battery of tests extensive enough to detect many different neurotoxic mechanisms of action. Such a test battery will be somewhat imprecise with regard to specifying the mechanism of action of agents, but it allows much more rapid screening than would be possible with a more analytical approach. Our logic is to develop a quick, but sensitive, screen for neurotoxicants, without regard to identifying the underlying mechanism of action. However, a practical and conceptual advantage of the hippocampal slice preparation is that it can be used during both phases of assessment, both as the primary method of screening and, following screening, as an analytical tool for more accurately determining the mechanism of action of neurotoxins. One additional advantage of this arrangement is that results of screening with the hippocampal slice preparation can provide initial hypotheses to guide work in the analytical stage of research.

The hippocampal slice screen we propose can be used to assess neurotoxic effects of chemicals on a well-studied CNS circuit containing excitatory, inhibitory, and plastic properties. In the studies reported here, paired-pulse stimulation was used throughout monitoring to assess the status of excitatory and inhibitory systems mediated primarily by pyramidal cells and basket cells in hippocampal area CA1. In principle, any deleterious effect of a chemical on this *in vitro* neural network will be reflected in changes in the electrophysiological properties of the tissue assessed by this measure. In addition, we have proposed that one other test be incorporated into a hippocampal slice screen, namely, a test to assess the plasticity of the system [cf. (12)]. The latter test is thought to provide information regarding the status of systems underlying learning and memory processes in the normal brain (25,26). Such a test battery, though consisting of only a few tests, should be broadly sensitive to a multitude of neurotoxic mechanisms by assessing the status of the primary functions of neural tissue, namely, excitatory transmission of information, inhibition, and plastic change. Our results to date from hippocampal slice studies of the electrophysiological effects of exposing slices to various known or suspected neurotoxins have illustrated the utility of the hippocampal slice screen we propose.

FUTURE DIRECTIONS

There are clearly a number of questions yet to be answered before the hippocampal slice screen concept could be adopted for general neurotoxicity screening. First, how well will the hippocampal slice screen predict the neurotoxic potential of a broader range of agents? Many more agents of known neurotoxic potential should be tested using the hippocampal slice preparation to determine the limits of the method. Second, how will we manage the problems common to many *in vitro* screening methods that must also be solved for the hippocampal slice preparation? For example, the problem of biotransformation of agents by organs or tissues outside the CNS must be addressed (e.g., the liver) [cf. (12)]. Finally, can the hippocampal slice preparation detect the neurotoxicity of chemicals that have specific effects on neuronal plasticity? The method for assessing neurotoxic effects on plasticity likewise should be tested with a broad, representative set of neurotoxic chemicals and non-neurotoxic controls.

We do have reason to be optimistic. Initial evidence suggests that the cDRF procedure may be useful for rapidly obtaining dose-response information in screening while reducing animal use. This can be accomplished by exposing the same hippocampal slice to many doses of an agent using the cDRF procedure. Though many questions remain unanswered regarding the utility of this approach, our initial results with ACR, MBA, and MTA (Figure 5), PbAc and TEL (Figure 6), and methylmercury (Figure 7) are promising and suggest that we should continue exploring the use of this methodology in conjunction with the hippocampal slice preparation. The results continue to favor the view that an *in vitro* hippocampal slice screen may prove to be a valid method of neurotoxicity screening.

ACKNOWLEDGMENTS

We thank Timothy J. Teyler for many useful discussions and ideas regarding conceptual and technical issues related to the continued development of the hippocampal slice screen concept, in particular regarding the cDRF procedure as a component of the approach. We also thank Bonnie S. Toner and Andrew W. Proctor for assistance in data collection. This research was supported by a grant from the Johns Hopkins Center for Alternatives to Animal Testing.

REFERENCES

1. ALGER, B.E., and NICOLL, R.A. (1983). Ammonia does not selectively block IPSPs in rat hippocampal pyramidal cells. *J. Neurophysiol.* **49**, 1381-1391.

2. ALLEN, C.N., and FONNUM, F. (1984). Trimethyltin inhibits the activity of hippocampal neurons recorded *in vitro*. *Neurotoxicol.* **5**, 23-30.

3. ANDERSEN, P., ECCLES, J.C., and LOYNING, Y. (1964). Pathway of postsynaptic inhibition in the hippocampus. *J. Neurophysiol.* **27**, 608-619.

4. ARMSTRONG, D.L., READ, H.L., CORK, A.E., MONTEMAYOR, F., and WAYNER, M.J. (1987). Effects of trimethyltin on evoked potentials in mouse hippocampal slices. *Neurotox. Teratol.* **9**, 359-362.

5. BUZSAKI, G. (1984). Feedforward inhibition in the hippocampal formation. *Progr. Neurobiol.* **22**, 131-153.

6. CARLEN, P.L., and CORRIGALL, W.A. (1980). Ethanol tolerance measured electrophysiologically in hippocampal slices and not in neuromuscular junctions from chronically ethanol-fed rats. *Neurosci. Letters* **17**, 95-100.

7. DUNWIDDIE, T.V. (1986). The use of in vitro brain slices in neuropharmacology. In *Electrophysiological Techniques in Pharmacology*. Edited by H. M. Geller. pp. 65-90. Alan R. Liss, New York.

8. DUNWIDDIE, T.V., ROBERSON, N.L., and WORTH, T. (1982). Modulation of long-term potentiation: Effects of adrenergic and neuroleptic drugs. *Pharm. Biochem. Behav.* **17**, 1257-1264.

9. FOUNTAIN, S.B., HENNES, S.K., and TEYLER, T.J. (1988). Aspartame exposure and *in vitro* hippocampal slice excitability and plasticity. *Fundam. Appl. Toxicol.* **11**, 221-228.

10. FOUNTAIN, S.B., and TEYLER, T.J. (1987). Characterizing neurotoxicity using the *in vitro* hippocampal slice preparation: Heavy metals. In *Model Systems in Neurotoxicology: Alternative Approaches to Animal Testing*. Edited by A. Shahar and A. M. Goldberg. pp. 19-31. Alan R. Liss, New York.

11. FOUNTAIN, S.B., TING, Y.-L.T., HENNES, S.K., and TEYLER, T.J. (1988). Triethyltin exposure suppresses synaptic transmission in area CA1 of the rat hippocampal slice. *Neurotoxicol. Teratol.* **10**, 539-548.

12. FOUNTAIN, S.B., TING, Y.-L.T., and TEYLER, T.J. (1992). The *in vitro* hippocampal slice preparation as a screen for neurotoxicity. *Toxic. in Vitro* **6**, 77-87.

13. FRENCH, E., and ZIEGLGANSBERGER, W. (1982). The excitatory response of *in vitro* hippocampal pyramidal cells to normorphine and methionine-enkephalin may be mediated by different receptor populations. *Exp. Brain Res.* **48**, 238-244.

14. GALVAN, M., KUPSCH, A., and TEN BRUGGENCATE, G. (1987). Actions of MPTP and MPP^+ on synaptic transmission in guinea-pig hippocampal slices. *Exp. Neurol.* **96**, 289-298.

15. GROVER, L.M., and TEYLER, T.J. (1989). Effects of extracellular potassium concentration and postsynaptic membrane potential on calcium-induced potentiation in area CA1 of rat hippocampus. *Brain Res.* in press.

16. HAYASHI, M., TANII, H., HORIGUCHI, M., and HASHIMOTO, K. (1989). Cytotoxic effects of acrylamide and its related compounds assessed by protein content, LDH activity and cumulative glucose consumption of neuron-rich cultures in a chemically defined medium. *Arch. Toxicol.* **63**, 308-313.

17. KURODA, Y. (1980). Brain slices, assay systems for the neurotoxicity of environmental pollutants and drugs on mammalian central nervous system. In *Mechanisms of Toxicity and Hazard Evaluation*. Edited by B. Holmstedt, R. Lauwerys, M. Mercier, and M. Roberfroid. pp. 59-62. Elsevier/North Holland Biomedical Press, Amsterdam.

18. LANGMOEN, I.A., and ANDERSEN, P. (1981). The hippocampal slice *in vitro*. A description of the technique and some examples of the opportunities it offers. In *Electrophysiology of Isolated Mammalian CNS Preparations*. Edited by G. A. Kerkut and H. V. Wheal. pp. 51-105. Academic Press, New York.

19. NEWBERRY, N.R., and NICOLL, R.A. (1984). A bicuculline-resistant inhibitory postsynaptic potential in rat hippocampal pyramidal cells *in vitro*. *J. Physiol.* **348**, 239-254.

20. NOWICKY, A.V., TEYLER, T.J., and VARDARIS, R.M. (1987). The modulation of long-term potentiation by delta-9-tetrahydrocannabinol in the rat hippocampus, *in vitro*. *Brain Res. Bull.* **19**, 663-672.

21. PREISENDORFER, V., ZEISE, M.L., and KLEE, M.R. (1987). Valporate enhances inhibitory postsynaptic potentials in hippocampal neurons *in vitro*. *Brain Res.* **435**, 213-219.

22. ROWAN, M.J. (1985). Central nervous system toxicity evaluation *in vitro*: Neurophysiological approach. In *Neurotoxicology*. Edited by K. Blum and L. Manzo. pp. 585-612. Dekker, New York.

23. SCHWARTZKROIN, P.A., and ALTSCHULER, R.L. (1977). Development of kitten hippocampal neurons. *Brain Res.* **134**, 429-444.

24. TEYLER, T.J. (1980). Brain slice preparation: Hippocampus. *Brain Res. Bull.* **5**, 391-403.

25. TEYLER, T.J., and DISCENNA, P. (1987). Long-term potentiation. *Ann. Rev. Neurosci.* **10**, 131-161.

26. TEYLER, T.J., and FOUNTAIN, S.B. (1987). Neuronal plasticity in the mammalian brain: Relevance to behavioral learning and memory. *Child Dev.* **58**, 698-712.

27. TING, Y.-L.T., FOUNTAIN, S.B., and TEYLER, T.J. (1988). Extracellular Ca^{2+} modulation of triethyltin neurotoxicity in area CA1 of the rat hippocampal slice. *Toxic. in Vitro* **6**, 159-164.

28. YAMAMOTO, C., and MCILWAIN, H. (1966). Electrical activities in thin sections from the mammalian brain maintained in chemically defined media *in vitro*. *J. Neurochem.* **13**, 1333-1343.

A4

An *In Vitro* Model for Human Peripheral Nerve Demyelination

J. LYNN RUTKOWSKI and GIHAN I. TENNEKOON

Division of Pediatric Neurology
University of Michigan
Ann Arbor, MI 48109-0570

ABSTRACT

Cell lines able to achieve a mature, differentiated phenotype should improve the reliability of *in vitro* neurotoxicity testing. We have generated both rat and human Schwann cell lines using a synthetic, metal-responsive promoter to regulate the expression of a viral oncogene. Transcription of the inserted oncogene was initiated and maintained with zinc, and the Schwann cells proliferated continuously. When zinc was omitted from the medium, expression of the oncogene declined to undetectable levels, and immortalized rat Schwann cells in coculture with embryonic neurons were able to surround axons with a normal myelin sheath. These results demonstrate that complete differentiation is possible when oncogene expression is tightly regulated. We are now generating cell lines from embryonic neurons, and eventually hope to establish myelinating coculture systems using both neuronal and glial cell lines. The validity of this coculture system for neurotoxicity testing can then be evaluated with either human or rodent cell lines.

INTRODUCTION

The peripheral nervous system (PNS) is particularly sensitive to environmental toxins and peripheral neuropathy is a common side-effect of therapeutic drugs. Neurotoxic agents can cause a peripheral neuropathy by damaging either neurons or Schwann cells (15), and because of their mutual interdependence, injury to one cell type often triggers secondary changes in the other (4). Toxins including n-hexane, acrylamide, carbon disulfide, arsenic, and mercury primarily affect neurons with subsequent myelin breakdown and Schwann cell proliferation. Conversely, exposure to agents such as isoniazid, hexachlorophene, triethyltin, and tellurium, by disrupting Schwann cell metabolism or attacking myelin membranes, subsequently reduce nerve conduction velocity. Moreover, it can often be difficult to determine whether neurons or Schwann cells are the primary target of a particular neurotoxin based on functional or histologic parameters, and both cell types may be affected.

In the PNS, all axons are embedded within a continuous string of Schwann cells. Smaller diameter axons are surrounded by a single layer of Schwann cell plasma membrane, while the larger axons are wrapped with a multilamellar myelin sheath which permits saltatory conduction of action potentials. Bunge and coworkers (9, 10) pioneered a model for *in vitro* myelination using rat dorsal root ganglia (DRG). Because many features of the intricate relationship between neurons and Schwann cells are retained, this model has enabled an understanding of key molecular events in the process of myelin formation and more recent efforts have been direct toward utilizing DRG cultures for neurotoxicity testing. Moreover, it is possible to culture both human DRG neurons (14) and human Schwann cells (20) so that the response of human cells can be examined *in vitro*.

A study of the effects of heavy metals on rat DRG cultures illustrates the utility of this model (28). The dose-response relationship of neurons and Schwann cells was compared by simple observation at the light microscopic level, i.e., measuring the radius of the neuritic halo and counting the number of myelin sheaths. Mercury and arsenic were much more potent inhibitors of neurite extension than lead and thallium which parallels their predilection for neurons rather than glial cells *in vivo*. Lead completely blocked myelin sheath formation at micromolar concentrations whereas millimolar concentrations were required to block neurite outgrowth. These findings are consistent with the effects of chronic lead intoxication in adult rats which causes segmental demyelination with complete sparing of axons in the PNS. However, considerable age and species variability exists in response to lead exposure with central rather than peripheral damage occurring in neonatal rats and a motor neuropathy predominating in adult humans (19, 29).

Schwann cells produce myelin only when contacting axons, therefore, more complex coculture systems like DRG explants are required to identify toxins which may affect the integrity of the myelin sheath. Since cultures can be treated with a suspected neurotoxin during the period of myelin initiation or after extensive myelination has occurred, it might be possible to predict developmental differences in susceptibility. DRG explants also provide a good model in which to assess neuronal sensitivity to toxins since sensory neurons are frequent targets of toxins, related at least partly to a deficient blood-nerve barrier (16). However, some toxins preferentially affect motor axons or neurons of the autonomic nervous system when the sensory system is unaffected (15). Because biochemical differences between neuronal types contributes to their selective vulnerability, the response of sensory neurons to a particular agent cannot be generalized to other neuronal populations. Nevertheless, the DRG model offers the potential for evaluating neurotoxic susceptibility based on differences in cell type, stage of development, and degree of cellular differentiation, but extensive validation remains to be done.

METHODS and RESULTS

Myelinating cocultures of Schwann cells and DRG neurons

By far, the most serious limitation to developing the DRG culture model for neurotoxicity testing is the technical difficulty of establishing the culture system. Ganglia dissected from mid-gestation embryos are attached to a collagen substratum and treated for two weeks with antimitotic drugs to eliminate fibroblasts which interfere with neurite extension (Fig. 1a). Antimitotics also kill the Schwann cells, so a pure population is obtained from the sciatic nerves of neonatal rats and then added back to the cultures. The Schwann cells are allowed to proliferate along the neurites for about two weeks before myelination is initiated with the addition of serum and ascorbic acid to the medium. Ascorbic acid serves as a cofactor for collagen synthesis, and Schwann cells must first assemble collagen into a basal lamina before elaborating a myelin sheath (10). The cultures are maintained for an additional two weeks while the myelin sheaths form and thicken (Fig. 1b).

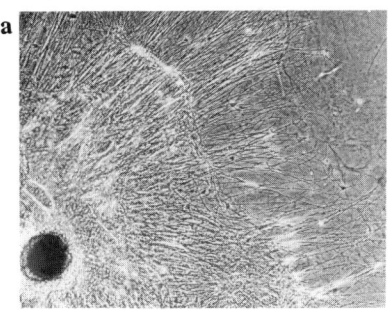 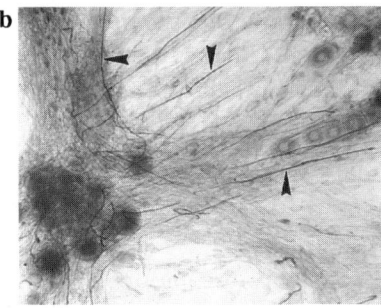

Fig. 1
a) Low power micrograph of a rat dorsal root ganglia culture showing neurite outgrowth during anti-mitotic treatment. (Magnification = 25x)
b) Sudan black staining of myelin sheaths (arrows) made by rat Schwann cells in coculture with neurons. (Magnification = 280x)

The use of cell lines could greatly simplify this culture model. The most difficult and time-consuming procedures, such as dissecting embryos, culturing primary cells, and purifying specific cell populations, would be eliminated. Many cell lines have already been derived from neural tumors but they express only a few properties of particular neurons or glia, and most are not capable of more complex interactions. For example, cells isolated from Schwannomas or spontaneously transformed Schwann cells do not produce myelin, and neuroblastoma or pheochromocytoma cells, when induced to extend neurites, do not trigger normal Schwann cells to myelinate them. Cell lines have also been established from many cell types by introducing viral oncogenes in culture. Since oncogenes are not subject to normal control mechanisms, the cell lines typically remain in a proliferative state and their ability to differentiate is impaired.. However, by replacing a continuously-active viral promoter with an inducible promoter to act as a switch, it might be possible to control oncogene expression and improve the capacity for a cell line to differentiate.

Generating rat Schwann cell lines with an inducible oncogene

Metallothionein (MT) genes are transcriptionally activated by heavy metals including zinc, cadmium, mercury, manganese, lead, cobalt, nickel, and vanadium (8). This family of genes is expressed in most tissues and cells in cultures from drosophila to man, and the metal-binding proteins are thought to be involved in zinc homeostasis and protection against heavy metal toxicity. To study oncogene regulation by a metal-inducible promoter, a plasmid was modified to contain the large tumor (T) antigen of simian virus 40 (SV40) downstream from the mouse MT-1 promoter, and an additional gene was inserted for neomycin resistance (17). T antigen was selected because it is able to immortalize and transform many different cell types in culture. Cultured rat Schwann cells were transfected with this plasmid, and cell lines were established as outlined in the Fig 2. Zinc was included in the medium to induce T antigen expression which stimulates cell proliferation. Foci formed from the progeny of cells in which the plasmid had stably integrated into the genome during mitosis. Neomycin (G418) was then added to eliminate the normal, untransfected cells, and individual colonies were expanded into cell lines.

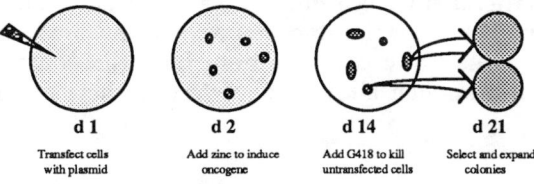

d 1	d 2	d 14	d 21
Transfect cells with plasmid	Add zinc to induce oncogene	Add G418 to kill untransfected cells	Select and expand colonies

Fig. 2 Procedure for etablishing Schwann cell lines with a metal-inducible oncogene.

The cell lines were serially passaged in the presence of zinc for at least 50 population doublings, well past their normal life-span, before their properties were studied (26). When zinc was removed from the medium, T antigen levels decreased by approximately 50%, but the cells continued to express a significant amount of the oncoprotein. The cells also exhibited properties of a transformed phenotype including an accelerated growth rate, abnormal morphology, decreased levels of differentiated markers, and loss of contact inhibition, which were unaffected by the removal of zinc. Thus, under the control of the wild-type MT promoter, zinc regulated T antigen levels up and down rather than on and off. The continued presence of the oncoprotein was likely interfering with differentiation and the Schwann cells were only able to interact with DRG neurons in coculture to a limited extent (18).

Oncogene regulation by a synthetic, metal-responsive promoter

In the intact animal, MT genes are induced by glucocorticoid hormones and cytokines in addition to heavy metals. Regulation of transcription is a complex process involving the interaction of multiple factors, and *in vitro* mutational analyses have identified some of the functional elements of MT gene promoters including a glucocorticoid response element (12), binding sites for cellular transcription factors (3, 6), a basal enhancer (11), and several homologous 15-base-pair motifs which responded to heavy metals (24). Gene transfer experiments showed that these metal-regulatory elements (MREs) could function in a heterologous promoter and that a minimum of two MREs were required for significant metal induction (5, 23). The mouse MT-1 gene contains five MREs (represented in Fig. 3a), and the isolated "d" element was found to produce the strongest gene induction (23). This work implied that it might be possible to synthesize an efficient promoter selectively responsive to metals.

We replaced the wild type MT promoter in the original immortalizing plasmid with a synthetic promoter (designated D4 or D5, shown in Fig. 3b) consisting of either four or five tandem MRE "d" elements upstream from the TATA sequence of the thymidine kinase gene (17). Only the cellular factor(s) that requires metal ions to associate with the MRE to activate transcription (2, 3) and the transcription initiation complex (22) should bind to this promoter, therefore, the promoter should be silent without metals. Rat Schwann cell lines were established with T antigen regulated by the synthetic promoters as describe above and the properties of these cells were examined.

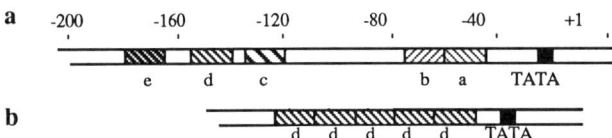

Fig. 3 a) Schematic arrangement of the five metal regulatory elements (a-d) within the 'wild-type' mouse metallothionein I promoter (from DNA sequence in ref. 24). b) The D5 synthetic promoter containing five tandem repeats of the "d" element.

A rat Schwann cell line generated with the synthetic D4 promoter regulating T antigen produced only 1/10 the amount of the oncoprotein compared to cells generated with wild type MT promoter (17). This level of T antigen was sufficient to immortalize the cells, albeit with reduced efficiency. When zinc was removed from the medium, T antigen expression decreased to undetectable levels, and the cells exhibited many characteristic traits of the parental cells including the ability to produce myelin when coculture with DRG neurons (18). The cells were not transformed as judged by standard *in vitro* criteria since cell growth was contact inhibited, and serum- and anchorage-dependent. Thus a synthetic, metal-inducible promoter enabled tight oncogene regulation. By controlling the extracellular zinc concentration, the cells could be maintained in an indefinite state of proliferation and then allowed to revert to their normal phenotype when desired.

Generating human Schwann cell lines

The ultimate goal of *in vitro* neurotoxicity testing is to predict the consequences of human exposure. Since data obtained with rodents often cannot be extrapolated to humans due to species-specific responses to toxins, an *in vitro* model using human cells would offer a distinct advantage. Therefore, we optimized the conditions for isolating and culturing human Schwann cell (20) and subsequently established human cell lines. Major methodological challenges included obtaining adequate numbers of viable cells from adult tissues, inhibiting fibroblast contamination, and stimulating Schwann cell mitosis. Intact nerve biopsies were found to exhibit a typical injury response with a burst of Schwann cell proliferation when held in explant culture for about 7-10 days. Large numbers of mitotically-active human Schwann cells were then released from the tissue with enzymes, and agents that increase intracellular cyclic AMP were used to suppress fibroblast growth. We then established human cell lines by transfecting plasmids carrying T antigen regulated by either the synthetic D4 promoter or the SV40 viral promoter. T antigen expression was regulated in human Schwann cell lines generated with the synthetic promoter but those using the SV40 promoter continually expressed high levels of the oncogene as shown by immunofluorescent staining (Fig. 4).

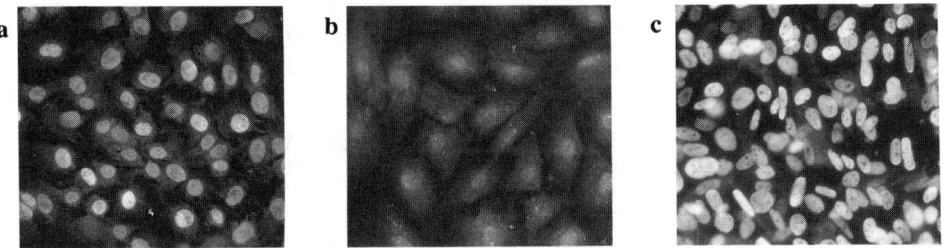

Fig. 4   Immunofluorescent staining of T antigen in the nucleus of human Schwann cells. Cells transfected with the T antigen gene regulated by the synthetic, metal-responsive promoter (a) maintained on zinc and (b) 7 days after zinc was removed from the medium. c) Cells transfected with the T antigen gene driven by its own viral promoter. (Magnification = 280x)

To test the ability of the human Schwann cell lines to differentiate, we cocultured them with rat DRG since human Schwann cells appear able to recognize and interact with rodent neurons. Segments of human nerve have been transplanted into the sciatic nerve of immunosuppressed mice, and the human Schwann cells within the transplant were able to form myelin (1). However, under *in vitro* conditions which permitted myelination by rat Schwann cells, neither primary human Schwann cells or the human Schwann cell lines produced myelin. Apparently, human Schwann cells have additional unknown requirements. While optimal conditions are being defined, we can test the ability of human Schwann cell lines to form myelin by transplanting the cells into the rodent nervous system.

CONCLUSIONS

A synthetic, metal-inducible promoter enables tight regulation of an oncogene such that transcription occurs only when zinc is included in the culture medium. Schwann cells immortalized with SV40 T antigen, a potent transforming oncogene, were able to revert to a normal phenotype when zinc was omitted from the medium. Although significant strides have been made in developing differentiating cell lines, the persistent problem of genetic instability due to spontaneous or oncogene-induced mutations still remains. Culture conditions must be carefully controlled to maintain selective pressure in favor of the differentiating phenotype. With vigilant care, a line maintained for over 500 population doublings was still able to differentiate. Zinc and G418 were always included in the medium. Zinc stimulates oncogene production which in turn maintains the mitotic rate of the differentiating cells close to that of any unregulated cells which may arise and otherwise overtake the cultures, while G418 eliminates cells in which plasmid sequences become rearranged. Also, the cultures were not allowed to reach confluence. Differentiating cells are contact inhibited but transformed cells are not, and would gain a selective growth advantage in confluent cultures. Environmental stresses resulting from nutrient depletion, pH imbalance, or bacterial toxins, for example, will favor the survival of the transformed phenotype and cultures were discarded if any stress had occurred. Cell lines can be recloned if necessary, however, it may be possible reduce the rate at which the transformed phenotype arises. Mutations in the SV40 T antigen gene which result in a transformation-defective protein that retains immortalizing activity have been identified (7, 25, 27). We plan to immortalize rat Schwann cells with various mutant forms of T antigen regulated by the synthetic, metal-responsive promoter to determine if these cell lines are more genetically stable.

REFERENCES

1. AGUAYO, A.J., KASARJIAN, J.K., SKAMENE, E., KONGSHAVN, P., and BRAY, G.M., (1977), Myelination of mouse axons by Schwann cells transplanted form normal and abnormal human nerves. Nature. 268(5622):753-755.

2. ANDERSON, R.D., TAPLITZ, S.J., OBERBAUER, A.M., CALAME, K.L., and HERSCHMAN, H.R. (1990), Metal-dependent binding of a nuclear factor to the rat metallothionein-I promoter. Nucleic Acid Res. 18(20):6049-6055.

3. ANDERSON, R.D., TAPLITZ, S.J., WONG, S., BRISTOL, G., LARKIN, B., and HERSCHMAN H.R., (1987), Metal-dependent binding of a factor in vivo to the metal-responsive elements of the metallothionein 1 gene promoter. Mol. Cell Biol. 7(10):3574-3581.

4. BRAY, G.M., RASMINSKY, M., AGUAYO, A.J., (1981), Interactions between axons and their sheath cells. Ann. Rev. Neurosci. 4:127-162.

5. BRINSTER, R.L., CHEN, H.Y., WARREN, R., SARTHY, A., and PALMITER, R.D., (1982) Regulation of metallothionein-thymidine kinase fusion plasmids injected into mouse eggs. Nature. 296:39-42.

6. CARTHEW, R.W., CHODOSH, L.A., and SHARP, P.A., (1987), The major late transcription factor binds to and activates the mouse metallothionein I promoter. Genes Dev. 1(9):973-980.

7. CHANG, L., PAN, S., PATER, M.M., and MAYORCA, G.D., (1985), Differential requirement for SV40 early genes in immortalization and transformation of primary rat and human embryonic cells. Virology 146:246-261.

8. DURNAM, D.M. and PALMITER, R.D., (1981), Transcriptional regulation of the mouse metallothionein-gene by heavy metals. J. Biol. Chem. 256(11):5712-5716.

9. ELDRIDGE, C.F., BUNGE, M.B., and BUNGE, R.P., (1989), Differentiation of axon-related Schwann cells in vitro: II. Control of myelin formation by basal lamina. J Neurosci. 9(2):625-638.

10. ELDRIDGE, C.F., BUNGE, M.B., BUNGE, R.P., and WOOD, P.M., (1987), Differentiation of axon-related Schwann cells in vitro. I. Ascorbic acid regulates basal lamina assembly and myelin formation. J Cell Biol. 105:1023-1034.

11. KARIN, M.A., HASLINGER, H., HEGUY, A., DIETLIN, T., and COOKE, T., (1987), Metal Responsive elements act as positive modulators of human metallothionein-II_A enhancer activity. Mol. Cell Biol. 7(2):606-613.

12. KARIN, M.A., HASLINGER, H., HOLTGREVE, R.I., RICHARDS, P., KRAUTER, H., WESTPHAL and BEATO, M., (1984), Characterization of DNA sequences through which cadmium and glucocorticoid hormones induce human metallothionein-II_A gene. Nature. 308:513-519.

3. MAYO, K.E., and PALMITER, R.D., (1982), Glucocorticoid regulation of the mouse metallothionein I gene is selectively lost following amplification of the gene. J. Biol. Chem. 257(6):3061-3067.

4. MORETTO, G., MONACO, S., PASSARIN, M.G., BENEDETTI, M.D., and RIZZUTO, N., (1991), Cytoskeletal changes induced by 2,5-hexanedione on developing human neurons in vitro. Arch Toxico 65(5):409-13.

5. NORTON, S., (1980), Toxic responses of the central nervous system, Toxicology: The Basic Science of Poisons, J. Doull, C.D. Klaassen, M.O. Amdur (Ed.) Macmillan Publishing Co., Ltd., 193-197.

6. OLSSON, Y., (1984), Vascular permeability in the peripheral nervous system, Peripheral Neuropathy, P.J. Dyck (Ed.) W.B. Saunders Company, 579-587.

7. PEDEN, K.W., CHARLES, C., SANDERS, L., and TENNEKOON, G.I., (1989), Isolation of rat Schwann cell lines: Use of SV40 T antigen gene regulated by synthetic metallothionein promoters. Exper. Cell Res. 185:60-72.

8. PEDEN, K.W., RUTKOWSKI, J.L., GILBERT, M., and TENNEKOON, G.I., (1990), Production of Schwann cell lines using a regulated oncogene. Annals of the New York Academy of Sciences, Volume 605: Myelination and Dysmyelination, I.D. Duncan, R.P. Skoff, and D. Colman (Ed.) New York Academy of Sciences, 286-293.

9. PENTSCHEW, A., and GARRO, F., (1966), Lead encephalo-myelopathy of the suckling rat and its implications on the porphyrinopathic nervous diseases. Acta Neuropathologica. 6:266-277.

20. RUTKOWSKI, J.L., TENNEKOON, G.I., and MCGILLICUDDY J.E., (1992), Selective culture of mitotically active human Schwann cells form adult sural nerves. Ann. Neurol. 31:727-733.

21. SEARLE, P.F., DAVISON, B.L., STUART, G.W., WILKIE, T.M., NORSTEDT, G., and PALMITER, R.D., (1984), Regulation, linkage, and sequence of mouse metallothionein I and II genes. Mol. Cell Biol. 4(7):1221-1230.

22. SHARP, P.A., (1992), TATA-binding protein is a classless factor. Cell. 68:819-821.

23. STUART, G.W., SEARLE, P.F., and PALMITER, R.D., (1985), Identification of multiple metal regulatory elements in mouse metallothionein-I promoter by assaying synthetic sequences. Nature. 317:828-831.

24. STUART, G.W., SEARLE, P.F., CHEN, H.Y., BRINSTER, R.L., and PALMITER, R.D., (1984), A 12-base-pair DNA motif that is repeated several times in metallothionein gene promoters confers metal regulation to a heterologous gene. Proc. Nat'l Acad. Sci. 81:7318-7322.

25. SUGANO, S., and YAMAGUCHI, N., (1984), Two classes of transformation-deficient, immortalization-positive simian virus 40 mutants constructed by making three-base insertions in the T antigen gene. J of Virology. 52(3):884-891.

26. TENNEKOON, G.I., YOSHINO, J., PEDEN, K.W., BIGBEE, J., RUTKOWSKI, J.L., KISHIMOTO, Y., DEVRIES, G.H., and MCKHANN, G., (1987), Transfection of neonatal rat Schwann cells with SV40 large T Antigen gene under control of the metallothionein promoter. J of Cell Biol. 105:2315-2325.

27. TEVETHIA, M.J., PIPAS, J.M., KIERSTEAD, T., and COLE, C., (1988), Requirements for immortalization of primary mouse embryo fibroblasts probed with mutants bearing deletions in the 3' end of SV40 gene A. Virology. 162:76-89.

28. WINDEBANK, A.J., (1986), Specific inhibition of myelination by lead in vitro; comparison with arsenic, thallium, and mercury. Exp. Neurol. 94:203-212.

29. WINDEBANK, A.J., MCCALL, J.T., and Dyck, P.J., (1984), Metal neuropathy, Peripheral Neuropathy, P.J. Dyck (Ed.) W.B. Saunders Company, 2133-2140.

B. Mechanisms of Dermatotoxicity

B1

In Vitro Models to Evaluate Agents that Contribute to Cutaneous Carcinogenesis

STUART H. YUSPA

Laboratory of Cellular Carcinogenesis and Tumor Promotion
National Cancer Institute
Bethesda, MD 20892

ABSTRACT

The induction of epithelial skin cancer is a multistage process. The initiating event is commonly a genetic change that alters the response of epidermal cells (keratinocytes) to signals that induce terminal differentiation. This is generally caused by specific mutagenic agents termed initiators. Genetically altered neoplastic keratinocytes are recognized when non-carcinogenic tumor promoters disturb cutaneous homeostasis by producing wounds, inflammation or hyperproliferation. These conditions favor the growth of neoplastic cells, and this population expands clonally to produce premalignant tumors. Malignant conversion occurs when further genetic changes develop in a cell in the premalignant population. Malignant conversion is rare, but the frequency is enhanced when premalignant cells are exposed to specific mutagens called converting agents. Thus, two specific genetic changes are sufficient to change a normal keratinocyte into a malignant tumor cell. The probability that two rare, relevant, genetic changes will occur in the same cell is very small. Clonal selection of premalignant cells by noncarcinogenic promoting agents greatly enhances the risk for subsequent genetic changes in this population. Thus, promoting agents determine the cancer incidence rate. Cellular and molecular changes have been identified, which characterize each stage of skin carcinogenesis. These have guided the development of in vitro assays to detect initiating, promoting and converting agents, and to further define molecular changes responsible for the multistage origin of epidermal tumors.

INTRODUCTION

The induction of epithelial skin cancer is a multistage process (1). The initiating event is commonly a genetic change that alters the response of epidermal cells (keratinocytes) to signals that induce terminal differentiation. This is generally caused by specific mutagenic agents termed initiators. Genetically altered neoplastic keratinocytes are recognized when non-carcinogenic tumor promoters disturb cutaneous homeostasis by producing wounds, inflammation or hyperproliferation. These conditions favor the growth of neoplastic cells, and this population expands clonally to produce premalignant (benign) tumors. Benign tumors, therefore, represent a monoclonal expansion of single initiated cells. Malignant conversion occurs when further genetic changes develop in a cell in the premalignant population. Malignant conversion is rare, but the frequency is enhanced when premalignant cells are exposed to specific mutagens called converting agents. Thus, two specific genetic changes are sufficient to change a normal keratinocyte into a malignant tumor cell. The probability that two rare, relevant, genetic changes will occur in the same cell is very small. Clonal selection of premalignant cells by noncarcinogenic promoting agents greatly enhances the risk for subsequent genetic changes in this population. Thus, promoting agents determine the cancer incidence rate. Cellular and molecular changes have been identified that characterize each stage of skin carcinogenesis (1). These have guided the development of in vitro assays to detect initiating, promoting and converting agents, and to further define molecular changes responsible for the multistage origin of epidermal tumors.

A MODEL TO STUDY INITIATORS OF SKIN CARCINOGENESIS

Basal epidermal cells can be selectively maintained as a monolayer in culture medium containing a low ionic Ca^{2+} concentration of 0.05 - 0.10 mM (2). These cells have a high proliferation rate, sustained growth potential and express protein markers characteristic of epidermal basal cells in vivo. Cessation of proliferation, expression of differentiation markers and shedding of squamous sheets can be induced in this population by increasing the Ca^{2+} concentration above 0.1 mM. Thus the Ca^{2+} models reflects changes characteristic of normal epidermal differentiation in vivo. Studies of benign epidermal tumors indicate that initiated cells are characterized by an altered differentiation phenotype whereby suprabasal cells continue to proliferate and differentiation marker expression is suppressed (3,4). We, therefore, predicted that changes in the phenotypic response to Ca^{2+} might follow exposure to carcinogens in vitro. Support for this hypothesis was provided by the observation that malignant epidermal cells continued to proliferate when switched from low to high Ca^{2+} medium (5). Tumor cells could thus be selected from a mixture including a large excess of normal cells which did not survive after induced differentiation. When primary epidermal cells cultured in low Ca^{2+} medium were treated on day 3 with a chemical carcinogen and then switched to higher Ca^{2+} growth conditions, epithelial colonies resisted the induction of differentiation by the Ca^{2+} signal and persisted to form stainable foci (6,7). Colony number was proportional to carcinogen dose for a variety of carcinogens tested. Cells obtained from colonies in treated cultures demonstrated characteristic epidermal morphology and keratinization, and could be subcultured, but did not grow in agar. Subsequent testing of a number of cell lines in vivo by subcutaneous inoculation or skin grafting revealed that selected foci could produce normal skin, papillomas or carcinomas. Thus, the assay selected for a property associated with an early change in skin neoplasia, but additional changes in some cells in vitro led to the fully malignant phenotype (8). When a series of carcinogens were tested in this assay, their ability to induce foci in vitro strongly correlated to their potency as initiators in vivo for mouse skin (7). This study, therefore, revealed a fundamental property of neoplastic keratinocytes and provided a screening method to evaluate skin carcinogens.

AN ANALYSIS OF TUMOR PROMOTION IN VITRO

Tumor promoters cause selective clonal expansion of initiated cells by several mechanisms in vivo all of which rely on differential response patterns of normal and neoplastic cells (9). The most potent skin tumor promoter, 12-O-tetradecanoylphorbol-13-acetate (TPA), provided the paradigm upon which the mechanism of promotion was elucidated (10). In skin, this promoter is a strong inducer of terminal differentiation for normal cells, but initiated cells are resistant and thus exhibit selected growth with each promoter treatment (10,11).

To facilitate the study of skin tumor promotion, a cell culture model system with characteristics analogous to initiated mouse epidermis was established. Cells of the keratinocyte cell line 308, derived from adult mouse skin initiated with 7,12-dimethylbenz[a]anthracene, display the initiated phenotype, since papillomas are produced when the cells are grafted to the backs of athymic mice. These cells are resistant to the induction of differentiation by Ca^{2+} and TPA in vitro (12,13). Coculture of a small number of 308 cells with confluent normal primary keratinocytes resulted in the inhibition of growth of colonies of 308 cells (14). Addition of fresh keratinocytes each week was required to sustain the inhibition for 3 - 4 weeks. Growth of 308 cells was not inhibited by coculture with confluent fibroblasts or by medium conditioned by either keratinocytes or fibroblasts. During continuous exposure of the cocultures to tumor promoters, 308 cell colonies became apparent within 2-3 weeks. A series of promoters have been tested in this model system and 12-O-tetradecanoylphorbol-13-acetate, 12-O-retinoylphorbol-13-acetate, mezerein, and benzoyl peroxide were all active (14). The number of colonies that developed during promoter exposure in cocultures showed a dose-response curve that differed from the dose-response curve for stimulation of growth of 308 colonies in the absence of normal keratinocytes. Simultaneous treatment with 12-O-tetradecanoylphorbol-13-acetate and known inhibitors of skin tumor promotion, such as retinoic acid, fluocinolone acetonide, and bryostatin 1, blocked colony formation of 308 cells in cocultures but not in cultures with only 308 cells. Thus in this model system, the actions of promoters and inhibitors both appear to be mediated by normal keratinocytes (14).

Further studies compared promoters with differing mechanisms of action such as those of TPA-type (those with protein kinase C as receptor) and those of non-TPA-type promoters in the coculture model. The TPA-type promoters, teleocidin and aplysiatoxin, show activity comparable to that of TPA. Exposure of cocultures to oleoyl-2-acetyl glycerol, a diacylglycerol activator of protein kinase C, also induces focal outgrowth of initiated cells, suggesting that protein kinase C is likely to be involved in the mechanism of action of these compounds. However, involvement of alternative pathways (not involving protein kinase C directly) for clonal selection are evident since the non-TPA-type promoters okadaic acid, staurosporine and thapsigargin are also active in the assay. Thus, this keratinocyte coculture model differs from fibroblast models of normal and neoplastic cocultures in which only TPA-type promoters are active. In further contrast to certain fibroblast cocultures, TPA did not inhibit cell-cell communication under conditions that suppress focus formation. The keratinocyte coculture model has broad application for detecting skin tumor promoters, and may be useful for dissecting the mechanism by which normal epidermal cells suppress the growth of initiated cells.

AN IN VITRO ASSAY TO STUDY MALIGNANT CONVERSION

While initiation and promotion in mouse skin carcinogenesis produce multiple benign tumors, only a few squamous cell carcinomas develop. The spontaneous conversion from the benign to the malignant phenotype occurs over many months and in stages, but induced malignant conversion can be accomplished more rapidly by exposure of papilloma-bearing mice to mutagens or by transfection of papilloma cell lines with specific oncogenes (15-18). The analysis of genetic targets responsible for carcinogen-induced neoplastic progression would be facilitated by the development of in vitro models where the process is rapid, focal and quantitative. To this end, primary newborn mouse keratinocytes were initiated in vitro by the introduction of the v-$\underline{ras}^{Ha}$ oncogene (v-ras-keratinocytes) via a defective retrovirus. Since recipient cells produce squamous papillomas, have a high proliferation rate in culture medium with 0.05 mM Ca^{2+}, and do not terminally differentiate in medium with high Ca^{2+}, they fulfill the criteria of initiated cells. However, v-$\underline{ras}$ keratinocytes have a very low proliferation rate in medium with high Ca^{2+} and thus differ from malignant keratinocytes which grow rapidly in such medium (19). When v-$\underline{ras}^{Ha}$-keratinocytes were exposed to mutagens in vitro, highly proliferative foci emerged after culture in 0.5 mM Ca^{2+} for 4 weeks (20). These foci stained intensely red with rhodamine stain, could be easily quantitated, and readily incorporated bromodeoxyuridine confirming their high proliferative capacity in 0.5mM Ca^{2+}. Dose-response studies with several mutagens indicated that the number of foci increased with concentration to a point until excessive cytotoxicity developed. Mutagens varied in potency for producing foci in the following order: cis-diamminedichloroplatinum $\geq$ benzo[a]pyrene diolexpoxide I > N-methyl-N'-nitro-N-nitrosoguanidine $\geq$ 4-nitroquinoline N-oxide > N-acetoxyacetyl-aminofluorene. The tumor promoters 12-O-tetradecanoylphorbol-13-acetate and benzoylperoxide were inactive in the assay. A subset of cell lines derived from foci produced malignant tumors in vivo, while others were not tumorigenic. Analysis of DNA from cell lines and tumors revealed that most tumorigenic cell lines maintained the v-ras^{Ha} genome, whereas the viral sequences were deleted in non-tumorigenic cell lines. Immunohistochemical analysis indicated that proliferative foci and quiescent v-ras^{Ha} keratinocytes expressed keratin 8, a marker of v-ras^{Ha} expression in cultured keratinocytes. Cells in foci, but not v-ras^{Ha} control cells, expressed keratin 13, a marker that is strongly associated with malignant progression of skin tumors in vivo. This in vitro assay provides a quantitative model to study chemically-induced focal neoplastic progression at the cellular level, and to identify agents that may be selective for enhancing malignant conversion.

CONCLUSION

Skin carcinogenesis studies have provided considerable insight into stages of carcinogenesis. The in vitro analogues I have described have extended the understanding of this process to a cellular and molecular level. Furthermore, they have provided convenient tools to assay for agents which are potential initiators, promoters, antipromoters and converting agents. Skin is a model for lining epithelial carcinogenesis in general. Thus cancer pathogenesis and experimental cancer induction in gastrointestinal, urogenital, and bronchial epithelium may have similar properties. Thus, these models are likely to reveal important information for major target sites for human cancer mortality and morbidity

REFERENCES

1. Yuspa, S.H. and Dlugosz, A.A. (1991), Cutaneous carcinogenesis: natural and experimental, *Physiology Biochemistry and Molecular Biology of The Skin*, L. Goldsmith (ed.) Oxford University Press, New York, 1365-1402.

2. Hennings, H., Michael, D., Cheng, C., Steinert, P., Holbrook, K. and Yuspa, S.H. (1980), Calcium regulation of growth and differentiation of mouse epidermal cells in culture. Cell 19:245-254.

3. Roop, D.R., Krieg, T.M., Mehrel, T., Cheng, C.K. and Yuspa, S.H. (1988), Transcriptional control of high molecular weight keratin gene expression in multistage mouse skin carcinogenesis. Cancer Res. 48:3245-3252.

4. Huitfeldt, H.S., Heyden, A., Clausen, O.P.F., Thrane, E.V., Roop, D. and Yuspa, S.H. (1991), Altered regulation of growth and expression of differentiation-associated keratins in benign mouse skin tumors. Carcinogenesis 12:2063-2067.

5. Yuspa, S.H., Hawley-Nelson, P., Koehler, B. and Stanley, J.R. (1980), A survey of transformation markers in differentiating epidermal cell lines in culture. Cancer Res. 40:4694-4703.

6. Kulesz-Martin, M.F., Koehler, B., Hennings, H. and Yuspa, S.H. (1980), Quantitative assay for carcinogen altered differentiation in mouse epidermal cells. Carcinogenesis 1:995-1006.

7. Kawamura, H., Strickland, J.E. and Yuspa, S.H. (1985), Association of resistance to terminal differentiation with initiation of carcinogenesis in adult mouse epidermal cells. Cancer Res. 45:2748-2752.

8. Kulesz-Martin, M., Kilkenny, A.E., Holbrook, K.A., Digernes, V. and Yuspa, S.H. (1983), Properties of carcinogen altered mouse epidermal cells resistant to calcium-induced terminal differentiation. Carcinogenesis 4:1367-1377.

9. Yuspa, S.H. and Poirier, M.C. (1988), Chemical carcinogenesis: From animal models to molecular models in one decade. Adv. Cancer. Res. 50:25-70.

10. Yuspa, S.H. (1987), Tumor promotion, <u>Accomplishments in Cancer Research 1986</u>, J.F. Fortner and J.E. Rhoads (eds.) JB Lippencott Co, Philadelphia, 169-182.

11. Yuspa, S.H., Morgan, D., Lichti, U., Spangler, E.F., Michael, D., Kilkenny, A. and Hennings, H. (1986), Cultivation and characterization of cells derived from mouse skin papillomas induced by an initiation-promotion protocol. Carcinogenesis 7:949-958.

12. Strickland, J.E., Greenhalgh, D.A., Koceva-Chyla, A., Hennings, H., Restrepo, C., Balaschak, M. and Yuspa, S.H. (1988), Development of murine epidermal cell lines which contain an activated ras^{Ha} oncogene and form papillomas in skin grafts on athymic nude mouse hosts. Cancer Res. 48:165-169.

13. Hennings, H., Michael, D., Lichti, U. and Yuspa, S.H. (1987), Response of carcinogen-altered mouse epidermal cells to phorbol ester tumor promoters and calcium. J. Invest. Dermatol. 88:60-65.

14. Hennings, H., Robinson, V.A., Michael, D.M., Pettit, G.R., Jung, R. and Yuspa, S.H. (1990), Development of an <u>in vitro</u> analogue of initiated mouse epidermis to study tumor promoters and antipromoters. Cancer Res. 50:4794-4800.

15. Hennings, H., Shores, R., Wenk, M.L., Spangler, E.F., Tarone, R. and Yuspa, S.H. (1983), Malignant conversion of mouse skin tumors is increased by tumor initiators and unaffected by tumor promoters. Nature 304:67-69.

16. Hennings, H., Shores, R.A., Poirier, M.C., Reed, E., Tarone, R.E. and Yuspa, S.H. (1990), Enhanced malignant conversion of benign mouse skin tumors by cisplatin. J. Natl. Cancer Inst. 82:836-840.

17. Greenhalgh, D.A. and Yuspa, S.H. (1988), Malignant conversion of murine squamous papilloma cell lines by transfection with the fos oncogene. Mol. Carcinog. 1:134-143.

18. Harper, J.R., Roop, D.R. and Yuspa, S.H. (1986), Transfection of the EJ rasHa gene into keratinocytes derived from carcinogen-induced mouse papillomas causes malignant progression. Mol. Cell. Biol. 6:3144-3149.

19. Yuspa, S.H., Kilkenny, A.E., Stanley, J. and Lichti, U. (1985), Keratinocytes blocked in phorbol ester-responsive early stage of terminal differentiation by sarcoma viruses. Nature 314:459-462.

20. Morgan, D., Welty, D., Greenhalgh, D., Hennings, H. and Yuspa, S.H. (1992), The development of an in vitro model to study carcinogen-induced neoplastic progression of initiated mouse epidermal cells. Cancer Res. 52:3145-3156.

B2

Photoimmunology

STEPHEN E. ULLRICH

Department of Immunology (178)
The University of Texas, M.D. Anderson Cancer Center
1515 Holcombe Boulevard
Houston, TX 77030

INTRODUCTION

Photoimmunology is a study of the immunomodulatory function of electromagnetic energy, primarily in the ultraviolet-B (280-320 nm, UVB) region of the solar spectrum. Although the discipline of photoimmunology is about 15 years old, it can trace its origins to earlier observations made in fields as diverse as tumor immunology, photocarcinogenesis, dermatology and medicine. The association between the skin and the immune system and the observation that there is a link between UVB-induced skin cancer induction and the ability of UVB radiation to suppress the immune system triggered research in photoimmunology. These observations led to intensive study on the mechanisms involved in skin cancer induction and immunosuppression following UVB exposure. The importance and significance of these studies is underscored by recent evidence for the destruction of the protective atmospheric ozone layer by environmental pollutants. Besides the distinct possibility for increased incidence of non-melanoma skin cancers, depletion of the ozone layer may also effect other aspects of human health, due to the immunosuppressive properties of UVB radiation. The focus of this review will be to discuss the mechanisms involved in the suppression of the immune response by UVB radiation.

BACKGROUND

The realization that there was a relationship between photocarcinogenesis and the suppressive effects of UVB radiation was one of the initial observations in photoimmunology. UVB exposure causes skin cancers in mice (1). In a study of the immunologic properties of these tumors, Kripke, found that the UVB-induced skin tumors were highly antigenic (2). UVB-induced tumors were rejected when transplanted into normal syngeneic mice and were only capable of progressive growth when transplanted into immunosuppressed recipients. This observation lead to the question of how can these highly antigenic tumor cells develop in the primary UVB-irradiated host without being destroyed by the animal's immune system. The answer lies in the fact that in addition to being carcinogenic, UVB is also immunosuppressive. Long before the primary tumors develop in the UVB-irradiated animals these mice lose their ability to reject UVB-induced tumors (3). Studies by Kripke and co-workers, and Daynes and colleagues documented a number of important findings concerning the suppression of tumor immunity by UVB radiation. The suppression is systemic, UVB-induced tumors grow progressively regardless of whether they are injected at the site of irradiation or at a distant, non-irradiated site (3). The suppressor cells recognize common antigenic determinants on UVB-induced tumor cells (4) and play a role in both the induction of primary tumors (5) and the inability of UVB-irradiated mice to reject transplanted tumors (6-8). The suppression is specific and highly selective. While UVB-induced tumors grow progressively in UVB-irradiated mice, other chemically induced tumors are rejected (9). Furthermore, not all aspects of the immune response are suppressed in UVB-irradiated animals. Although these mice do not reject the highly antigenic UVB-induced tumors they do reject allogeneic skin grafts, generate antibodies following immunization, and have lymphocytes that respond normally to mitogenic and antigenic stimulation (10, 11).

Photoimmunology can also trace its roots to dermatology and medicine. Although Finsen received the 1903 Nobel prize for his observation that the skin lesions associated with tuberculosis infection often resolved after UVB exposure, the use of light and light activated drugs to treat skin diseases can trace its origins to ancient times. Early Egyptians recognized that a light activated compound present in the plant *Ammi majus* promoted sunburn and used this property to treat the patches of de-pigmentation seen in the skin disorder vitiligo. This ancient observation was reconfirmed in the 1940's by Abdel El Mofty at the University of Cairo who used an extract from *A. majus* and sunlight to treat vitiligo. The chemical purification of the active compound, 8-methoxypsoralen, and the use of artificial sources of UVA (320-400 nm) radiation propelled psoralen plus UVA radiation (PUVA) into the clinic where it is used to treat a variety of diseases, including, psoriasis, alopecia, lichen planus, vitiligo, mycosis fungoides, and cutaneous T cell lymphoma (12-17). Because PUVA-treatment results in the formation of bifunctional cross-links between adjacent strands of DNA, the beneficial effect of PUVA therapy on hyperproliferative diseases such as psoriasis is probably due to DNA damage. However, PUVA is also immunosuppressive. Patients undergoing chronic PUVA-treatment for psoriasis have impaired T cell function (18). Contact hypersensitivity is suppressed and antigen-specific suppressor T cells are present in PUVA-treated mice (8, 19). Indeed the immunosuppressive effects of PUVA photochemotherapy may explain its therapeutic effect, especially on non-proliferative diseases such as vitiligo.

Finally, the special association between the skin and the immune system, an association that has been recognized and used by immunologists for years has helped promote the discipline of photoimmunology. In 1983, Streilein, introduced the terminology, skin associated lymphoid tissue (SALT), to describe the special relationship that exists between the skin and elements of the immune system (20). The evidence for SALT comes from a number of observations. First, epidermal Langerhans cells and dermal dendritic cells function as *in situ* antigen-presenting cells. Second, activated keratinocytes produce a wide variety of immunomodulatory cytokines that may act locally or at distant sites. Third, epidermotrophic T cells can and do migrate to the skin from the peripheral blood to respond to locally processed antigen. Fourth, specialized endothelial cells appear to be present in the blood vessels of the dermis to promote the transport of skin seeking T lymphocytes. Thus, within the skin are all the elements required to recognize and respond to new antigens, recognize and respond to recall antigens and distinguish between self and non-self. Furthermore, exposure to environmental agents, such as UVB radiation, that impair the function of one or more of these elements, results in the loss of immunologic protection and the induction of immunologic suppression.

Mechanisms involved in the immunosuppression seen following UVB exposure

Historically, investigators working in photoimmunology tend to divide the suppression induced by UVB radiation into two categories, local and systemic. Local suppression refers to the model originally described by Toews and colleagues in which the contact allergen is applied directly to the site of UV exposure (21). In systemic suppression, as exemplified by the experiments of Noonan et al (22), the contact allergen is applied at a distant non-irradiated site.

Local suppression of immunity by UVB radiation The model of local suppression, refers to a situation where mouse skin is irradiated on four consecutive days with a dose of UVB radiation equivalent to the amount that induces moderate erythema in normal human skin (400 J/m^2). Immediately after the last exposure the contact allergen is applied directly onto the irradiated skin. Six days later the mice are challenged by applying the contact allergen on the ears, and the resulting ear swelling reaction is used to measure contact hypersensitivity (CHS). Toews et al (21) found that sensitization of mice through irradiated skin prevented the induction of CHS. Langerhans cell density at the site of sensitization appeared to be a critical determinant for the induction of non-responsiveness. UVB exposure caused a decrease in Langerhans cell number and altered their morphology. The unresponsiveness did not reflect a "null event" because UVB-irradiated mice were unable to respond to a second application of the same hapten, suggesting the induction of suppressor cells. Elmets et al (23) subsequently demonstrated the appearance of hapten-specific suppresser T cells in the spleens of the UV-irradiated animals. The effect was local, irradiation at one site, with sensitization at a distant site, resulted in a vigorous CHS response.

The destruction of Langerhans cells at the site of sensitization suggests that they are the relevant targets for UVB in this model system and two pieces of evidence support this hypothesis. The first comes from a study by Cruz et al (24). In these experiments a relatively "pure" population of Langerhans cells was obtained by sorting Ia+ epidermal cells with the fluorescence activated cell sorter. These cells were irradiated with UVB, derivatized with hapten *in vitro*, and injected intravenously into normal syngeneic mice. The animals were challenged six days later, and CHS measured the next day. Mice injected with non-irradiated, hapten-conjugated, Ia+, epidermal cells had a CHS response that was identical to that seen in control non-irradiated animals. When UVB-irradiated hapten-conjugated Langerhans cells were used to immunize the mice, CHS was significantly depressed, and these animals did not respond to resensitization, suggesting the induction of suppressor cells.

Simon et al (25) also measured the ability of *in vitro* irradiated Langerhans cells to present antigen. The design of this study took advantage of the fact that there are at least two different subclasses of CD4+ T cells, distinguished by the pattern of cytokines released upon activation. T helper 1 cells (Th1) release interleukin (IL)-2, gamma-interferon (IFN-γ) and lymphotoxin after antigenic-stimulation, whereas T helper 2 cells (Th2) produce IL-4, 5, 6, and 10. Th1 cells help cellular immune reactions such as CHS, whereas, Th2 cells are much more efficient in helping B cells during antibody formation (26). Simon et al used sorter purified Langerhans cells to present antigen to either Th1 or Th2 clones. They found that although normal Langerhans cells presented antigen to either Th1 or Th2 cells, UVB-irradiated Langerhans cells would only present to Th2 cells. These authors suggest the UVB-irradiated Langerhans cells suppress CHS by two distinct mechanisms. The first mechanism involves suppressing Th1 cell activation, thus inhibiting the cells responsible for the induction of CHS. The second mechanism involves increased production of IL-10, cytokine synthesis inhibitory factor, by Th2 cells. IL-10 feeds back and prevents the production of IFN-γ by Th1 cells, thus further limiting CHS. In a subsequent report, Simon et al demonstrate that Th1 cells become anergic following interaction with UVB-treated Langerhans cells (27).

In addition to the damaging effect of UVB radiation directly on Langerhans cell function there also appears to be a role for tumor necrosis factor alpha (TNF-α) in the local suppression model (28). Because TNF-α is released by keratinocytes following UVB exposure (29) and studies on the genetics of local UVB-induced suppression suggested a link between TNF-α production and UVB susceptibility (30), Yoshikawa and Streilein examined the role of TNF-α in the induction of suppression. They found that intradermal injection of TNF-α mimicked the effects of UVB and suppressed the induction of CHS. Furthermore, injecting anti-TNF-α antibodies overcame the suppressive effects of UVB (28). Their results suggest that the local release of TNF-α may play a role in the induction of local suppression, perhaps by interfering with Langerhans cell function at the site of irradiation.

Studies from our laboratory demonstrated that applying contact allergens through PUVA-treated skin also suppressed the induction of CHS (31). In this study two different classes of psoralen were used. 8-methoxypsoralen, a classic bifunctional psoralen that cross-links opposing strands of DNA after exposure to UVA radiation, and angelicin, a monofunctional psoralen, which does not cross-link opposing strands of DNA but rather forms photoadducts on the same strand of DNA. Monofunctional psoralens are interesting compounds because they are much less erythemogenic and mutagenic than bifunctional psoralens. Mice treated with 8-methoxypsoralen and UVA (PUVA) have severe epidermal phototoxicity and a significant reduction in the numbers of Ia+ Langerhans cells at the site of irradiation. Although we saw no evidence of skin phototoxicity, application of angelicin and UVA radiation caused a significant reduction in the numbers of epidermal Langerhans cells. Application of the contact sensitizer, dinitroflurobenzene, through either PUVA- or angelicin and UVA-treated skin resulted in a significant suppression CHS with an associated induction of splenic suppressor cells. This study confirmed the observation of others that application of contact allergens through PUVA-treated skin could suppress CHS (32). Furthermore these findings suggest that the phototoxicity and inflammation associated with topical PUVA-treatment is not a requirement for the induction of immunological unresponsiveness, but damage to epidermal Langerhans cells is.

Systemic suppression of immunity by UVB radiation The model of systemic suppression, as originally described by Jessup and colleagues (33), and Noonan et al (34) refers to a situation where mice are irradiated with a single dose of UVB radiation and sensitized with the contact allergen at a distant non-irradiated site. Langerhans cell damage at the site of sensitization is not involved (35), but associated with the induction of systemic suppression by UVB radiation is a defect in splenic antigen-presenting cell capability (36, 37) and the induction of antigen-specific suppressor T cells (34).

Over the past years the local and systemic models of UVB-induced suppression have also been differentiated based on the dose of UVB used to suppress CHS. Generally, lower doses of UVB have been used to induce suppression in the local model (1.4 kJ/m^2 versus 30-40 kJ/m^2). Recently, however, Noonan and De Fabo (38) reported induction of systemic suppression with a relatively small dose of UVB (2.2 kJ/m^2). They point out that the dose of UV needed to cause suppression varies with the strain of mouse tested, and that there appears to be no correlation between the dose of UV used and the induction of systemic versus local suppression. Therefore, using the terms low-dose or high-dose to describe local or systemic suppression appears to be in error and should be discontinued.

Studies on the systemic suppression of contact and delayed hypersensitivity essentially grew from experiments designed to measure the immunologic profile of tumor-susceptible UV-irradiated mice. A great deal of information concerning the mechanisms involved in the induction of suppression and suppressor cells by UVB radiation has been generated from these experiments. A wide variety of antigens can be used to induce suppressor cells. Sensitization of UVB-irradiated mice with contact allergens, TNP-coupled spleen cells, protein antigens, foreign erythrocytes, viral, fungal and bacterial antigens, parasites and allogeneic histocompatibility antigens results in the induction of suppression, and in most cases tested, antigen-specific suppressor T cells (36, 39-44). Once induced the suppressor T cells can regulate multiple immunologic pathways, T cell proliferation, the generation of cytotoxic T lymphocytes, and antibody formation are all suppressed, in an antigen-specific manner by the UV-induced suppressor T cells (45, 46).

We determined the target of the UVB-induced suppressor T cells by taking advantage of the observation that the suppressor cells could inhibit antibody formation. UVB-irradiated mice were sensitized with trinitrochlorobenzene (TNCB) to generate TNP-specific suppressor cells. The suppressor cells were then injected into normal recipients and these mice were immunized with either a T-dependent antigen (TNP-coupled to erythrocytes) or a T-independent antigen (TNP conjugated to LPS). Mice injected with the suppressor cells did not generate antibodies against the T-dependent antigen but did produce a vigorous response after immunization with the T-independent antigen. Because T cell help is required to make antibody following immunization with T dependent but not T-independent antigens, these findings indicate that the target of the UVB-induced suppressor cell is the helper T cell. Moreover, the suppressor cell inhibited IL-2 production *in vitro* and its suppressive activity *in vivo* was abrogated by the injection of IL-2 (47). Similarly, Romerdahl and Kripke reported that the UVB-induced suppressor lymphocyte that interfered with tumor immunity targeted T helper cell activity (48, 49).

Although exposure to UV radiation is a unique way to induce suppressor cells, it appears that once induced the suppressor cells use a common mechanism to suppress the immune response; the elaboration of suppressive factors. Steele et al (50) have described a monoclonal antibody that recognizes a common determinant on a variety of first-order suppressive factors. We observed that injecting this antibody into UVB-irradiated mice inhibited the induction of suppression (51). These findings indicate that the UVB-induced suppressor T cells mediate their suppressive effects through the elaboration of a suppressive factor that shares common antigenic epitopes with other first order T cell suppressor factors.

The role of soluble factors in the induction of systemic suppression following UVB exposure One of the most intriguing questions concerning the induction of systemic suppression by UVB-radiation concerns how the suppressive signal is transmitted from the skin to the rest of the body. As mentioned above, Langerhans cells at the site of sensitization are normal (35) so the mechanism appears to differ from that described in the local model of suppression (24, 25). Although a variety of hypothesis have been proposed over the years to deal with the systemic induction of suppression (22), most of the evidence collected to date support a role for UVB-induced suppressive photoproducts. Serum-factors from UV-irradiated mice, cis-urocanic acid, IL-1, contra-IL-1, TNF-α, PGE$_2$, and keratinocyte-derived cytokines that suppress CHS and/or DTH have all been described as playing a major role in the induction of suppression following UVB radiation.

Serum Factors In 1984, Swartz reported that serum from UVB-irradiated mice could transfer the suppression of CHS when injected into normal recipients (52). Similarly, Harriott-Smith and Halliday (53) found that serum from UVB-irradiated animals could suppress CHS and the *in vitro* leukocyte-adherence assay. Other than crude estimates of the molecular weights of these factors (1-10 kDa for Swartz and >15 kDa for Harriott-Smith and Halliday), little is known about the biochemistry of these factors.

Cis-urocanic acid A provocative paper published by De Fabo and Noonan generated great interest and a fair amount of research into the role of cis-urocanic acid in the induction of immunosuppression following UVB exposure (54). An action spectrum for the suppression of CHS by UVB was constructed and compared to the known UVB-absorption spectrum of compounds within the skin. On the basis of this analysis, the two best candidates for the UVB photoreceptor were DNA and urocanic acid. Because urocanic acid is located superficially in the stratum corneum, De Fabo and Noonan removed the stratum corneum by tape stripping and examined the effect this procedure had on the induction of suppression. Suppression was significantly abrogated if the stratum corneum was removed before exposure to *monochromatic short wave UVC light* (254 nm). From these data, De Fabo and Noonan concluded that the *UVB photoreceptor* must be urocanic acid since it is located superficially. Furthermore, they suggested that the photo-isomerization of trans-urocanic to cis-urocanic acid by UVB, and the subsequent release of cis-urocanic acid is the initiating event in the induction of systemic suppression following UVB-exposure.

The latter hypothesis is supported by data presented by Ross et al (55). Painting cis-urocanic acid onto the skin of mice, or injecting cis-urocanic acid into the subcutis, 3-5 days prior to immunization with herpes simplex virus caused a significant suppression of anti-viral DTH. Moreover, antigen-specific suppressor T lymphocytes were found in the spleens of the treated animals, and the phenotype of the suppressor cells was identical to those previously observed by this group in the spleens of UV-irradiated mice (56). Injecting cis-urocanic acid intravenously yielded similar results (57).

Cis-urocanic acid has also been shown to depress splenic antigen-presenting cell activity (58). The proliferative response of antigen-primed T cells to antigen-pulsed dendritic cells isolated from cis-urocanic injected mice was significantly lower than that observed when the antigen was presented on normal dendritic cells or cells isolated from mice injected with trans-urocanic acid. As mentioned above, a systemic defect in antigen-presentation has been found after UVB exposure, so the depressed antigen-presentation seen in this study supports the hypothesis that the release of cis-urocanic acid is involved in the induction of systemic suppression following UVB exposure.

Although the accumulated evidence supports a role for cis-urocanic acid in the induction of systemic suppression by UVB-irradiation, the claim that trans-urocanic acid is the photoreceptor for UVB radiation has been questioned. Morison and Kelly (59) sought to reproduce the data supporting the claim that the photoreceptor is located superficially. They removed the stratum corneum by tape stripping and examined the effect this treatment had on the ability to suppress CHS. While tape stripping was very efficient at removing the stratum corneum, as verified by HPLC analysis, it was also very efficient at suppressing CHS. Compared to normal controls, tape stripped animals had a 57% reduction in their CHS reaction. When these mice were exposed to UVC radiation, Morison and Kelly observed a further reduction in the CHS response. Unlike the results reported by De Fabo and Noonan, Morison and Kelly found that the suppression in tape stripped UVC-irradiated animals was identical to that seen in mice exposed only to UVC. These observations suggest that the photoreceptor is not located in the stratum corneum.

Applegate et al (60) arrived at a similar conclusion using entirely different methods. This study took advantage of the fact that the cells of the South American opossum, *Monodelphis domestica* contain the enzyme that repairs UVB-induced DNA pyrimidine dimers. Exposing the marsupial cells to visible light after UVB irradiation activates the enzyme, which repairs the dimers, and restores the DNA to its original configuration. Applegate and colleagues found that exposing the marsupials to UVB radiation suppressed CHS, and the suppression was reversed if the animals were treated with photoreactivating visible light immediately after UVB exposure. The photoreactivating light had no suppressive effect by itself, and exposing the animals to the photoreactivating light prior to UVB did not reverse the suppression. Because of the exquisite specificity of the photoreactivating enzyme for DNA dimers, these findings suggest that DNA and not urocanic acid is the target of UVB radiation.

IL-1 and TNF-α Activated keratinocytes release a wide variety of cytokines and epidermal-cell derived thymocyte activating factor, a substance that has been since shown to be biologically, biochemically and immunologically identical to IL-1, was the first keratinocyte-derived cytokine described [reviewed by Sauder, (61)]. Elevated serum levels of IL-1 after UV-exposure (62) prompted Robertson et al to ask if IL-1 was responsible for the induction of suppression following UVB-irradiation (63). Injecting rIL-1 into mice did depress their ability to respond to contact allergens. Treating the mice with the prostaglandin synthetase inhibitor, indomethacin, blocked the suppression, indicating a role for PGE_2. Although suppressor cells were found in the spleens of the rIL-1 injected mice, these cells suppressed the elicitation but not the induction of CHS, a situation contrary to that seen after UV exposure (19). Similarly, injecting rTNF-α also suppressed CHS, but since the effect was on the efferent and not the afferent limb of CHS, it appears that the mechanism involved is different from that seen following UV exposure (64). The authors suggest that the suppression of CHS observed in these studies reflects a normal feedback mechanism.

Contra-CHS and Contra-IL-1 Because the penetrating power of UVB radiation is such that most of the energy is absorbed in the epidermis and upper layers of the dermis (65), Schwarz and colleagues anticipated that the site of initiation for the UVB-induced immunosuppression would be the epidermis. To test this hypothesis, primary epidermal cell cultures, or a transformed murine keratinocyte cell line, were exposed to UV radiation. Supernatants were collected 18 to 24 hours later and injected into normal mice. The mice were then sensitized with a contact allergen and their ability to generate CHS was tested. Injecting supernatants from UV-irradiated keratinocytes but not UV-irradiated macrophages or fibroblasts suppressed CHS. Similar to the situation seen after total-body UV exposure, only the induction of CHS was suppressed, injecting the supernatants from the UV-irradiated keratinocytes had no effect on the elicitation of the response. Although separation of the suppressive material on HPLC indicated a fair amount of size heterogeneity, the majority of the suppressive activity migrated with a fraction that had a molecular weight of 20 kDa. Treating the keratinocytes with indomethacin had no effect on the ability to generate suppressive activity indicating that the suppressive activity was not due to the release of PGE_2 (66).

In addition to contra-CHS activity, a contra-IL-1 activity was also found in the supernatant fluid collected from UV-irradiated keratinocytes (67). When the supernatants from the UV-irradiated keratinocytes were fractionated on HPLC, the 40-kDa fraction inhibited the ability of IL-1 to activate murine thymocytes. The suppressive activity appeared to be specific for IL-1 since this material did not suppress spontaneous DNA synthesis nor did it inhibit the proliferation of IL-2 and IL-3 dependent cell lines. The factor was released after treating the keratinocytes with UVB radiation or phorbol myristate acetate (PMA), and de novo protein synthesis was required for the production of contra-IL-1 since cycloheximide treatment inhibited its production. The isoelectric point of contra-IL-1 was reported as 8.8.

The relationship between contra-IL-1 and contra-CHS remains an important issue. Is contra-IL-1 involved in the induction of systemic suppression of CHS following total-body UVB exposure? It is not clear but the presence of contra-IL-1 in the serum of UVB-irradiated mice lends support to this hypothesis (68). Contra-IL-1 activity, migrating with an apparent molecular weight of 40 kDa, and a pI of 9.0 was found in the serum of UV-irradiated but not normal mice. Serum contra-IL-1 did not suppress the proliferation of IL-2 or IL-3 dependent cell lines. Suppressive activity was found in the serum at 3 hours, peaked by 24 hours and was absent at 72 hours.

Furthermore, contra-IL-1 appears to suppress antigen-presenting cell activity. Krutmann et al (69) used human monocytes as accessory cells for autologous T cell activation. Addition of human HPLC-fractionated contra-IL-1 inhibited T cell proliferation in a dose dependent manner. When solid phase anti-CD3 was used to activate the T cells (accessory cell independent T cell activation), contra-IL-1 had no effect, indicating that contra-IL-1 was affecting monocyte accessory cell function and not the responding T cells. Krutmann et al suggest that systemic suppression of antigen-presenting cell function *in vivo* after UV exposure may result from the release of contra-IL-1.

UVB-induced Keratinocyte-derived suppressive factors that induce antigen-specific suppressor cells Over the past few years a major focus of my own research has concerned using UVB radiation to suppress unwanted immune reactions such as allograft rejection (70-73). The beauty of using UVB as an immunosuppressive agent is the specificity and selectivity of the suppression; the major drawback is the phototoxicity and potential risk of skin cancer development. While we were attempting to deal with these problems, we became aware of the exciting data generated by Thomas Schwarz and his colleagues in Vienna, so we modified our system to determine if factors from UVB-irradiated keratinocytes could be used to suppress the immune reaction to allogeneic histocompatibility antigens. Our preliminary studies were designed to answer two questions. First, would injecting the supernatant from UVB-irradiated keratinocytes suppress the immune response to alloantigens, in an antigen-specific manner? Second, would injecting the keratinocyte-derived suppressive cytokine mimic the effect of total-body UV exposure and induce a selective suppression of immunity?

Injecting supernatants from UVB-irradiated primary epidermal cell cultures, or UVB-irradiated keratinocyte cell lines suppressed the induction of DTH to alloantigen. The suppression was associated with the appearance of splenic $CD3^+$, $CD4^+$, $CD8^-$, suppressor T cells, and the suppressor cells were specific for the antigen used to sensitize the factor-injected mice. Treating the keratinocytes with indomethacin did not abrogate the suppressive activity, suggesting that the suppressive factor was not PGE_2. Treating the keratinocytes with cycloheximide or treating the supernatants with trypsin did remove all suppressive activity indicating the factor was a protein. Passing the suppressive material over a Concanavalin-A-agarose column depleted all suppressive activity indicating the suppressive material is glycosylated (74). Thus, injecting the suppressive factor from UV-irradiated keratinocytes mimicked the suppression induced following total-body UVB exposure. Furthermore, the characteristics of the suppressive cytokine resembled contra-CHS as described by Schwarz et al (66, 67).

It was when we began to study the selectivity of the suppression that we first had an indication that we were looking at a cytokine that differed from the one described by Schwarz et al. As mentioned above, the immunological profile of a UV-irradiated animal is unique. While some cellular immune reactions are suppressed (rejection of UVB-induced tumors, CHS and DTH) humoral immune reactions are normal in these mice. We anticipated that injecting the cytokine from UV-irradiated keratinocytes would yield a similar pattern of immunosuppression. While we could suppress the generation of DTH to hapten-modified self or alloantigen with supernatants from UVB-irradiated keratinocytes, we were unable to suppress CHS (75). At first this finding surprised us because it appeared that our methods were identical to those used by Schwarz and colleagues. Upon closer examination, however, it soon was apparent that the light sources used in our studies differed considerably in their spectral outputs. Schwarz et al used a lamp that produced primarily UVA radiation (68% UVA, 32% UVB) whereas the light source used in our study produced primarily UVB radiation (65% UVB, 35% UVA). Could different wavebands of UV radiation produce unique immunosuppressive factors that had different effects on CHS and DTH? To test this hypothesis we irradiated our keratinocytes with either UVB or pure (>99%) UVA radiation. We found that exposing the keratinocytes to UVB radiation produced a factor that suppressed DTH but not CHS, whereas UVA exposure produced a factor that suppressed CHS but not DTH. Neither factor suppressed antibody formation *in vivo*. Thus, it appears that different wavebands of UV radiation activate keratinocytes to produce at least two different immunosuppressive factors, one that suppresses DTH and one that suppresses CHS.

While the identity of the keratinocyte-derived factor that suppresses DTH is still unknown, lately we have directed our attention to a newly described cytokine, IL-10 (76). Why IL-10? Primarily because the biologic activity of IL-10 closely mimics the suppression found after UV exposure. IL-10 is not a pan-immunosuppressive cytokine, only cellular immune reactions, such as DTH are suppressed by IL-10, antibody formation is not suppressed by IL-10 (77). IL-10 also inhibits antigen-presenting cell function (78). Therefore, we wondered if UVB exposure activated keratinocytes to release IL-10 and could the release of IL-10 into the circulation initiate the systemic immunosuppression? To test this hypothesis we took a number of approaches. First, synthetic oligonucleotides were constructed based on the published cDNA sequence of T cell IL-10. The mRNA from UV-irradiated keratinocytes was then isolated and analyzed by Northern analysis. At various times after exposure (1, 3, 6 hours) IL-10 mRNA expression was enhanced. Second, Western blots using IL-10 specific monoclonal antibodies demonstrated that IL-10 was released by UV-irradiated keratinocytes. The keratinocyte-derived IL-10 was biologically active in that it suppressed IFN-γ production by antigen-activated Th1 cells. Finally treatment of the supernatant from the UV-irradiated keratinocytes with neutralizing anti-IL-10 antibody abrogated suppressive activity (Rivas and Ullrich, manuscript in preparation). Thus, these findings suggest that IL-10 is released by keratinocytes after UV exposure and IL-10 plays a role in the induction of suppression by keratinocyte-derived cytokines. Whether IL-10 also plays a role in the induction of suppression after whole-body UV exposure remains to be seen.

It is clear from a review of the literature that immunomodulatory factors released by epidermal cells after UVB exposure play an important role in the induction of systemic suppression. On the basis of their ability to mimic the *in vivo* suppression seen after UVB exposure (suppression of DTH or CHS, activation of suppressor cells, depression of antigen-presenting cell activity) cis-urocanic acid, contra-IL-1, and IL-10 must be considered as the primary mediators involved in transmitting the suppressive signal from the target organ, the skin, to the rest of the immune system.

Effects of UVB on infectious disease Cell-mediated immune reactions play a prominent role in protecting against many infectious agents. Because environmental exposure to UVB radiation will most certainly increase, due to the depletion of the atmospheric ozone layer, the UV-induced suppression of cellular immunity may become an important public health problem.

The effect of UVB radiation on the immune response to herpes simplex virus (HSV) is one area that has received considerable attention. For years the ability of sunlight to induce cold sores has been recognized. In 1985, Spruance demonstrated that UVB exposure triggered herpes lesions in patients with a history of herpes infection, in a dose dependent manner (78). Studies with mice suggest that this may be due to local impairment of immune function. UVB-irradiation at the site of intradermal HSV-2 injection increased the severity of disease (79). More lesions developed in UVB-irradiated mice compared to non-irradiated controls. Furthermore the time required for the lesion to heal was increased in UVB-irradiated mice and correlated with the dose of UVB used. UVB exposure inhibited the ability of Ia^+ epidermal cells to present viral antigen to T cells, and this depression was associated with the production of a soluble factor that inhibited T cell proliferation (80). Also associated with the increased severity of HSV-2 lesions in UVB-irradiated mice was a systemic defect in DTH to HSV-2 and the induction of antigen-specific suppressor T cells (81). Similar findings have been reported by Howie et al in regard to the effects of UVB radiation on the immune response to HSV-1 (40, 56, 82, 83).

Giannini has examined the effects of UVB exposure on cutaneous Leishmaniasis (47). After exposure to relatively low doses of UVB (<1 kJ/m^2) infected mice had skin lesions that were cosmetically less severe when compared to the lesions found on control non-irradiated mice. The effect of the UVB was on the skin of the host animals because there was no effect of the irradiation on parasite load or viability. Because the ulcer in cutaneous Leishmaniasis results from an immune reaction it appeared that the inhibition of skin pathology was due to a suppressed immune response. This was confirmed by measuring protective immunity against a subsequent re-infection at a distant non-irradiated site. Protective immunity was readily apparent in non-irradiated immunized mice. The skin lesions were considerably smaller in these animals than in the non-immunized controls. This contrasted with the situation found in UVB-irradiated animals, the skin lesions in these mice were indistinguishable from the lesions found in non-immunized mice. Moreover, the number of viable organisms at the site of challenge was significantly higher in UVB-irradiated mice when compared to non-irradiated immunized controls.

UVB exposure also suppresses immunity to the fungus, *Candida albicans* (41). The suppression was systemic in nature and both the induction and elicitation of DTH was inhibited in irradiated animals. The afferent suppression was associated with the induction of suppressor cells, whereas, no suppressor cell activity could be demonstrated in the suppression of elicitation of DTH by UVB radiation.

UVB has also been shown to suppress DTH to *Mycobacterium bovis* BCG. Exposing mice to a single large dose, or to multiple smaller doses of UVB, followed by sensitization at a distant, non-irradiated site with live BCG, significantly suppressed the induction of DTH. In addition, clearance of the bacteria from the lymphoid organs was impaired following UVB exposure (42, 84). The systemic suppression of DTH appears to associated with the release of suppressive cytokines from UVB-irradiated keratinocytes. Recently we observed that DTH to BCG was suppressed in mice injected with supernatants from UV-irradiated epidermal cells. Furthermore, macrophages isolated from mice injected with the suppressive cytokine or normal cells cultured *in vitro* with supernatants from UVB-irradiated keratinocytes were unable to ingest live BCG (85). Thus, these data suggest that the suppression of DTH, and depressed bacterial clearance seen after UVB exposure results from the release of suppressive cytokines by UVB-irradiated keratinocytes *in vivo*.

Clearly, UVB exposure suppresses the immune response to infectious agents in animal models. While it is impossible to predict with absolute confidence how UVB exposure will affect human immunity to infectious agents, it is important to keep a number of points in mind. First the suppression seen in all cases was systemic in nature. Second, the doses of UVB used in the above mentioned studies were relatively small and well within the range of human exposure (86). Third, as pointed out below, we do know that exposure to UVB radiation can cause systemic alterations in human immunity.

Consequences of UVB exposure on human health

Although much of the experimental work in photoimmunology has employed laboratory animals, there is data from a number studies concerning the effects of UV radiation on human health and human immunity [for an in depth review please see Morison (87)].

Skin Cancer. UVB radiation is the etiologic cause of the majority of non-melanoma skin cancer in humans (88). Is there is a link between the immunosuppressive and carcinogenic effects of UVB radiation in man, similar to what has been obesrved in mice? Data from a number of studies suggest that such a link exists. There is a documented increase in the incidence of skin cancers on the sun exposed sites of immunosuppressed transplant recipients, suggesting a link between immunosuppression, UVB radiation and the induction of skin cancers in humans (89, 90). Second, patients with the genetic disease xeroderma pigmentosum who are unable to repair UV-induced lesions in DNA have an increased number of skin cancers on sun-exposed areas of the body. Morison et al found that contact hypersensitivity was suppressed in these patients, and the magnitude of immunosuppression correlated with the severity of cutaneous disease (91). Third, it appears that susceptibility to the suppressive effects of UVB on CHS is one risk factor for the development of skin cancer in humans. In a study by Yoshikawa et al (92) the ability of biopsy-proven skin cancer patients and normal volunteers to respond to sensitization with a contact allergen was measured. The patients and volunteers were placed into two different categories, UVB-susceptible and UVB-resistant depending upon their ability to mount a CHS reaction following UVB-irradiation. Whereas, 60% of the volunteers were able to generate a vigorous CHS reaction when the contact allergen was applied to UVB-irradiated skin (UVB-resistant), almost all (92%) of the skin cancer patients failed to mount a response (UVB-susceptible). Moreover, 45% of the skin cancer patients remained unresponsive when resensitized with the contact allergen at a distant site, suggesting the induction of tolerance in these patents. Yoshikawa et al conclude that UVB-susceptibility, as they define it (unable to respond to a universally sensitizing dose of DNCB) may be a risk factor for the induction of human skin cancer. Unfortunately, UVB-susceptibility does not appear to be a universal risk factor for skin cancer induction in all patient populations tested. In a subsequent study, Vermeer et al (93) examined the effects of UVB on cutaneous immune reactions in deeply pigmented individuals. Because blacks rarely develop non-melanoma skin cancer the hypothesis that was tested was that melanin protected from the immunosuppressive effect of UVB radiation. They found that UVB radiation depleted Langerhans cells from highly pigmented or Caucasian skin to the same degree. Also UVB-susceptibility existed as a polymorphic trait in black and deeply tanned individuals similar to that seen in normal Caucasian subjects. Vermeer et al conclude that although UVB-susceptibility may function as a risk factor for skin cancer in Caucasians, it does not appear to function similarly in blacks. The authors suggest that since skin cancer is multifactorial in nature, the susceptibility to the suppressive effects of UVB on CHS is only one factor involved in the induction of skin cancer. They suggest that other factors play a role in the induction of skin cancer in deeply pigmented individuals.

Contact allergy Although the suppressive effect of UVB on CHS in mice is well documented, there are only a few studies showing a similar effect in humans. As mentioned above, Yoshikawa et al and Vermeer et al demonstrated the suppressive effect of UVB exposure on contact allergy. Previously, O'Dell et al (94) examined the effect that UVB radiation had on the elicitation of CHS in humans. Volunteers were sensitized with a contact allergen and then the challenge dose was applied to sun-damaged skin. Compared to non-irradiated controls, a depressed CHS reaction was observed when the contact allergen was applied to the UV-irradiated skin. What is it not clear is if this depressed reaction reflects suppressed immunity or decreased absorption of the contact sensitizer through the UV-damaged skin because studies using mice have demonstrated that UVB exposure suppresses the induction but not the elicitation of CHS (19). Hersey and colleagues found that exposing normal volunteers to radiation from a tanning solarium depressed DTH to skin test reagents, induced suppressor cells, altered lymphocyte subsets and depressed natural killer cell activity (95). Similar but less pronounced effects on natural killer cell activity and DTH skin test reactions were noted after exposure to sunlight (96).

Effects of UVB on immunocompetent cells within the epidermis Studies with human materials and human volunteers indicate that UVB exposure can affect the functioning of immunocompetent cells within the epidermis. Human Langerhans cells are sensitive to the deleterious effects of UVB radiation and UVB exposure does suppress Langerhans cells antigen-presenting cell function (97). Cooper and colleagues confirmed this finding and noted that immediately after UVB exposure the antigen-presenting capacity of CD1+, DR+, Birbeck granule positive, epidermal Langerhans cells was depressed (98). Soon after UVB exposure, however, epidermal antigen-presenting cell function increased to values greater than that seen in non-irradiated skin. The enhanced antigen-presenting cell function was not due to the re-appearance of epidermal Langerhans cells, but rather to the appearance of a CD1-, DR+, Birbeck granule negative, OKM1-OKM5+, melanophage (99). UV wavelengths in the UVB region of the spectrum maximally induced the CD1-, DR+ melanophage, with some activity by UVC radiation but no induction following exposure to UVA radiation (100). The function of this cell appears to be the induction of suppressor cells. Human CD4+ T cells can be subdivided into two populations based in the expression of a post-translational modification of CD45 to CD45R. CD45R is expressed on CD4 lymphocytes that provide help for the maturation of CD8+ suppressor cells (the so called suppressor-inducer subset of CD4 cells). CD45R- cells are found in the helper subset of CD4 cells (101, 102). The UV-induced CD1-, DR+, melanophages preferentially activated CD4+, CD45R+, T cells suggesting that these melanophages may be involved in the induction of suppression (103). To test this hypothesis, Baadsgaard and Cooper mixed the CD1-, DR+, epidermal cells with autologous peripheral blood T cells. The cells were cultured for 7 days, after which time the T cells were isolated. The T cells were then added to cultures of pokeweed mitogen-stimulated autologous blood mononuclear cells. T lymphocytes isolated from cultures containing CD1-, DR+, UV-irradiated epidermal melanophages suppressed immunoglobulin production by the mitogen-induced mononuclear cells compared to the levels seen when unstimulated T cells were added to the mononuclear cells, or when T cells from cultures containing non-irradiated epidermal cells were added (104). These findings suggest that UVB exposure induces antigen-presenting cells that preferentially activate suppressor T cells. It is of interest to note that Granstein and colleagues came to a similar conclusion when studying the effect of UVB-irradiation on antigen-presenting cell populations in murine epidermis (105-107).

Although the information concerning the effect of UVB radiation on human immunity is limited a number of conclusions can be drawn. First, the data suggest that there may be a link between the immunosuppressive effects of UVB radiation and the induction of skin cancer in humans. Second, UVB exposure suppresses CHS and DTH in humans. Although the response is polymorphic and not all human volunteers are UVB-susceptible to the same degree, it must be remembered that in mice the effects of UVB radiation vary from strain to strain (28, 30). Finally, UVB irradiation compromises the function of immunocompetent cells in human epidermis and induces an antigen-presenting cell that preferentially activates suppressor T cells.

Conclusions

Although photoimmunology is a relatively new field, during the past 15 years research in this area has been marked by exceptional activity and discovery. The driving force behind this activity was the realization that induction of skin cancer by UVB is associated with immunosuppression. The catalyst for future research will undoubtedly be concern over the increased potential for skin cancer due to the depletion of the ozone layer. The role of UVB radiation in the induction of both melanoma and non-melanoma skin cancers in humans is an area that requires further attention. However, it is also clear that UVB exposure causes immunologic alterations, including systemic suppression of cellular immune reactions. Will the consequence of increased UVB in our environment be an increased susceptibility to infectious disease? Animal studies support this possibility, unfortunately, we know little of the effects of UV radiation on human immunity to infectious agents. However, because the characteristics of the immunosuppression found in humans after UVB exposure are similar to those observed in mice it would appear unlikely that UVB exposure would suppress the response to infectious organisms in mice and not in men.

Like any new area of research photoimmunology has moved from a description of the phenomena, to elucidation of the mechanisms involved in modulation of the immune response by UVB radiation, to studies designed to understand at the molecular level how UVB interacts with the cellular machinery. Hopefully we can apply some of this knowledge to gain a better understanding of how other potential toxic environmental agents interact with the skin and the immune system. We know for instance, that chemical carcinogens and tumor promoters, also interact with the skin and cause systemic immunosuppression (108, 109). Are the mechanisms involved similar to those described over the past years for UVB-induced suppression? If so, perhaps the *in vitro* production of suppressive cytokines by human keratinocytes can serve as a test to screen for immunotoxicity by physical and chemical agents other than UVB.

REFERENCES

1. Blum, H. F. (1959) Carcinogenesis by Ultraviolet Light. Princeton Univ Press, Princeton, NJ.

2. Kripke, M. L. (1974) Antigenicity of murine skin tumors induced by UV light. J. Natl. Cancer Inst. 53:1333.

3. Kripke, M. L. and M. S. Fisher. (1976) Immunologic parameters of ultraviolet carcinogenesis. J. Natl. Cancer Inst. 57:211.

4. Roberts, L. K. (1986) Characterization of a cloned ultraviolet radiation (UV)-induced suppressor t cell line that is capable of inhibiting anti-UV tumor-induced responses. J. Immunol. 136:1908.

5. Fisher, M. S. and M. L. Kripke. (1982) Suppressor T lymphocytes control the development of primary skin cancers in UV-irradiated mice. Science 216:1133.

6. Fisher, M. S. and M. L. Kripke. (1977) Systemic alteration induced in mice by ultraviolet light irradiation and its relationship to ultraviolet carcinogenesis. Proc. Natl. Acad. Sci. USA. 74:1688.

7. Daynes, R. A. and C. W. Spellman. (1977) Evidence for the generation of suppressor cells by UV radiation. Cell. Immunol. 31:182.

8. Ullrich, S. E. and M. L. Kripke. (1984) Mechanisms in the suppression of tumor rejection produced in mice by repeated UV irradiation. J. Immunol. 133:2786.

9. Fisher, M. S. and M. L. Kripke. (1978) Further studies on the tumor-specific suppressor cells induced by ultraviolet radiation. J. Immunol. 121:1139.

10. Norbury, K. C., M. L. Kripke and M. B. Budman. (1977) *In vitro* reactivity of macrophages and lymphocytes from UV-irradiated mice. J. Natl. Cancer Inst. 59:1231.

11. Spellman, C. W., J. G. Woodward and R. A. Daynes. (1977) Modification of immunological potential by ultraviolet radiation. I. Immune status of short-term UV-irradiated mice. Transplantation 24:112.

12. Parrish, J. A., T. B. Fitzpatrick, L. Tanebaum and M. A. Pathak. (1974) Photochemotherapy with oral methoxsalen and long wave ultraviolet light. N. Engl. J. Med. 291:1207.

13. Weissmann, I., C. Hoffman, G. Wagner, G. Plewig and O. Braun-Flaco. (1978) PUVA-therapy for alopecia areata. An investigative study. Arch. Dermatol. Res. 262:333.

14. Ortonne, J. P., J. Thivolet and C. Sannwald. (1978) Oral photochemotherapy in the treatment of lichen planus. Br. J. Dermatol. 99:77.

15. Parrish, J. A., T. B. Fitzpatrick, C. Shea and M. A. Pathak. (1976) Photochemotherapy of vitiligo: use of orally administered psoralen and a high intensity long wave ultraviolet light source. Arch. Dermatol. 112:1531.

16. Gilchrest, B. A., J. A. Parrish, L. Tanebaum, H. A. Heyes and T. B. Fitzpatrick. (1976) Oral methoxsalen photochemotherapy of mycosis fungoides. Cancer 38:683.

17. Edelson, R., C. Berger, F. Gasparro, B. Jegasothy, P. Heald, B. Wintrob, E. Vonderheid, R. Knobler, K. Wolff, G. Plewig, G. McKiernan, Christiansen I, Oster M, Honigsmann H, H. Wilford, E. Kokoschka, T. Rehle, M. Perez, G. Stingl and L. Laroche. (1987) Treatment of cutaneous T-cell lymphoma by extracorporeal photochemotherapy. N. Engl. J. Med. 316:297.

18. Morison, W. L., J. Wimberly, J. A. Parrish and K. J. Bloch. (1985) Abnormal lymphocyte function following long-term PUVA therapy for psoriasis. Br. J. Dermatol. 108:445.

19. Kripke, M. L., W. L. Morison and J. A. Parrish. (1983) Systemic suppression of contact hypersensitivity in mice by psoralen plus UVA radiation (PUVA). J. Invest. Dermatol. 81:87.

20. Streilein, J. W. (1983). Skin-associated lymphoid tissues (SALT): Origins and functions. J. Invest. Dermatol. 80:12s.

21. Toews, G. B., P. R. Bergstresser and J. W. Streilein. (1980) Epidermal Langerhans cell density determines whether contact hypersensitivity or unresponsiveness follows skin painting with DNFB. J. Immunol. 124:445.

22. Noonan, F. P., E. C. De Fabo and M. L. Kripke. (1981) Suppression of contact hypersensitivity by ultraviolet radiation: an experimental model. Springer Semin. Immunopathol. 4:293.

23. Elmets, C. A., P. R. Bergstresser, R. E. Tigelaar, P. J. Wood and J. W. Streilein. (1983) Analysis of the mechanism of unresponsiveness produced by haptens painted on skin to low dose UV radiation. J. Exp. Med. 158:781.

24. Cruz, P. D., J. Nixon-Fulton, R. E. Tigelaar and P. R. Bergstresser. (1989) Disparate effects of *in vitro* UVB irradiation in intravenous immunization with purified epidermal cell subpopulations for the induction of CHS. J. Invest. Dermatol. 92:160.

25. Simon, J. C., P. C. Cruz, P. R. Bergstresser and R. E. Tigelaar. (1990) Low dose ultraviolet B-irradiated Langerhans cells preferentially activate CD4+ cells of the T helper 2 subset. J. Immunol. 145:2087.

25. Cherwinski, H., J. Schumacher, K. Brown and T. Mosmann. (1987) Two types of mouse helper T clones. III. Further differences in lymphokine synthesis between Th1 and Th2 clones. J. Exp. Med. 166:1229.

27. Simon, J. C., R. E. Tigelaar, P. R. Bergstresser, D. Edelbaum and P. D. Cruz. (1991) Ultraviolet B radiation converts Langerhans Cells from immunogenic to tolerogenic antigen-presenting cells: Induction of specific clonal anergy in CD4+ T helper 1 cells. J. Immunol. 146:485.

28. Yoshikawa, T. and J. W. Streilein. (1990) Tumor necrosis factor-alpha and ultraviolet light have similar effects on contact hypersensitivity in mice. Regional Immunol. 3:139.

29. Oxholm, A., P. Oxholm, B. Staberg and K. Bendtzen. (1988) Immunohistological detection of IL-1-like and TNF in human epidermis before and after UVB-irradiation. Br. J. Dermatol. 118:369.

30. Yoshikawa, T. and J. W. Streilein. (1990) Genetic basis of the effects of ultraviolet B light on cutaneous immunity. Evidence that polymorphism at the Tnfa and Lps loci governs susceptibility. Immunogenetics 32:298.

31. Alcalay, J., S. E. Ullrich and M. L. Kripke. (1989) Local suppression of contact hypersensitivity in mice by a monofunctional psoralen plus UVA radiation. Photochem. Photobiol. 50:217.

32. Horio, T. and H. Okamoto. (1982) The mechanisms of inhibitory effect of 8-methoxypsoralen and longwave ultraviolet light on experimental contact sensitization. J. Invest. Dermatol. 78:402.

33. Jessup, J. M., N. Hanna, E. Palaszynski and M. L. Kripke. (1978) Mechanisms of depressed reactivity to dinitrochlorobenzene and ultraviolet-induced tumors during ultraviolet carcinogenesis in BALB/c mice. Cell. Immunol. 38:105.

34. Noonan, F. P., E. C. De Fabo and M. L. Kripke. (1981) Suppression of contact hypersensitivity and its relationship to UV-induced suppression of tumor immunity. Photochem. Photobiol. 34:683.

35. Morison, W. L., C. Bucana, and M. L. Kripke. (1984) Systemic suppression of contact hypersensitivity in mice is unrelated to the UVB-induced alterations in the morphology and number of Langerhans cells. Immunology 52:299.

36. Greene, M. I., M. S. Sy, M. L. Kripke and B. Benacerraf. (1979) Impairment of antigen-presenting cell function by UV radiation. Proc. Natl. Acad. Sci. USA. 76:6591.

37. Noonan, F. P., M. L. Kripke, G. M. Pedersen and M. I. Greene. (1981) Suppression of contact hypersensitivity by UV radiation is associated with defective antigen presentation. Immunology 43:527.

38. Noonan, F. P. and E. C. De Fabo. (1990) Dose response curves for local and systemic immunosuppression are identical Photochem. Photobiol. 52:801.

39. Ullrich, S. E., E. Azizi and M. L. Kripke. (1986) Suppression of the induction of delayed hypersensitivity reactions in mice by a single exposure to UV radiation. Photochem Photobiol. 43:633.

40. Howie, S. E. M., M. Norval and J. Maingay. (1986) Exposure to low dose UVB light suppresses delayed type hypersensitivity to herpes simplex virus in mice by suppressor cell induction. J. Invest. Dermatol. 86:125.

41. Denkins, Y., I. J. Fidler and M. L. Kripke. (1989) Exposure of mice to UVB radiation suppresses delayed hypersensitivity to *Candida albicans*. Photochem. Photobiol. 49:615.

42. Jeevan, A. and M. L. Kripke. (1989) Effect of a single exposure to Ultraviolet radiation on *Mycobacterium bovis* Bacillus Calmette-Guerin infection in mice. J. Immunol. 143:2837.

43. Giannini, M. S. H. (1986) Suppression of pathogenesis in cutaneous Leishmaniasis by UV irradiation. Infect. Immun. 51:838.

44. Ullrich, S. E., E. Azizi and M. L. Kripke. (1986) Suppression of the induction of delayed hypersensitivity reactions in mice by a single exposure to UV radiation. Photochem Photobiol. 43:633.

45. Ullrich, S. E. (1985) Suppression of lymphoproliferation by hapten-specific suppressor T lymphocytes from mice exposed to UV radiation. Immunology 54:343.

46. Ullrich, S. E., G. K. Yee and M. L. Kripke. (1986) Suppressor lymphocytes induced by epicutaneous sensitization of UV-irradiated mice control multiple immunological pathways. Immunology 58:185.

47. Ullrich, S. E. (1987) The effect of ultraviolet radiation-induced suppressor cells on T cell activity. Immunology 60:353.

48. Romerdahl, C. A. and M. L. Kripke. (1986) Regulation of the immune response against UV-induced skin cancers: Specificity of helper cells and their susceptibility to UV-induced suppressor cells. J. Immunol. 137:3031.

49. Romerdahl, C. A. and M. L. Kripke. (1988) Role of helper T-lymphocytes in rejection of UV-induced murine skin cancers. Cancer Res. 48:2325.

50. Steele, J. K., H. Kawaski, V. K. Kuchroo, M. Minami, J. G. Levy and M. E. Dorf. (1987) A monoclonal antibody raised to tumors-specific T cell-derived suppressor factors also recognizes T suppressor inducer factors of the 4-Hydroxy-3-Nitrophenyl acetyl hapten suppressor network. J. Immunol. 139:2629.

51. Yee, G. K., J. G. Levy, M. L. Kripke and S. E. Ullrich. (1990) The role of suppressor factors in the regulation of the immune response by UV-induced suppressor T lymphocytes. III. Isolation of a suppressor factor with the B16G monoclonal antibody. Cell. Immunol. 126:255.

52. Swartz, R. P. (1984) Role of UVB-induced serum factors in suppression of contact hypersensitivity in mice. J. Invest. Dermatol. 83:305.

53. Harriott-Smith, T. G. and W. J. Halliday. (1986) Circulating suppressor factors in mice subjected to UV irradiation and contact hypersensitivity. Immunology 57:207.

54. De Fabo, E. C. and F. P. Noonan. (1983) Mechanism of immune suppression by ultraviolet irradiation *in vivo*. I. Evidence for the existence of a unique photoreceptor in skin and its role in photoimmunology. J. Exp. Med. 157:84.

55. Ross, J. A., S. E. M. Howie, N. M., J. Maingay and T. J. Simpson. (1986) Ultraviolet-irradiated urocanic acid suppresses delayed type hypersensitivity to herpes simplex virus in mice. J. Invest. Dermatol. 87:630.

56. Howie, S. E. M., M. Norval, J. Maingay and J. A. Ross. (1986) Two phenotypically distinct T cells (Lyt 1+2- and Lyt 1-2+) are involved in ultraviolet-B light induced suppression of the efferent DTH response to HSV-1 *in vivo*. Immunology 58:653.

57. Ross, J. A., S. E. M. Howie, M. Norval and J. Maingay. 1988. Systemic administration of urocanic acid generates suppression of the delayed type hypersensitivity response to herpes simplex virus in a murine model of infection. Photodermatology 5:9.

58. Noonan, F. P., E. C. De Fabo and H. Morrison. (1988) Cis-urocanic acid, a product formed by UVB irradiation of the skin, initiates an antigen presentation defect in splenic cells *in vivo*. J. Invest. Dermatol. 90:92.

59. Morison, W. L. and S. P. Kelly. (1986) Urocanic acid may not be the photoreceptor of contact hypersensitivity. Photodermatology 3:98.

60. Applegate, L. A., R. D. Ley, J. Alcalay and M. L. Kripke. (1989) Identification of the molecular target for the suppression of contact hypersensitivity by UV radiation. J. Exp. Med. 170:1117.

61. Sauder, D. N. (1989) Interleukin-1. Arch. Dermatol. 125:679.

62. Gahring, L. C., M. Baltz, M. B. Pepys and R. A. Daynes. (1984) The effect of UV radiation of the production of ETAF/IL-1 *in vivo* and *in vitro*. Proc. Natl. Acad. Sci. USA. 81:1198.

63. Robertson, B., L. Gahring, R. Newton and R. A. Daynes. (1987) *In vivo* administration of IL-1 to normal mice decreases their capacity to elicit contact hyper-sensitivity responses: Prostaglandins are involved in this modification of the immune response. J. Invest. Dermatol. 88:380.

64. Robertson, B., K. Dostal and R. A. Daynes. (1988) Neuropeptide regulation of inflammatory and immunologic responses. The capacity of α-melanocyte-stimulating hormone to inhibit tumor necrosis factor and IL-1 inducable biological responses. J. Immunol. 140:4300.

65. Evertt, M. A., E. Yeargers, R. M. Sayre and R. L. Olson. (1966) Penetration of epidermis by ultraviolet rays. Photochem. Photobiol. 5:533.

66. Schwarz, T., A. Urbanska, F. Gschnait and T. A. Luger. (1986) Inhibition of the induction of contact hypersensitivity by a UV-mediated epidermal cytokine. J. Invest. Dermatol. 87:289.

67. Schwarz, T., A. Urbanska, F. Gschnait and T. A. Luger. (1987) UV-irradiated epidermal cells produce a specific inhibitor of IL-1 activity. J. Immunol. 138:1457.

68. Schwarz, T. S., A. Urbanski, R. Kirnbauer, A. Kock, F. Gschnait and T. A. Luger. (1988) Detection of a specific inhibitor of Interleukin-1 in sera of UVB-treated mice. J. Invest. Dermatol. 91:536.

69. Krutmann, J., T. Schwarz, R. Krinbauer, A. Urbanska and T. A. Luger. (1990) Epidermal cell-contra-interleukin 1 inhibits human accessory cell function by specifically blocking interleukin 1 activity. Photochem. Photobiol. 52:738.

70. Ullrich, S. E. (1986) Suppression of the immune response to allogeneic histocompatibility antigen by a single exposure to UV radiation. Transplantation 42:287.

71. Ullrich, S. E. and M. J. Magee. (1988) Specific suppression of allograft rejection after treatment of recipient mice with UV radiation and allogeneic spleen cells. Transplantation 46:115.

72. Magee, M. J., M. L. Kripke and S. E. Ullrich. (1989) Suppression of the elicitation of the immune response to alloantigen by ultraviolet radiation. Transplantation 47:1008.

73. Magee, M. J., M. L. Kripke and S. E. Ullrich. (1989) Inhibition of the immune response to alloantigen in the rat by exposure to ultraviolet radiation. Photochem. Photobiol. 50:193.

74. Ullrich, S. E., B. W. McIntyre and J. M. Rivas. (1990) Suppression of the immune response to alloantigen by factors released from ultraviolet-irradiated keratinocytes. J. Immunol. 145:489.

75. Kim, T.-Y., M. L. Kripke and S. E. Ullrich. (1990) Immunosuppression by factors released from UV-irradiated epidermal cells: selective effects on the generation of contact and delayed hypersensitivity after exposure to UVA or UVB radiation. J. Invest. Dermatol. 94:26.

76. Mosmann, T. R. (1991) Regulation of Immune responses by T cells with different cytokine secretion phenotypes: Role of a new cytokine, cytokine synthesis inhibitory factor (IL10). Int. Arch. Allergy and Appl. Immunol. 94:110.

77. Fiorentino, D. F., A. Zlotnik, P. Viera, T. R. Mosmann, M. Howard, K. W. Moore and A. O'Garra. (1991). IL-10 acts on the antigen-presenting cell to inhibit cytokine production by Th1 cells. J. Immunol. 146:3444.

78. Spruance, S. (1985) Pathogenesis of Herpes Simplex labialis: experimental induction of lesions with UV light. J. Clin. Microbiol. 22:366.

79. Yasumoto, S., Y. Hayashi and L. Aurelian. (1987) Immunity to herpes simplex virus type 2: suppression of virus induced immune responses in ultraviolet B irradiated mice. J. Immunol. 139:2788.

80. Hayashi, Y. and L. Aurelian. (1986) Immunity to Herpes Simplex Virus type 2: viral antigen-presenting capacity of epidermal cells and its impairment by ultraviolet irradiation. J. Immunol. 136:1087.

81. Aurelian, L., S. Yasumoto and C. Smith. (1988) Antigen specific immune suppressor factor in Herpes Simplex type 2 infections of UVB-irradiated mice. Am. Soc. Micro. 62:2520.

82. Howie, S. E. M., M. Norval, J. Maingay and J. A. Ross. (1987) *In vivo* modulation of antigen presentation generates Ts rather than Tdth in HSV-1 infection. Immunology 60:419.

83. Howie, S. E. M., M. Norval and J. P. Maingay. (1986) Alterations in epidermal handling of HSV-1 antigens *in vitro* induced by *in vivo* exposure to UV-B light. Immunology 57:225.

84. Jeevan, A. and M. L. Kripke. (1990) Alteration of the immune response to *Mycobacterium bovis* BCG in mice exposed chronically to low dose UV radiation. Cell. Immunol. 130:32.

85. Jeevan, A., S. E. Ullrich, V. V. Dizon and M. L. Kripke. (1992) Supernatants from UV-irradiated keratinocytes decrease the resistance and delayed type hypersensitivity response to *Mycobacterium bovis* BCG in mice and impair the phagocytic ability of macrophages. Photodermatology, Photoimmunology & Photomedicine *in press*.

86. Giannini, S. H. (1992) Effects of Ultraviolet B irradiation on cutaneous Leishmaniasis. Parasitology Today 8:44.

87. Morison, W. L. (1989) Effects of ultraviolet radiation on the immune system in humans. Photochem. Photobiol. 50:515.

88. Urbach, F. (1978) Evidence and epidemiology of UV-induced carcinogenesis in man. Natl. Cancer Inst. Monogr. 50:5.

89. Penn, I. (1984) Depressed immunity and skin cancer. Immunology Today 5:291.

90. Penn, I. (1987) Cancers following cyclosporine therapy. Transplantation 43:32

91. Morison, W. L., C. Bucana, N. Hashem, M. L. Kripke, E. Cleaver and J. L. German. (1985) Impaired immune functions in patients with xeroderma pigmentosum. Cancer Res. 45:3229.

92. Yoshikawa, T., V. Rae, W. Bruins-Slot, J. W. vand-den-Berg, J. R. Taylor and J. W. Streilein. (1990) Susceptibility to effects of UVB radiation on induction of contact hypersensitivity as a risk factor for skin cancer in humans. J. Invest. Dermatol. 95:530.

93. Vermeer, M., G. J. Schmieder, T. Yoshikawa, J.-W. van-den Berg, M. Metzman, S. Taylor and J. W. Streilein. (1991) Effects of ultraviolet B light on cutaneous immune responses of humans with deeply pigmented skin. J. Invest. Dermatol. 97:729.

94. O'Dell, B. L., R. T. Jessen, L. E. Beeker, R. T. Jackson and E. D. Smith. (1980) Diminished immune response in sun-damaged skin. Arch. Dermatol. 116:559.

95. Hersey, P., G. Haran, E. Hansic and A. Edwards. (1983) Alteration of T cell subsets and induction of suppressor T cell activity in normal subjects after exposure to sunlight. J. Immunol. 131:171.

96. Hersey, P., E. Hansic, A. Edwards, B. M., G. Haran and W. H. McCarthy. (1983) Immunological effects of solarium exposure. The Lancet 1:545.

97. Aberer, W., G. Stingl, L. A. Stingl-Gazze and K. Wolff. (1982) Langerhans cells as stimulator cells in the immune primary epidermal cell lymphocyte reaction: Alteration by UVB irradiation. J. Invest. Dermatol. 79:129.

98. Cooper, K. D., P. Fox, G. R. Neises and S. I. Katz. (1985) Effects of UVR on human epidermal cell alloantigen presentation: initial depression of Langerhans cell dependent function is followed by the appearance of T6-DR+ cells that enhance epidermal alloantigen presentation. J. Immunol. 134:129.

99. Cooper, K. D., G. R. Neises and S. I. Katz. (1986) Antigen-presenting OKM5+ melanophages appear in human epidermis after ultraviolet radiation. J. Invest. Dermatol. 86:363.

100. Baadsgaard, O., K. D. Cooper, S. Lisby, H. C. Wulf and G. L. Wantzin. (1987) UVB and UVC, but not UVA, induce the appearance of T6-DR+ antigen-presenting cells in human epidermis. J. Invest. Dermatol. 89:113.

101. Morimoto, C., N. L. Letvin, J. A. Distaso, W. R. Aldrich and S. F. Schlossman. (1985) The isolation and characterization of human suppressor inducer T cell subset. J. Immunol. 134:1508.

102. Takeuchi, T., S. F. Schlossman and C. Morimoto. (1987) The 2H4 molecule but not T3-receptor complex is involved in suppressor inducer signals in the AMLR system. Cell Immunol. 107:107.

103. Baadsgaard, O., D. A. Fox and K. D. Cooper. (1988) Human epidermal cells from ultraviolet light-exposed skin preferentially activate autoreactive CD4+2H4+ suppressor-inducer lymphocytes and CD8+ suppressor/cytotoxic lymphocytes. J. Immunol. 140:1783.

104. Baadsgaard, O., B. Salvo, A. Mannie, B. Dass, D. Fox and K. C. Cooper. (1990) *In vivo* ultraviolet-exposed human epidermal cells activate T suppressor cell pathways that involve CD4+CD45RA+ suppressor-inducer T cells. J. Immunol. 145:2854.

105. Granstein, R. D., M. Askari, D. Whitaker and G. F. Murphy. (1987) Epidermal cells in the activation of suppressor lymphocytes: further characterization. J. Immunol. 138:4055.

106. Granstein, R. D. (1985) Epidermal I-J-bearing cells are responsible for transferable suppressor cell generation after immunization of mice with ultraviolet radiation-treated epidermal cells. J. Invest. Dermatol. 84:206.

107. Granstein, R. D., A. Lowy and M. I. Greene. (1984) Epidermal antigen-presenting cells in activation of suppression: identification of a new functional type of UV-resistant epidermal cell. J. Immunol. 132:563.

108. Halliday, G. M. and H. K. Muller. (1987) Sensitization through carcinogen-induced Langerhans cell-deficient skin activates specific long-lived suppressor cells for both cellular and humoral immunity. Cell. Immunol. 109:206.

109. Kodari, E., A. Pavone and J. J. Reiners. (1991) Induction of suppressor T cells and inhibition of contact hypersensitivity in mice by TPA and its analogs. J. Invest. Dermatol. 96:864.

B3

The Epidermal Response to Retinoic Acid in Cell Culture and *In Vivo*

DEAN S. ROSENTHAL,[1] CHRISTOPHER E.M. GRIFFITHS,[2]
JOHN J. VOORHEES,[2] and STUART H. YUSPA[3]

[1]*Department of Biochemistry and Molecular Biology*
Georgetown University School of Medicine, Silver Spring, MD 20906

[2]*Department of Dermatology*
University of Michigan Medical Center, Ann Arbor, MI 48109

[3]*Laboratory of Cellular Carcinogenesis and Tumor Promotion*
National Cancer Institute, Bethesda, MD 20892

Abstract

A number of studies have shown that vitamin A and its derivatives (retinoids) have a profound influence on the coordinated program of gene expression in cultured keratinocytes. Removal of retinoids from the culture medium induces morphological changes, cross-linking of the cornified envelope by epidermal transglutaminase, and the expression of markers associated with terminal differentiation, including the keratin pair K1/K10. Conversely, when retinoids are added to the medium, these events associated with terminal differentiation are suppressed. Retinoid excess has also been shown to induce the basal cell-specific keratin pair K5/K14, the hyperproliferation-specific pair K6/K16, and the expression of two keratins not normally associated with epidermal differentiation, keratins K13 and K19. To examine the similarities between the in vitro and in vivo models, skin biopsies derived from volunteers treated topically with 0.1% all-trans retinoic acid nightly for 4 months or under occlusion for 4 days, were examined histologically and immunocytochemically for markers of differentiation. Our results indicate that for all markers except loricrin, the major component of the cornified envelope, the changes induced by acute and chronic treatment were similar. Furthermore, many of the changes induced in vivo differ from those in cultured cells, suggesting that alterations in the dermis or other skin components may play an important role in the epidermal response to retinoic acid

Introduction

Epidermal differentiation comprises a number of morphological and biochemical changes resulting in a well organized stratified squamous epithelium. In normal skin, proliferation is restricted to a single layer of basal cells; these cells cease to divide as they lose contact with the basement membrane and enter the spinous layer. The destructive phase becomes apparent in the granular layer, where keratinocytes begin to lose their nuclei and cytoplasmic organelles. In the outermost layers, termed the stratum corneum, the terminally differentiated epidermal cells or "squames" consist almost entirely of bundles of keratins within the cross-linked envelopes. As squames are sloughed from the skin, new cells generated from the basal layer replenish the supply. The differentiation program of keratinocytes is the result of a tightly regulated program of gene expression, and each cell layer within the epidermis can be characterized by the expression of a specific set of proteins. The most abundant proteins synthesized during differentiation are the keratins, a family of proteins encoded by at least 20 different genes. Keratins can be grouped into two classes based upon size, isoelectric point, and sequence homology. As in all epithelial cells, type I and type II keratins are expressed as specific pairs within epidermis. In mammalian basal cells the keratin pair K5/K14 comprises the bulk of the intermediate filament network (1), whereas the K1/K10 pair forms the predominant filaments of the suprabasal layers (1-3). Other non-keratin proteins associated with the terminal stages of epidermal differentiation include filaggrin, which promotes keratin filament aggregation (4), as well proteins involved in the formation of the cornified envelope (5): epidermal transglutaminase (6), as well as its substrates, loricrin (7) and involucrin (8) are all expressed in the most superficial layers of the epidermis.

The cell culture model

Factors that regulate the morphological and biochemical changes associated with differentiation have been defined primarily in the cell culture model. A number of these *in vitro* studies have implicated both calcium and retinoids as important regulators of epidermal differentiation. In cultured keratinocytes, the calcium concentration in the cell culture medium can select for either a basal or suprabasal cell phenotype. In low calcium medium (<0.05 mM), mouse keratinocytes proliferate rapidly, express K5 and K14, and do not cornify, while higher calcium (0.10 mM) induces squamous differentiation, including the induction of keratins K1 and K10, filaggrin, and loricrin (9). The strict calcium dependence of marker expression is demonstrated in experiments in which primary mouse epidermal cells were cultured in low calcium and then switched to either .05, 0.12 or 1.4 mM calcium. Western analysis shows that the four epidermal differentiation-specific markers: K1, K10 loricrin, and filaggrin are all induced maximally in 0.12 mM calcium (9). Retinoids also clearly play an important role in the coordinated program of gene expression. In cultured mouse and human keratinocytes, retinoids suppress a variety of morphological and biochemical properties of differentiation. The in vitro effects of retinoids include suppression of markers of differentiation (10-13), including the keratin K1/K10 pair, loricrin, filaggrin, and epidermal transglutaminase; and the induction of markers not normally associated with keratinocytes, such as keratins 13 and 19, which are expressed in internal epithelia (10,14,15). Physiological markers, such as rates of proliferation and desquamation, are also altered by retinoids. An example of marker suppression by retinoids can be shown at the level of individual cells, using monospecific antibody to K1. In high calcium, many mature squames express K1. When keratinocytes are pre-incubated with retinoic acid, the endogenous gene is almost completely suppressed by 10^{-6} M retinoic acid, except for rare positive cells.

Independent pathways for regulation of keratin K1 by calcium and retinoids

We took two approaches to examine the role of retinoids in epidermal differentiation. The first was to use primary keratinocytes derived from mice containing the retinoid-sensitive human keratin 1 transgene to examine the mechanism for retinoid suppression. Transgenic mice containing the coding sequence, along with 5' and 3' flanking sequences in the 11 kb human genomic fragment were used to establish lines of transgenic mice. These mice expressed both mouse and human keratin 1 specifically in the epidermis. Epidermal cells were derived from these mice and induced to differentiate by elevated calcium. Western analysis using species-specific antibodies to the endogenous mouse K1, or the transgenic human K1, showed a strong calcium dependence for induction of human and mouse K1 (16). This indicated that a calcium-responsive genetic element was located within the genomic fragment used to establish the transgenic mice. When the transgenic cells were pre-incubated with retinoic acid prior to a calcium shift, the endogenous gene is completely suppressed by 10^{-8} M retinoic acid. However, the human gene was not suppressed by retinoic acid pretreatment, suggesting that the DNA element that mediates retinoid suppression was not within the human K1 genomic fragment. These results suggested that K1 and perhaps all epidermal differentiation-specific genes are controlled by both positive and negative regulatory elements, which can function independently. The positive element is induced by calcium, while the negative element, missing from the transgene, is regulated by retinoids. The model also postulates that when the positive and negative elements are both present, retinoids exert a dominant suppressive effect on gene expression.

The in vivo response to topical retinoic acid

The second approach we took was to test this model in vivo, since little was known about the applicability of these observations in cell culture to the response of human skin to topical retinoids (17,18). We obtained 10 sets of skin punch biopsies that were derived from volunteers treated with a single topical application of vehicle with or without 0.1% RA cream under a plastic wrap occlusion for 4 days. Histologic examination of all RA-treated skin showed epidermal thickening, due to an increased number of cell layers, as well as an increase in the size of some of the individual cells. Based on epidermal thickness, patients could be categorized as weak or strong responders. Strong responders also demonstrated significant granular layer thickening. Immunofluorescent staining with K1- specific antibody shows that the overall pattern of staining is the same in control and RA-treated epidermis. This is therefore in sharp contrast to the model in cell culture in which K1 is completely suppressed by retinoids. Using antibodies to K1 and K10, coexpression of K1 and K10 was observed in all suprabasal layers in both Retin-A and control epidermis of all 10 individuals. This is also in contrast with the situation in vitro, in which K10 is suppressed by retinoids.

To test whether a longer treatment period was necessary to suppress markers of differentiation in vivo, we obtained samples derived from 25 volunteers treated nightly with 0.1% retinoic acid for 4 months. H and E staining showed that these patients also exhibited epidermal thickening, and fell into weak and strong responder groups. However, all 25 individuals in the 4 month treatment group showed the same pattern of expression of K1 in the suprabasal layers, with no noticeable suppression. Furthermore, in situ hybridization revealed that for two individuals examined, there was no difference in K1 between control and treatment groups at the RNA level. Likewise, K10 was not suppressed in any of the 25 individuals. We then examined late markers of differentiation to see if these genes were suppressed by retinoic acid. Both involucrin and filaggrin are expressed primarily in the granular in control epidermis. In cell culture, filaggrin is suppressed at both the pre- and posttranslational levels (11). On the other hand, filaggrin is expressed in more layers in retinoic acid treated skin, as is involucrin. We obtained the same results for the 4 month and 4 day treatment group. In normal skin, transglutaminase is expressed in the cell membranes of the granular layer. However, in the 4 month RA-treated epidermis, expression is observed precociously. The response after 4 days was the same. Enzyme activity was also higher in RA-treated epidermis than controls (19). Again, this is the opposite of the in vitro system in which epidermal transglutaminase levels are suppressed by retinoic acid (19).

One marker that behaved similarly in vivo and the cell culture model, was loricrin, the major component of the cornified envelope. In control epidermis, loricrin is expressed in a contiguous plane in the granular layer. In the 4 day treatment group, loricrin was suppressed. However, in the 4 month treatment group, loricrin expression was actually enhanced.

Another marker that showed a similar response in vitro and in vivo is keratin K13. K13 is normally expressed only in internal stratified epithelia, such as esophagus, and in squamous cell carcinomas, but not in normal epidermis or cultured keratinocytes, except in retinoid excess. K13 was induced in vivo in individuals in both the 4 day and the 4 month treatment groups. Expression was patchy and limited to the suprabasal layers as it is in internal stratified epithelia.

We postulated that some of the observed changes might be due to a state of hyperproliferation induced by retinoids. An increased number of mitotic figures in the basal layer suggested that this was the case. We therefore examined the distribution of keratin K6 which is normally confined to the outer root sheath of the hair follicle, and only expressed in interfollicular epidermis under hyperproliferative conditions, such as wound healing and neoplasia (20,21). In control epidermis, K6 is confined to the hair follicle. However, K6 is induced in the interfollicular epidermis in most of the strong responders from both the chronic and acute treatment groups. In the acute treatment group, expression was in most of the suprabasal cells, while in the chronic treatment group expression is patchy. We are currently examining which of the observed retinoid-induced changes in marker expression can also be induced by SDS, another agent that induces hyperplasia.

In summary, only two of these changes: suppression of loricrin in the acute treatment group, and the induction of K13 in both acute and chronic treatment groups were predicted from the cell culture model. The other changes were dissimilar or opposite to those observed in vitro, including expanded expression of epidermal transglutaminase, involucrin, filaggrin, and loricrin, and the lack of suppression of K1 and K10.

Conclusions

We have found that in cultured keratinocytes, retinoids and calcium act through independent pathways to control expression of keratin 1. In the presence of both negative and positive DNA response elements, retinoids exert a dominant suppressive effect on markers of differentiation. Most of the retinoic acid-induced changes in marker expression in the cell culture model are not observed in vivo following 4 day or 4 month treatment of human skin with retinoic acid.

The differential effects of RA on marker expression in vivo and in culture may ultimately stem from the interaction of keratinocytes with a vast network of other epidermal and dermal components, and some degree of caution should be exercised when attempting to predict the in vivo response to RA by extrapolation of results from cell culture experiments.

References

1. WOODCOCK-MITCHELL, J., EICHNER, R., NELSON, W.G., ET AL. (1982), Immunolocalization of keratin polypeptides in human epidermis using monoclonal antibodies. J. Cell Biol. 95:580.

2. ROOP, D.R., HAWLEY-NELSON, P. CHENG, C.K., ET AL. (1983), Keratin gene expression in mouse epidermis and cultured epidermal cells. Proc. Natl. Acad. Sci. USA 80:716.

3. SCHWEIZER, J., KINJO, M., FURSTENBERGER, G., ET AL. (1984), Sequential expression of mRNA-encoded keratin sets in neonatal mouse epidermis: basal cells with properties of terminally differentiating cells. Cell 37:159.

4. DALE, B.A., HOLBROOK, K.A., and STEINERT, P.M. (1978), Assembly of stratum corneum basic protein and keratin filaments in macrofibrils. Nature 276:729.

5. RICE, R.H., and GREEN, H. (1977), The cornified envelope of terminally differentiated human epidermal keratinocytes consists of cross-linked protein. Cell 11:417.

6. THACHER, S.M., and RICE, R.H. (1985), Keratinocyte-specific transglutaminase of cultured human epidermal cells: relation to cross-linked envelope formation and terminal differentiation. Cell 40: 685.

7. MEHREL, T., HOHL, D., ROTHNAGEL, J.A., ET AL. (1990), Identification of a major keratinocyte cell envelope protein, loricrin. Cell 61: 1103.

8. WATT, F.M. (1983), Involucrin and other markers of keratinocyte terminal differentiation. J. Invest. Dermatol. 81: 100S.

9. YUSPA, S.H., KILKENNY, A.E., STEINERT, P.M., and ROOP, D.R. (1989). Expression of murine epidermal differentiation markers is tightly regulated by restricted extracellular calcium concentrations in vitro. J. Cell Biol. 109: 1207.

10. FUCHS, E., and GREEN H. (1981), Regulation of terminal differentiation of cultured human keratinocytes by vitamin A. Cell 25: 617.

11. ASSELINEAU, D., DALE, B.A., and BERNARD, B. (1990), Filaggrin production by cultured human epidermal keratinocytes and its regulation by retinoic acid. Differentiation 45: 221.

12. HOHL, D., LICHTI, U., BREITKREUTZ, D., STEINERT, P.M., and ROOP, D.R. (1991), Transcription of the human loricrin gene in vitro is induced by calcium and cell density and suppressed by retinoic acid. J. Invest. Dermatol. 96: 414.

13. MICHEL, S., REICHERT, U., ISNARD, J.L., SHROOT, B., and SCHMIDT, R. (1989), Retinoic acid controls expression of epidermal transglutaminase at the pre-translational level. FEBS letters 258: 35.

14. ECKERT, R.L., and GREEN, H. (1984), Cloning of cDNAs specifying vitamin-A-responsive human keratins. Proc. Natl. Acad. Sci. USA 88: 4582.

15. KOPAN, R., TRASKA, G., and FUCHS, E. (1987), Retinoids as important regulators of terminal differentiation: examining keratin expression in individual epidermal cells at various stages of keratinization. J. Cell Biol. 105: 427.

16. ROSENTHAL, D.S., STEINERT, P.M., CHUNG, S., ET AL. (1991), a human epidermal differentiation-specific keratin gene is regulated by calcium but not negative modulators of differentiation in transgenic mouse keratinocytes. Cell Growth and Differentiation 2: 107.

17. ROSENTHAL, D.S., ROOP, D.R., HUFF, C.A., ET AL. (1990), Changes in photo-aged human skin following topical application of all-trans retinoic acid. J. Invest. Dermatol. 95: 510.

18. ROSENTHAL, D.S., GRIFFITHS, C.E.M., YUSPA, ET AL. (1992), Acute or chronic topical retinoic acid treatment of human skin in vivo alters the expression of epidermal transglutaminase, loricrin, involucrin, filaggrin, and keratins 6 and 13 but not keratins 1, 10, and 14. J.Invest. Dermatol. 95:510.

19. GRIFFITHS, C.E.M., ROSENTHAL, D.S., REDDY, A., ET AL. (1992), Short-term retinoic acid treatment increases in vivo, but decreases in vitro, epidermal transglutaminase K enzyme activity and immunoreactivity. J.Invest. Dermatol. In press.

20. MOLL, R., FRANKE, W.W., SCHILLER, D.L., ET AL. (1982), The catalog of human cytokeratins: patterns of expression in normal epithelia, tumors and cultured cells. Cell 31: 11.

21. STARK, H.J., BREITKREUTZ, D., LIMAT, A., ET AL. (1987), Keratins of the human hair follicle: "hyperproliferative" keratins consistently expressed in outer root sheath cells in vivo and in vitro. Differentiation 35: 236.

C. Development of New Biological Components for Toxicity Testing Systems

C1

Immortalization of Cells

HARRIET C. ISOM and JIAN-MING HU

Department of Microbiology and Immunology
The Milton S. Hershey Medical Center
The Pennsylvania State University
College of Medicine
500 University Drive
Hershey, PA 17033

ABSTRACT

Rat hepatocytes were immortalized with the goal of generating cell lines that maintain specific properties of normal hepatocytes in particular liver-like levels of albumin gene expression. Nonreplicating primary rat hepatocytes maintained on a rat tail collagen coated dish were transfected with recombinant DNA containing the simian virus 40 (SV40) genome or the adenovirus E1A and E1B genes. At 4 to 12 weeks post transfection, colonies containing replicating epithelial cells were observed. Depending upon the culture medium, the cell colonies arose amidst a background of dying cells or a layer of viable nonreplicating hepatocytes. Albumin expressing cell lines were obtained when immortalization was mediated by SV40 DNA but not when immortalization was mediated by adenovirus DNA. The ability to generate stable immortalized cell lines that maintained differentiation required multiple rounds of selection of high albumin producing colonies. The SV40-immortalized hepatocyte cell lines established grow in a chemically defined medium in the absence of serum or epidermal growth factor (EGF) and on tissue culture dishes in the absence of extracellular matrix. We have used the SV40-immortalized hepatocyte cell lines to study regulation of expression of albumin and acute phase genes. The SV40-immortalized hepatocyte cell lines can be transiently transfected and have been used to examine expression of regulatory DNA sequences for liver-specific genes including the Hepatitis B Virus (HBV) X gene, the albumin promoter and the albumin enhancer. It is also possible to transfect SV40-immortalized hepatocyte cell lines with the neomycin resistance gene and an exogenous gene of choice, select in the presence of G418 and generate new cell lines expressing the exogenous gene. Using this procedure, we have introduced the activated c-Ha-*ras* gene into SV40-immortalized hepatocyte cell lines and developed a model for multistep hepatocarcinogenesis. SV40-immortalized hepatocyte cell lines can also be used to study liver cell injury including injury caused by the chronic presence of HBV gene products. We have introduced the HBsAg under control of the albumin enhancer/promoter sequences or HBV X gene under the control of its own enhancer/promoter into SV40-immortalized hepatocyte cell lines to generate two series of cell lines that express the HBsAg polypeptides and HBV X transcripts respectively. These cell lines can be used to determine the effects of HBV gene expression on hepatocytes, in particular, on the expression of liver-specific genes. In conclusion, we have derived a series of cell lines that have been and will continue to be useful for understanding normal and abnormal function of hepatocytes.

INTRODUCTION

Immortalization of cells from a variety of tissues has been the object of investigation in numerous laboratories. The subject of this paper will be limited to a discussion of immortalization of rat hepatocytes. Hepatocytes in the liver of the intact host produce numerous gene products that are expressed solely or predominantly by this cell type. In addition, hepatocytes can respond to numerous external stimuli including growth factors, hormones, cytokines, drugs, etc. resulting in altered expression of gene products. Hepatocytes can also replicate normally or abnormally. Hepatocytes can be removed from the rat to yield primary rat hepatocyte cultures. The placement of rat hepatocytes in culture does not spontaneously yield a primary cell line. In fact, it is necessary to provide the cells with a substratum for attachment, composed either of rat liver epithelial cells or extracellular matrix components, and specialized medium for the primary hepatocytes to survive and remain differentiated *in vitro*. In response to treatment with specific hormones and drugs, primary hepatocytes can be induced to undergo DNA synthesis and a limited number of rounds of cell division. The purpose of this study was to establish well-differentiated immortalized rat hepatocyte cell lines that would replicate in a chemically defined medium in the absence of extracellular matrix and added growth factor (EGF, transforming growth factor-α hepatocyte growth factor, acidic and basic fibroblast growth factors), would respond to external stimuli, and could be used to study regulation of gene expression at a molecular level.

MATERIALS AND METHODS

Primary hepatocyte cultures. Hepatocytes were isolated by *in situ* collagenase perfusion of male Fischer F344 rats (180-200g) as described (1-3). Isolated hepatocytes were plated at a density of 1-2 x 10^6 cells, cultured on 60-mm plastic cell culture dishes coated with rat tail collagen (4) and fed RPCD medium (5) referred to as CDM. CDM was used alone or supplemented with EGF (25 ng/ml) and/or DMSO (2%).

Cell lines. Immortalized hepatocyte cell lines and stable transfectants derived from immortalized hepatocyte cell lines were maintained on 100-mm plastic cell culture dishes and fed fresh RPCD medium every 3 days. When cultures became confluent, the cells were trypsinized and subcultured at dilutions ranging from 1:3 to 1:10 depending upon the cells using RPCD medium supplemented with 5% FCS to eliminate residual trypsin activity and to aid cell attachment. Approximately 4 h after plating, cells were fed fresh RPCD medium without serum.

Transfection of SV40-immortalized hepatocyte cell lines. Cell were grown to 50 to 60% confluence in RPCD in 60-mm cell culture dishes, at which time the cells were washed and fed L-15 medium (3). Cells maintained in L-15 medium for 2 to 3 h were transfected by the calcium phosphate procedure (5-7). Cultures were transfected with 1 µg of SV2-*neo* DNA and 10 µg DNA of the gene to be introduced. Control cultures were transfected with only the DNA for the *neo* gene. At 3 h after transfection, the cells were washed and fed serum-supplemented medium. The day after transfection, the cultures were washed with serum-free RPCD medium and fed RPCD medium. When the cells reached 80-90% confluence, the cultures were fed RPCD medium supplemented with G418. Colonies of G418 resistant cells were detectable by 3 to 4 weeks after transfection.

Transient transfection. Plasmid DNA transfections were performed by the calcium phosphate precipitation method (6). The initial steps of the procedure were similar to those described above for generation of stably transfected cell lines. No drug resistance gene such as *neo* was used in these studies. The amount of plasmid DNA used was predetermined to be within the linear range of DNA uptake and chloramphenicol acetyltransferase (CAT) expression. For most studies, 15 µg of DNA were used per 100-mm dish. The cells from several plates were harvested 48 h after transfection and pooled. A portion of the cells were frozen and thawed for protein extraction and the protein extract assayed for CAT activity (8). The remainder of the pooled harvested cells was lysed to extract plasmid DNA (9). Southern blot hybridization analysis was carried out (10)) using as probe a nick-translated 1 kb fragment containing the CAT coding sequence. CAT activity from each transfection was normalized to the amount of protein used and the CAT plasmid DNA level in the transfected cells.

RESULTS AND DISCUSSION

The importance of the properties of the primary hepatocytes to the outcome of the immortalization process. We have previously reported that transfection of primary rat hepatocytes with SV40 DNA yielded the outgrowth of colonies of replicating epithelial cells and it was possible to establish hepatocyte cell lines from some of these colonies (5, 11). Primary rat hepatocytes were plated on a rat tail collagen coated plated at a density of 1-2 x 10^6 cells/60-mm dish and fed CDM, CDM+EGF or CDM+EGF+DMSO. The cells were transfected with SV40 DNA and observed. Media samples were collected and analyzed for rat albumin secretion (12 13). Hepatocytes plated in CDM or CDM+EGF lost the ability to produce detectable levels of albumin by 15 and 26 days after plating, respectively, while hepatocytes fed CDM+EGF+DMSO continued to produce high levels of albumin for at least 60 days (Fig. 1; 14, 15). At 3 to 4 weeks after transfection, the outgrowth of colonies of replicating epithelial cells was observed in cultures transfected with SV40 DNA but not in those transfected with carrier DNA. In cultures fed CDM or CDM+EGF, the primary hepatocytes had died by this point and the colonies arose in the absence of any viable background cells. The total number of colonies was higher in plates fed CDM+EGF than in those fed CDM alone. In plates fed CDM+EGF+DMSO, the colonies of replicating

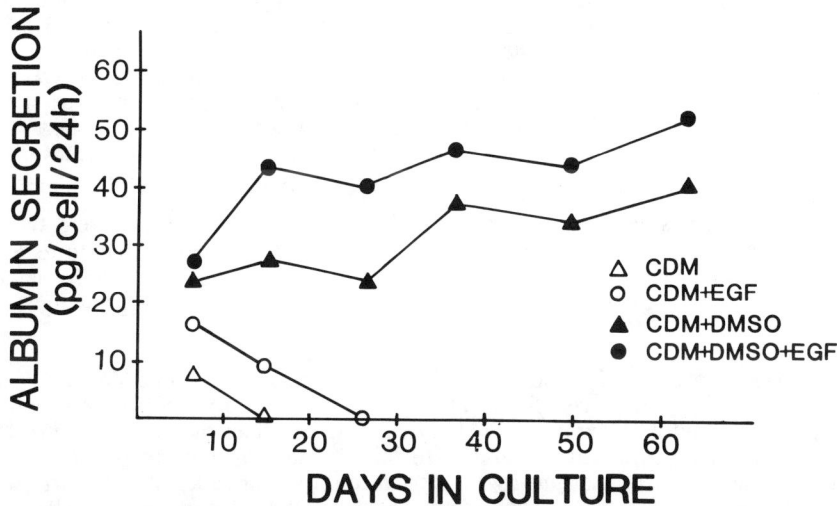

Figure 1. Effect of composition of culture media on maintenance of albumin secretion by primary hepatocytes. Primary rat hepatocytes plated on rat tail collagen coated dishes were fed CMD with or without EGF and/or DMSO as indicated. Culture medium was collected 24 h after cell feeding and analyzed for rat albumin content using rocket immunoelectrophoresis (12).

epithelial cells arose amidst islands of nonreplicating well-differentiated, highly functional hepatocytes. Within any one culture dish, the colonies that arose differed in size and shape and were composed of cells of varying morphology. The different types of colonies and cell types were present in all culture dishes and were independent of the composition of the culture medium. Cultures were overlaid with a sterile agarose gel containing antibody to albumin in order to identify colonies containing cells that produced albumin (5, 16, 17). The number of colonies containing albumin producing was 50% in cultures fed CDM+EGF+DMSO and was higher than that in cultures fed CDM cells or CDM+EGF (5). In general, albumin producing colonies were small with smooth borders and contained tightly packed small cells while the albumin negative colonies were usually large, diffuse with irregular borders and contained larger cells with fewer cell-cell contacts.

Albumin positive colonies were picked (in the absence of trypsin treatment) and transferred to fresh culture dishes. Less than 5% of the picked colonies survived. In cultures in which the cells grew, the cells initially grew as colonies and not a monolayer. The culture was then rescreened for albumin positive colonies by immuno-overlay and the strongest albumin producing colonies reseeded. This process was repeated 3-5 times. The colonies which were all morphologically identical and albumin positive were then trypsinized to form a cell line. If the colonies were trypsinized at an earlier time point in this process, it was not possible to establish a cell line. Colonies that arose in dishes fed CDM+EGF+DMSO were fed CDM+EGF since DMSO inhibited cell growth. Cell lines were initially established in CDM+EGF. After it was established that growth in the absence of EGF had no effect on albumin production, the cell lines were routinely cultured in CDM.

Well-differentiated high albumin expressing immortalized cell lines were successfully derived from colonies that arose in cultures fed CDM, CDM+EGF, or CDM+EGF+DMSO. These findings indicated that maintenance of albumin expression for a minimum of 10 days was sufficient time for SV40 immortalization to occur. We previously observed that high albumin producing immortalized cell lines could not be derived using hepatocytes fed L-15 medium supplemented with FCS. These cells stopped producing detectable levels of albumin prior to 10 days in culture. It appears from these studies that in order to generate an immortalized cell line which retains the ability to express a specific gene, the target cell must express that gene *in vitro* for as long as it is necessary for the immortalization event to occur. Additional support for this statement comes from the finding that primary hepatocytes cultured in CDM+EGF+DMSO lose the ability to produce $\alpha_{2\mu}$-globulin between 6 and 12 days post plating (15) and SV40-immortalized hepatocytes do not express $\alpha_{2\mu}$-globulin. One critical aspect for maintenance of differentiation by the SV40-immortalized hepatocyte cell lines was the use of the immuno-overlay to repeatedly isolate colonies containing cells producing high levels of albumin. In the absence of selection, we would have most likely generated cell lines composed of more rapidly growing poorly-differentiated cells.

We have derived and characterized eleven albumin positive and one albumin negative SV40-immortalized hepatocyte cell lines (11, 18). Each cell line is unique with regard to morphology (Fig. 2) and gene expression (11, 19). These cell lines maintained expression of multiple liver-specific genes and the ability to be regulated by hormones and cytokines (11, 18, 19). Some of the cell lines underwent spontaneous transformation with *in vitro* passage (18). Two of the cell lines that did transform spontaneously produced well-differentiated hepatocellular carcinomas when the cells were injected subcutaneously into newborn syngeneic hosts (18). SV40-immortalized hepatocytes have already been used in many ways to further understand liver function and have numerous other potential uses (Table 1).

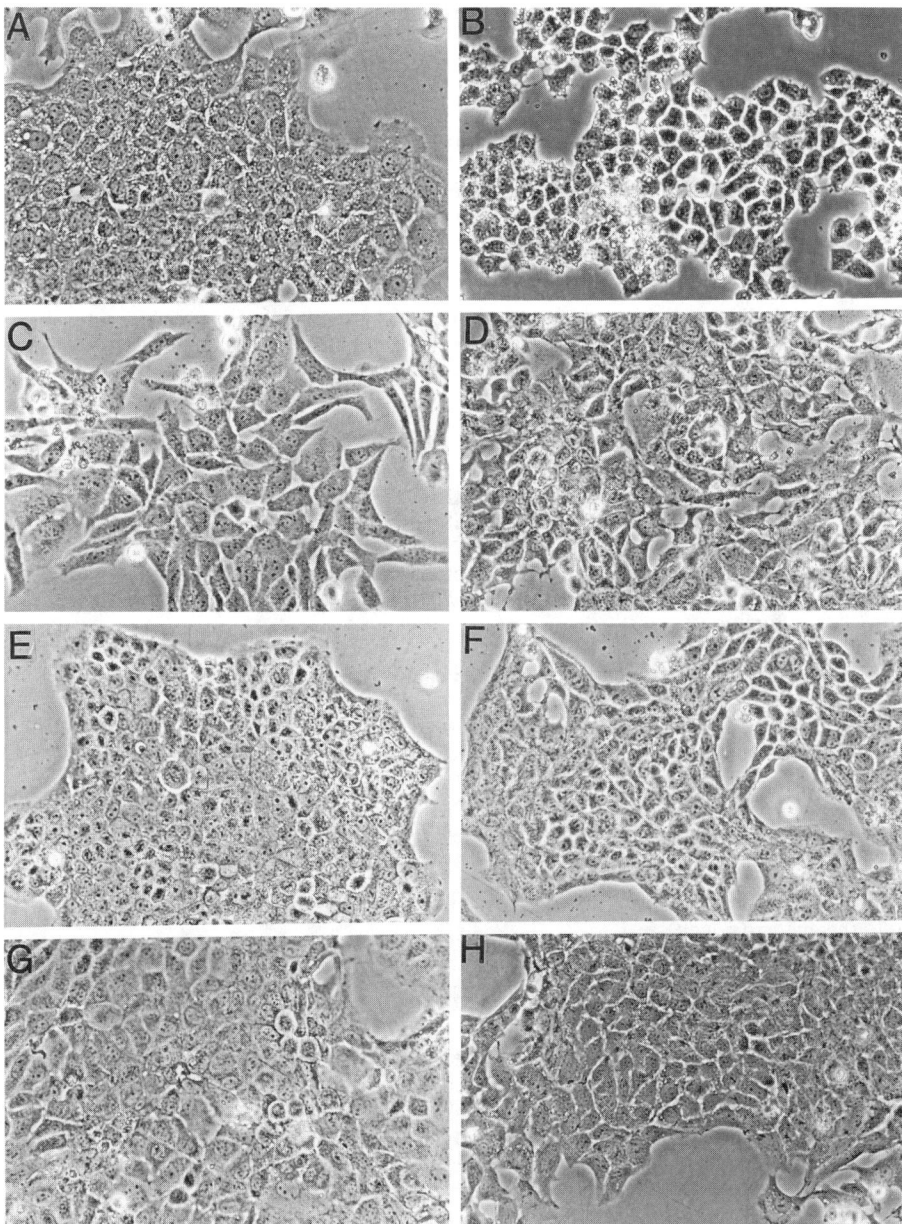

Figure 2. Photomicrograph of hepatocyte cell lines CWSV1 (A), CWSV2 (B), CWSV8 (C), CWSV14 (D), CWSV16 (E), CWSV17 (F), N4 (G), NAd4 (H). CWSV1, CWSV2, CWSV14, CWSV16, and CWSV17 are albumin positive SV40-immortalized hepatocyte cell lines. CWSV8 is an SV40-immortalized hepatocyte cell line that lost albumin expression at early passage and is used as a negative control. N4 is a *neo* transfectant derived from CWSV1 and is albumin positive. NAd4 is a *neo*+E1A+E1B transfectant derived from CWSV1 and is albumin negative.

Table 1

Uses for SV40-immortalized Hepatocyte Cell Lines

I. To understand mechanisms of normal function of hepatocytes

   A. Cell lines can be directly characterized for expression of serum proteins, acute phase proteins, enzymes, cytochrome p450s, growth factors, extracellular matrix proteins, proteins that mediate cell-cell and cell-extracellular matrix adhesion, etc.

   B. Cell lines can be treated with hormones, growth factors, cytokines, etc. to study regulation of expression of genes in hepatocytes at the RNA and protein level or at the functional level (enzyme activity, binding, etc.).

   C. Cell lines can be transiently transfected with genetically engineered DNA constructs to functionally map regulatory elements of liver-specific genes; extracts can be prepared from cell lines to structurally map regulatory elements of liver-specific genes.

   D. Cell lines can be stably transfected with expression vectors encoding specific genes or with antisense DNA constructs to understand normal function.

II. To determine how external agents injure hepatocytes

   A. Cell lines can be treated with drugs or toxins or exposed to physical agents to study cell injury.

   B. Cells can be infected with viruses or stably transfected with virus genes (such as HBsAg and HBV X gene) to study cell injury by virus gene products.

III. To develop *in vitro* models for studying malignant transformation (hepatocarcinogenesis).

   A. Immortalized cells can be examined with *in vitro* passage for spontaneous transformation.

   B. Viral genes or oncogenes can be added by infection or transfection to transform the already immortalized cell line.

   C. Immortalized cell lines can be treated with promoting or progression-inducing chemicals and observed for transformation.

Effect of the immortalizing agent on the ability to establish high albumin producing well-differentiated immortalized hepatocyte cell lines. Transfection of primary hepatocytes fed CDM+EGF+DMSO with the adenovirus E1A and E1B genes led to the outgrowth of replicating epithelial cells at 3 to 4 months post transfection (20). In contrast to the results obtained with SV40, we were unable to obtain albumin positive colonies in adenovirus-transfected cultures fed CDM or CDM+EGF. Our studies indicate that immortalization of hepatocytes by adenovirus E1A and E1B genes takes approximately twice as long as immortalization by SV40. For this reason, it was necessary to use culture conditions that enable primary hepatocytes to remain viable for more than 4 to 5 weeks in order to use the E1A and E1B genes to immortalize a hepatocyte that continues to produce albumin. Using the same procedures used for deriving high albumin producing SV40-immortalized hepatocyte cell lines, it was not possible to derive high albumin producing hepatocyte cell lines immortalized by the E1A and E1B genes. We were able to derive two adenovirus immortalized cell lines that produced low levels of albumin, levels that were at most 10% of the levels that we observed for SV40-immortalized hepatocyte cell lines. These findings suggested that expression of the E1A and/or E1B genes down regulate albumin expression. To test this hypothesis, we transfected the CWSV1 cell line, a high albumin producing SV40-immortalized cell line with E1A and E1B genes and the neomycin resistance gene (*neo*). The cells were then treated with G418, and 9 *neo*+E1A+E1B transfected cell lines were derived (Table 2). Eight of the 9 transfected cell lines were negative for albumin production by

Table 2

Albumin Secretion by Ad Transfectants of CWSV1 Cells

Cell line	Albumin secretion (pg/cell/24 h) with passage[a]							
	p2[b]	p3	p4	p5	p6	p7	p8	p9
N1[c]		22	22	15		7	25	11
N2		30	15	22			12	13
N3		37	14	31				
N4			25		66	13	15	16
N5	37	13	14	11				
N6	73	45	33	18				
NAd1[d]		0	3	0				
NAd2	0	0	0					
NAd4	0	0	0	0				
NAd5	8	6	4	0	0	0	0	
NAd6	0	0						
NAd7		0	0					
NAd8	27	21						
NAd9	0	0						
NAd10		11	0					

[a]The concentration of rat albumin in the culture medium was determined by rocket immunoelectrophoresis. The amount of albumin secreted per cell in 24 h was then determined by dividing the amount of albumin secreted by a culture by the number of cells in the culture.

[b]Passage 2.

[c]N1, N2, etc. are *neo* transfectants derived from CWSV1.

[d]NAd1, NAd2, etc. are *neo*+E1A+E1B transfectants derived from CWSV1.

passage 6. When similar experiments were carried out with *neo* alone or the activated c-Ha-*ras* gene in combination with *neo*, the transfectants continued to produce high levels of albumin similar to those produced by CWSV1 (Table 2; 13). We conclude from these studies that the immortalizing agent can affect gene expression in the cell type being immortalized.

Transfection of SV40-immortalized hepatocyte cell lines. The usefulness of a cell line for current molecular studies of gene expression and gene regulatory elements is enhanced if the cell line can be transfected. We knew from the studies we carried out to generate immortalized hepatocyte cell lines that primary rat hepatocytes could be transfected using the calcium phosphate precipitation method (5). It was important to determine whether we could co-transfect SV40-immortalized hepatocyte cell lines with a specific gene driven by its own promoter or a heterologous promoter and the *neo* gene, treat the cultures with G418 and generate stably transfected cell lines that expressed the added gene. Using this procedure, we have successfully established cell lines that express the activated c-Ha-*ras* gene (13), the adenovirus E1A and E1B genes (as discussed above), the *Bgl*IIA fragment of the HBV genome driven by the mouse albumin enhancer/promoter (Isom, *et al.*, unpublished data) and the HBV X gene driven by its own enhancer/promoter (Isom, *et al.*, unpublished data). Generation of these cell lines was possible for several reasons. First, the cell lines were capable of taking up DNA using calcium phosphate precipitation. Second, the SV40-immortalized cell lines were killed by treatment with G418. CWSV1 cells were killed after 5-7 days of treatment with G418 (0.5 mg/ml). Third, the regulatory sequences driving the specific genes being introduced were functional in CWSV1 cells. We have also determined that the Rous sarcoma virus (RSV) promoter is active in CWSV1 cells. Therefore, if the endogenous promoter of the gene to be added to an immortalized hepatocyte cell line is not functional in the cell line, then we can generate a construct using a heterologous promoter such as the RSV promoter or albumin enhancer/promoter to drive the gene of interest. We initially established stable transfectants using CWSV1 cells and have recently also generated stably transfected cell lines from CWSV2 cells. We have also demonstrated that a second gene can be added to a *neo* resistant immortalized hepatocyte cell line by transfection of the cells with the second gene inserted in a hygromycin containing vector followed by selection in hygromycin (Serra and Isom, unpublished data).

We also wanted to determine whether immortalized hepatocyte cell lines could be transiently transfected with regulatory DNA sequences driving a reporter gene. Specifically, one of our goals was to transiently transfect SV40-immortalized hepatocyte cell lines with various DNA constructs driving a CAT gene in order to evaluate the function of the *cis*-acting sequences controlling albumin gene expression. In order to establish the assay conditions, we used varying amounts of protein extracts (ranging from 0.2 to 200 µg protein) from CWSV1 cells transfected with albumin enhancer/promoter sequences driving the CAT gene to establish the relationship between µg protein extract and amount of CAT conversion (Fig. 3). In order to correct for variation in transfection efficiency between individual experiments, different plasmids, and cell lines, we quantitated the plasmid DNA level in the transfected cells so we could directly compare the reporter gene expression relative to the introduced gene copy number. In agreement with previous reports (21), we found this approach to be accurate and highly reproducible. For example, when a plasmid containing albumin enhancer/promoter sequences driving CAT, was transfected into CWSV1 cells and the DNA uptake was deliberately increased by glycerol shock, a two fold (from 4.0 to 8.3%) increase in CAT expression was observed in glycerol shocked cells (Fig. 4). Similarly, a two fold increase in uptake of plasmid DNA was observed (0.15 to 0.3 OD). When the CAT activity was corrected for variation in level of DNA uptake, the resulting normalized CAT activities became essentially the same (27.0 compared to 26.4). Similar results were obtained for NR4T-1 cells except that a ten fold (from 0.3-3.5%) increase in CAT expression was observed in glycerol shocked cells.

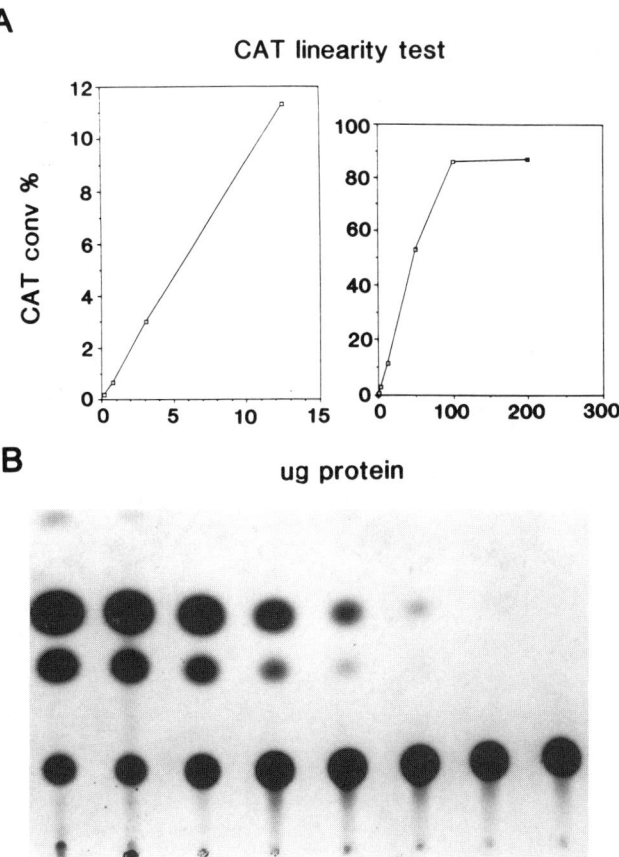

Figure 3. Relationship between amount of protein in CAT assay and percent CAT conversion. CWSV1 cells were transfected with albumin enhancer/promoter sequences driving the CAT gene using the calcium phosphate precipitation method. Precipitates were removed 4-5 h after transfection and the cells were fed fresh media. The cells were harvested 48 h after transfection and protein extract was prepared. Protein concentrations were determined using the Bio-Rad (Richmond, California) protein assay. 0, 0.2, 0.8, 3.2, 12.5, 50, 100, and 200 μg of protein extract were assayed for CAT activity as described (8). A. CAT conversion plotted against μg protein extract used in the assay. B. Autoradiograph of CAT activity with increasing amounts of protein from right to left.

Using transient transfection, we have shown that the hepatitis B virus (HBV) enhancer 5' to the X gene is functional in CWSV1 cells (22). This finding was significant because it demonstrated that this viral enhancer was not species (human) specific and could function in rat cells. Using transient transfection, we have carried out mapping experiments of the albumin enhancer and compared the ability of the albumin enhancer and promoter to function in immortalized and transformed hepatocyte cell lines and cell lines derived from tumors produced by transformed hepatocyte cell lines (Hu, *et al.*, unpublished data).

Advantages and disadvantages of using immortalized hepatocyte cell lines. The usefulness of an immortalized cell line depends upon how closely it resembles its *in vivo* counterpart with regard to the question being addressed. For example, the SV40-immortalized hepatocyte cell lines we have established are highly appropriate for studying the molecular mechanisms for expression and regulation of expression of albumin but are not of value for studying α2μ-globulin.

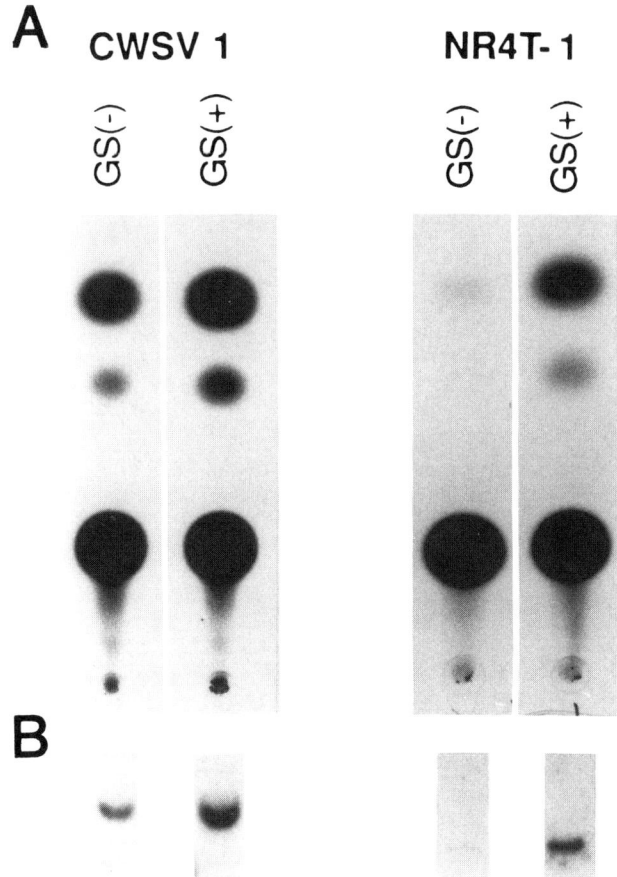

Figure 4. Standardization of transfection efficiency by quantitation of plasmid DNA uptake. CWSV1 cells were transfected with 15 μg of plasmid DNA containing the mouse albumin promoter and enhancer driving CAT in the presence (GS+) or absence GS(-) of 15% glycerol shock. NR4T-1 cells were transfected with 15 μg of plasmid DNA containing the albumin promoter driving CAT in the presence (GS+) or absence GS(-) of 15% glycerol shock. A. CAT assays. The substrate was [^{14}C]-chloramphenicol. The reaction products were separated by thin layer chromatography and the radioactive spots from the thin layer plates were cut out and counted in a liquid scintillation counter to quantitate the conversion rate of chloramphenicol to the acetylated products. B. Hirt DNA was prepared and quantitated by Southern blotting. Plasmid DNA bands were quantitated by densitometric scanning.

Testing the effects of hormones and drugs on the function of a hepatocyte can be best carried out using primary hepatocytes or immortalized hepatocyte cell lines. The disadvantage of using whole animals for these studies is that it is difficult to target the compound to the hepatocyte without it potentially being altered within the intact animal. Possible disadvantages of using primary hepatocytes or immortalized cell lines for these studies is that these cells *in vitro* may have lost receptors for the compounds or the ability to appropriately transport or metabolize the compound.

One disadvantage of using SV40-immortalized hepatocyte cell lines is that they express the SV40 T antigen, a multi-functional protein. Therefore, studies on these cell lines are subject to the criticism that T antigen may be having some unknown effect on gene expression or liver cell function.

Manipulation of a cell by the addition of specific genes to that cell type can be carried out most easily by generating stable transfectants from immortalized cell lines. Genes can be added to whole animals by generating transgenic animals and expression of that gene can be targeted to a specific cell type by using the appropriate promoter. However, generation and characterization of transgenic animals is costly and time consuming. Genes cannot be added to primary hepatocytes by using drug selection (neomycin, hygromycin resistance, etc) because primary hepatocytes do not replicate.

Fine mapping of regulatory elements for liver-specific genes cannot be carried out in the intact liver of a rat and can be more appropriately carried out in primary cells or an immortalized cell line than in transgenic animals. We have found that the ability of the albumin enhancer to increase albumin promoter driven CAT activity can be measured in CWSV1 cells, *neo* transfectants of CWSV1 cells, CWSV2 cells, and primary hepatocytes in CDM+EGF+DMSO (Hu, *et al.*, unpublished data). Although the enhancement is approximately two fold higher in primary hepatocytes than in the immortalized hepatocyte cell lines, the enhancer mapping studies can be carried out more efficiently using the immortalized cells for several reasons. (1) The immortalized cells replicate and, therefore, large numbers of cells can be readily obtained. (2) The immortalized cells replicate in the absence of a substratum and/or EGF. (3) The immortalized cells take up more DNA during transfection than the primary hepatocytes. (4) Transcription of albumin as measured in a nascent chain extension assay (15) using nuclei isolated from CWSV1 cells is approximately the same level as in nuclei from liver while transcription using nuclei isolated from primary hepatocytes in CDM+EGF+DMSO is only about 22% the level in nuclei from liver.

ACKNOWLEDGMENT

The investigation was supported in part by Public Health Service grant CA23931 from the National Cancer Institute. We thank T. Miller for expert technical assistance and T. Grierson for help with photography.

REFERENCES

1. BERRY, M.N. and FRIEND, D.S. (1969), High-yield preparation of isolated rat liver parenchymal cells. J. Cell. Biol., 43:506-520.
2. FELDHOFF, R.C., TAYLOR, J.M., and JEFFERSON, L.S. (1977), Synthesis and secretion of rat albumin *in vivo*, in perfused liver, and in isolated hepatocytes. J. Biol. Chem., 252:3611-3616.
3. ISOM, H. C. (1980), DNA synthesis in isolated hepatocytes infected with herpesviruses. Virology, 103:199-216.
4. ELDSDALE, T. and BARD, J. (1972), Collagen substrata for studies on cell behavior. J. Cell Biol., 54:626-637.
5. WOODWORTH, C., SECOTT, T., and ISOM, H.C. (1986), Transformation of rat hepatocytes by transfection with simian virus 40 DNA to yield proliferating differentiated cells. Cancer Res, 46:4018-4026.
6. GRAHAM, F.L. and VAN DER EB, A.J. (1973), A new technique for the assay of infectivity of human adenovirus 5 DNA. Virology, 52:456-467.
7. WIGLER, M., PELLICER, A., SILVERSTEIN, S., AXEL, R., URLAUB, G., and CHASIN, L. (1979), DNA-mediated transfer of the adenine phosphoribosyltransferase locus into mammalian cells. Proc. Natl. Acad. Sci. USA, 76:1373-1376.
8. GORMAN, C.M., MOFFAT, L.F., and HOWARD, B.H. (1982), Recombinant genomes which express chloramphenicol acetyltransferase in mammalian cells. Mol. Cell. Biol., 2:1044-1051.

9. HIRT, B. (1967), Selective extraction of polyoma DNA from infected mouse cell cultures. J. Mol. Biol., 26:365-369.
10. MANIATIS, T., FRITSCH, E., and SAMBROOK, J. (1982), Molecular Cloning: A Laboratory Manual, Cold Spring Harbor.
11. WOODWORTH, C.D., and ISOM, H.C. (1987), Regulation of albumin gene expression in a series of rat hepatocyte cell lines immortalized by simian virus 40 and maintained in chemically defined medium. Mol. Cell. Biol., 7:3740-3748.
12. LAURELL, C.B. (1966), Quantitative estimation of proteins by electrophoresis in agarose gel containing antibodies. Anal. Biochem., 15:45-52.
13. ISOM, H.C., WOODWORTH, C.D., MENG, Y., KREIDER, J., MILLER, T., and MENGEL, L. (1992), Introduction of the *ras* oncogene transforms a simian virus 40-immortalized hepatocyte cell line without loss of expression of albumin and other liver-specific genes. Cancer Res., 52:940-948.
14. ISOM, H.C., SECOTT, T., GEORGOFF, I., WOODWORTH, C., and MUMMAW, J. (1985), Maintenance of differentiated rat hepatocytes in primary culture. Proc. Natl. Acad. Sci. USA, 82:3252-3256.
15. ISOM, H., GEORGOFF, I., SALDITT-GEORGIEFF, M., and DARNELL, Jr., J.E. (1987), Persistence of liver-specific messenger RNA in cultured hepatocytes: different regulatory events for different genes. J. Cell Biol., 105:2877-2885.
16. SAMMONS, D.W., SANCHEZ, E., and DARLINGTON, G.J. (1980), Immuno-overlay: a method for identification of hepatoma cell colonies that secrete albumin. In Vitro, 16:918-924.
17. ISOM, H.C. and GEORGOFF, I. (1984), Quantitative assay for albumin-producing liver cells after simian virus 40 transformation of rat hepatocytes maintained in chemically defined medium. Proc. Natl. Acad. Sci. USA, 81:6378-6382.
18. WOODWORTH, C.D., KREIDER, J.W., MENGEL, L., MILLER, T., MENG, Y., and ISOM, H. C. (1988), Tumorigenicity of simian virus 40-hepatocyte cell lines: Effect of *in vitro* and *in vivo* passage on expression of liver-specific genes and oncogenes. Mol. Cell. Biol., 8:4492-4501.
19. LIAO, W.S.L., MA, K.-T., WOODWORTH, C.D., MENGEL, L., and ISOM, H.C. (1989), Stimulation of the acute-phase response in simian virus 40-hepatocye cell lines. Mol. Cell. Biol., 9:2779-2786.
20. WOODWORTH, C.D. and ISOM, H.C. (1987), Transformation of differentiated rat hepatocytes with adenovirus and adenovirus DNA. J. Virol., 61:3570-3579.
21. ALWINE, J.C. (1985), Transient gene expression control: Effects of transfected DNA stability and *trans*-activation by viral early proteins. Mol. Cell. Biol., 5:1034-1042.
22. PATEL, N.U., SHAHID, J., ISOM, H., and SIDDIQUI, A. (1989), Interactions between nuclear factors and the hepatitis B virus enhancer. J. Virol., 63:5293-5301.

C2

Steps in Development of an *In Vitro* Nasal Toxic Response Assay: Comparison of Carboxylesterase in Human and Rat Nasal Tissue

PAMELA M. MATTES[1] and WILLIAM B. MATTES[2]

[1]*Department of Pediatrics*
University of Connecticut School of Medicine
Farmington, CT 06032

[2]*Environmental Health Center*
CIBA-GEIGY Corporation
Farmington, CT 06032

Introduction

Inhalation of certain gaseous and particulate pollutants leads to functional impairment and in some cases carcinoma of the nasal cavity (1-5). Current methods for nasal toxicity assessment rely on retrospective epidemiological studies and animal models such as the rat. While inhalation by rodents of a variety of vapors common in industrial settings produces site-specific lesions in the nasal cavity (e.g. 6), it is not clear that the rat upper airway model is valid for determining toxicity of inhaled vapors to the human nasal cavity (7). Our objective, therefore, is to develop an *in vitro* human nasal cell culture assay system to screen for potentially harmful effects of inhaled toxicants to the nasal cavity.

Inhalation of toxic vapors by animals can result in high nasal tissue concentrations and inflammation, ulceration, and necrosis of the nasal mucosa. An obvious risk factor for nasal lesions is that the nasal cavity is the primary interface for contact with inhaled pollutants, thus receiving the ultimate dose of toxicant. Less evident is the fact that the nasal cavity serves to protect the lower respiratory tract by absorbing or "scrubbing" the incoming airstream of toxic chemicals (8), resulting in high tissue concentrations and therefore high potential for toxic injury. It is also clear that the site and extent of damage from exposure to a particular toxicant is often determined by the presence (or absence) of toxicant-activating enzymes or detoxication pathways in particular cell types lining the nasal cavity (9). Xenobiotic-metabolizing enzyme activities which are expressed at high levels in the nasal cavity and which strongly influence nasal sensitivity to metabolites include cytochrome P450 monooxygenases (10,11), aldehyde dehydrogenase (12), rhodanese (13), epoxide hydrolases (14), and carboxylesterases (15). Because metabolism plays a key role in the mechanism of nasal toxicity for certain inhaled chemicals *in vivo*, it is desirable that cultured cells in *in vitro* test systems also be capable of biotransforming test xenobiotics.

We are focusing on the effects of inhaled toxic esters on the nasal cavity, and modeling those effects *in vitro* using differentiated nasal epithelial cells in culture. *In vivo*, inhalation exposure to ethyl acrylate (16), propylene glycol monomethyl ether acetate (17), and dibasic ester vapors (18) leads to selective degeneration of the olfactory epithelium of the rodent nasal cavity. Injury results from hydrolysis of the compounds to acid metabolites by olfactory tissue carboxylesterase *in situ*. This conclusion is supported by the the findings that 1) *in vivo* exposure to acid and not alcohol metabolites of esters causes olfactory damage similar to that of the parent compound (19), 2) administration of a carboxylesterase inhibitor to rats prior to their exposure to a toxic ester prevents the toxic response (20); 3) in rodents, cell types of the olfactory neuroepithelium contain the highest levels of carboxylesterase in the nasal cavity (21). Carboxylesterase expression is central to nasal tissue toxic response to esters *in vivo*, thus its expression is also required *in vitro* to accurately predict the toxicity of novel inhaled esters.

To facilitate quantitation of carboxylesterase activity in nasal epithelial cell cultures we developed a highly sensitive spectrophotometric assay for carboxylesterase (22). The assay substrate is α-naphthyl butyrate, the substrate commonly used in the histochemical localization of carboxylesterase (21). Additionally we directly compared the substrate specificities of α-naphthyl butyrate esterases in human and rat nasal homogenates and found striking differences between the species. These findings are important to determining the minimum number substrates necessary to determine toxic ester-metabolizing potential of individual nasal cell lines, as well as to human risk assessment.

The source of tissue for human nasal test cells is nasal polyp specimens excised for therapeutic purposes. Nasal cell lines with enhanced lifespans (ELS) *in vitro* are derived from the primary cultures by infection with a recombinant Adenovirus5-SV40 virus (23). Since validation, i.e. direct comparison of toxic responses of cells *in vitro* with those of parent tissues *in vivo*, is an important step in development of *in vitro* assay systems, we derived nasal epithelial primary cultures and derivative differentiated ELS lines from F344 rat nasal cavity. These cells will 1) facilitate assessment of the importance of the normal microenvironment on nasal toxic response; 2) allow direct comparison of human and rat nasal sensitivities to toxicants, thus giving quantitative information on human risk assessment. This paper, then, discusses progress in three areas:

1.) Derivation and characterization of primary and ELS (Enhanced Life Span) epithelial cells from human and rat nasal cavity;
2.) Development of a sensitive spectrophotometric assay for carboxylesterase;
3.) Comparison of carboxylesterase substrate specificities in rat and human nasal tissue.

1.) Derivation and characterization of human and rat nasal cell cultures

Derivation of primary cultures   Primary cultures of human nasal epithelial cells are derived from nasal polyp tissue discarded from nasal polypectomies performed for therapeutic purposes (24,25). Upon excision, tissue is placed in LHC basal medium (Biofluids, Rockville, MD) containing gentamycin, 50 μg/ml, and amphotericin B, 2.5 μg/ml. Subsequently, small pieces of tissue are anchored to tissue culture dishes prepared by incubation for at least 2 hours with LHC medium containing collagen, 30 μg/ml (Vitrogen, Collagen Corp.), human fibronectin, 10 μg/ml (Collaborative Research), and bovine serum albumin, 10 μg/ml (Miles). Dishes are filled with LHC-8e growth medium (26) and placed in a 37 incubator with a 5% CO_2 atmosphere. Alternatively, primary cultures are derived by incubating polyp tissue overnight at 4° in growth medium containing 0.1% Type XIV protease (Sigma) (25). Cell suspensions are subsequently plated on coated dishes.

Rat nasal primary cultures are obtained as previously described (27), by perfusing the nasal cavity of a euthanized F344 male rat with a protease solution and plating the resulting suspension in serum-free medium (28).

Derivation of ELS cultures   Human nasal ELS cell lines are obtained by infecting nasal primary cultures with the recombinant viral vector Adenovirus 5-SV40 (23). Adenovirus 5-SV40 is a recombinant hybrid consisting of the complete early region of the SV40 genome (ori-, origin defective) cloned into the early regions 1a and 1b of the helper independent Adenovirus 5 vector E1/X (23). The virus was kindly provided by Dr. Roger Reeves, Johns Hopkins University School of Medicine. For infections, primary cultures are plated in LHC-8e medium at a density of 2×10^5 per 60 mm dish. Two days later Adeno5-SV40 virus is added to dishes at multiplicities of infection ranging from 10 to 100. Control dishes (no virus) are treated identically. After 4 hours at 37°C medium is aspirated and replenished. Growth medium is changed every 3 days. 4-6 weeks later foci of rapidly dividing cells appeared over a background of flat, non-dividing cells, or no cells. From 1-11 foci were observed in 11 out of 17 dishes. No foci were observed in control dishes. Nasal ELS lines have been established from Adeno5-SV40 infection of 5 of 6 primary nasal cell cultures from different individuals.

Rat nasal ELS cultures were established as previously described (27), by infecting primary cultures with the same recombinant Adenovirus 5-SV40 virus used to establish human nasal ELS lines. Results of studies initiated to characterize rat nasal cultures and Adenovirus5-SV40 infected rat nasal lines are published (27).

Characterization of human primary and ELS nasal cells

General characteristics   Primary human nasal cultures on tissue culture plastic have a distinctive cuboidal "cobblestone" morphology. When cultures are 90% confluent they are trypsinized using .01% trypsin (Worthington) and passed, or frozen in liquid nitrogen for future use. In some cases explants attached to fresh dishes after original cell outgrowths had been trypsinized away from them produced additional cell monolayers. Primary cultures two weeks of age or less derived by the proteolytic digestion procedure frequently harbored cell groups with beating cilia, a phenotypic property of respiratory epithelial cells. In general human primary cultures grew well over two passages, and subsequently terminally differentiated. Figure 1 is a photomicrograph of a confluent monolayer of an human ELS nasal line recovered from Adeno5- SV40 infection of a primary culture. Using light microscopy the cells are morphologically indistinguishable from the parent primary culture. Transformed nasal lines are grown in culture in the same fashion as the parent primaries. Of course, an important advantage of these lines for *in vitro* toxic response studies is their extended lifespan in culture, 40 to 50 population doublings more than that of the primary cultures (Data not shown).

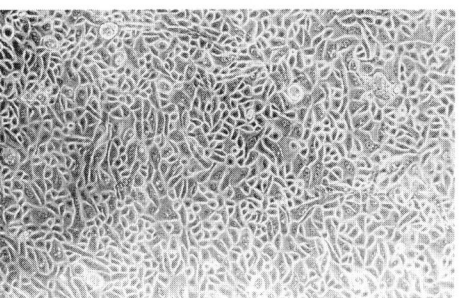

Figure 1. Human ELS nasal line.

SV40 T-antigen SV40 large T- antigen is expressed in the nuclei of SV40 transfected cells soon after infection. To confirm the presence of SV40 sequences in human ELS cultures *in vitro* and thus the origin of their enhanced lifespan, we tested for expression of SV40 large T antigen by indirect immunofluorescence techniques. Briefly, cells on coverslips were rinsed in PBS, fixed in cold (-20°C) 1:1 methanol/acetone, rinsed again, and then treated 30 minutes at 37°C with 30μl of 1:1600 dilution of mouse monoclonal antiserum to SV40 T-antigen (kindly provided by Dr. Keith Peden, Johns Hopkins School of Medicine). Coverslips were then rinsed, and treated with 30μl 1:80 dilution of fluorescein-conjugated goat anti-mouse IgG (Kirkeguard and Perry, Gaithersburg, MD) in 1% control serum. After 30 minutes at 37°C coverslips were rinsed and mounted using Mowiol 4-88 (Calbiochem). Slides were visualized with an Olympus microscope using epifluorescence illumination. Figure 2 shows a human ELS cell line stained for SV40 T-antigen. Positive nuclear staining suggests the presence of SV40 sequences in the cellular genome. Parent primary cultures were negative for nuclear staining (Data not shown).

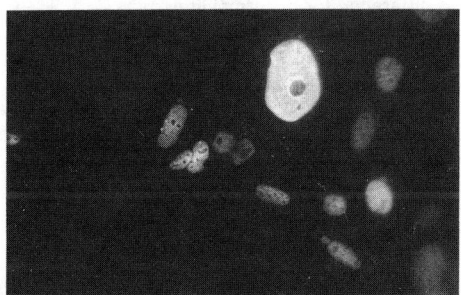

Figure 2. Human nasal ELS line stained for SV40 T-antigen.

Keratin expression Keratin is a protein which is prominent in the cytoskeleton of epithelial cells, but absent in fibroblasts. Assays for keratin were done essentially according to Sun and Green (29), using a rabbit polyclonal antiserum to keratin (provided by Dr. Susan Banks-Schlegel, NIH) and indirect immunofluorescent techniques. Figure 3 is a photomicrograph of cells from a human nasal ELS line stained for keratin. Keratin fibers are clearly visualized. Figure 3b shows results of staining a rat nasal ELS line (27) for keratin. As controls, both 1) parallel cultures treated with pre-immune rabbit serum instead of antiserum, and 2) human skin fibroblasts treated with anti-keratin antiserum were negative for staining (Data not shown).

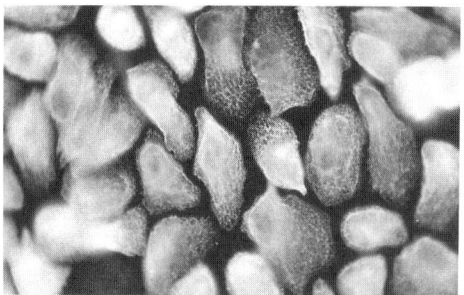

Figure 3a.
A human nasal ELS line stained for keratin.

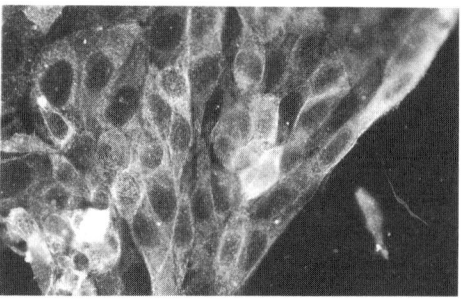

Figure 3b.
A rat nasal ELS line stained for keratin.

Transepithelial electrical measurements A major function of airway epithelium is maintainance of normal gradients of water and electrolytes across the epithelium *via* active transport processes. To test the ability of rat and human ELS nasal lines to perform this differentiated epithelial cell function we seeded cell lines on permeable collagen matrices attached to polycarbonate supports (30) and looked for the development of transepithelial electrical activity, using standard electrophysiological techniques (31). Results of measuring the time course of development of transepithelial voltage, short circuit current, and transepithelial resistance by a rat nasal ELS line grown on a collagen matrices have been reported (27). Human ELS nasal lines derived from normal individuals and those with cystic fibrosis (CF) and seeded on collagen matrices in LHC-8e medium supplemented with 6×10^{-4} M developed a transepithelial potential difference within 4 days which persisted for approximately 3 weeks. The mean maximum potential difference of 6 CF lines was -1.2 +/- 0.2 mV (SEM), and the mean maximum potential difference for 5 normal lines was -2.1 +/- 0.3 mV (SEM). We also tested the effect of amiloride, an apical membrane Na^+ channel blocker, upon the human nasal lines cultured upon collagen matrices. 1×10^{-6} M amiloride added to growth medium on the apical side of the cultured epithelia reversibly inhibited transepithelial voltage produced by CF and normal ELS cultures as well as normal primary cultures (see Table 1). Basolaterally applied amiloride had no effect on transepithelial voltage. Thus the human nasal ELS lines retain important differentiate functions of parent primary nasal cells, including tight junctions, membrane polarity, and functional amiloride-sensitive Na^+ channels on the apical membrane.

Table 1

Effect of 1 μM amiloride (apical dose) upon potential difference across normal human primary, normal human ELS and cystic fibrosis ELS nasal cells cultured on collagen matrices.

Cell Type	# of samples	Potential Difference (mV) ± S.E.M. Control	+ Amiloride	%Inhibition
Normal 1°	7	-6.5 ±2.0	-3.6 ±1.1	45 ±5.8
Normal ELS	4	-1.4 ±0.1	-0.6 ±0.1	58.6 ±9.3
CF ELS	2	-1.3	-0.65	52.6

In each case the amiloride effect was reversible and specific to the apical membrane.

2.) Development of a sensitive carboxylesterase assay

Expression of carboxylesterase is needed by an *in vitro* nasal culture system to predict toxicities of novel inhaled esters. Initially human and rat nasal ELS cell homogenates were assayed for carboxylesterase by the method of Bogdanffy et al. (32), in which rate of hydrolysis of dimethylsuccinate to monomethylsuccinate is monitored. Cultured cell carboxylesterase activities per mg cell protein were at least 50-fold lower than those of fresh rat nasal tissue homogenates (32), and were in fact below the method's limit of sensitivity. Thus we developed a more sensitive assay for carboxylesterase, using *α*-naphthyl butyrate as the substrate (22). This spectrophotometric assay permits quantitation of as little as 0.5 nmole of product, allowing accurate measurement of enzyme activity in relatively small numbers of cells. In addition, since a-naphthyl butyrate is the histochemical substrate for carboxylesterase (21), its use in a biochemical assay permits monitoring the enzyme in cells and tissues both biochemically and histochemically in parallel.

Before screening cultured nasal epithelial cells for a-naphthyl butyrate esterase activity we assayed homogenates prepared from human nasal polyp tissue and pooled F344 rat nasal tissue. Although nasal polyp tissue is by definition abnormal (34), it is the most readily obtainable human nasal tissue source. Homogenates were prepared and assayed as described (22).

Figure 4 is a Michaelis-Menten plot of the kinetics of a-naphthyl butyrate esterase in human and rat nasal homogenates. Kinetic constants describing hydrolysis of a-naphthyl butyrate were derived from Lineweaver-Burke double reciprocal plots (33). The mean apparent Michaelis constants (Km) for the rat and human activities are not different, 49.3 μM and 58.1 μM, respectively, and are 1 -2 orders of magnitude less than those reported for hydrolysis of the industrially important pollutants (15,32). On the other hand the mean apparent maximal velocity (Vmax) for the rat nasal enzyme activity, 4,030 nmol/min/ mg protein, was about 40-fold higher than that of the human activity, 108.9 nmol/min/mg These data suggest that (1) the affinities of the two species' nasal a-naphthyl butyrate esterase activities for the substrate are the same, and (2) human nasal mucosa contains less esterase activity than rat nasal tissue, per mg protein. The latter findings disagree with a recent

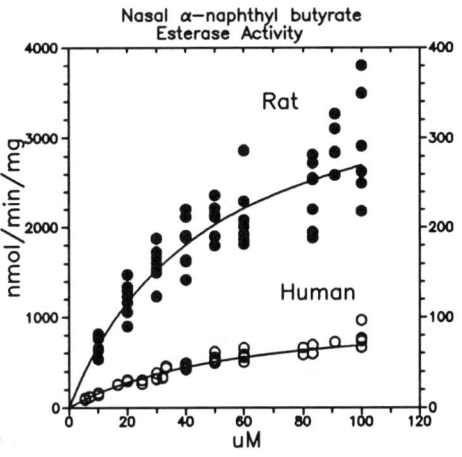

Figure 4. Kinetics of human and rat nasal a-naphthyl butyrate esterase

preliminary report (35) that carboxylesterase levels of homogenates of human nasal turbinate and rat nasal tissue are comparable, using p- nitrophenylbutyrate as the esterase substrate. Possible reasons for the discrepancy between the findings of the two laboratories include (1) difference in type of human nasal tissue tested, and (2) difference in substrate assayed. Direct comparison of carboxylesterase in parallel human and rat nasal tissue types is clearly central to human risk extrapolation from animal toxicity data.

3.) Carboxylesterase substrate specificities in human and rat nasal tissue

The purpose of the a-naphthyl butyrate esterase assay is to serve as a sensitive screen to identify nasal cell cultures and lines capable of metabolizing potentially toxic inhaled carboxylesters prevalent in industrial settings. To ascertain whether the assay fulfills the latter purpose it was necessary to demonstrate that nasal a-naphthyl butyrate esterase activity indeed hydrolyzes toxicologically significant industrial esters. Thus we assessed the effects of various carboxylesters upon the kinetics of human and rat nasal a-naphthyl butyrate esterase activities. The results of these studies have been reported in preliminary form (36).

Figures 5 through 8 are Lineweaver-Burke reciprocal plots of results of experiments in which the kinetics for rat and human nasal a-naphthyl butyrate esterase were determined in the presence and absence of each of four carboxylesters: p-nitrophenylbutyrate, the common biochemical assay substrate for carboxylesterase, figure 5; ethyl acrylate, an important compound in the plastics industry, figure 6; dimethylsuccinate, a solvent component in the paint industry, figure 7; and propylene glycol monomethyl ether acetate, another prominent industrial solvent, figure 8. As shown by the figures, rat nasal a-naphthyl butyrate esterase activity was competitively inhibited by each ester, suggesting that each competing ester is also a substrate for a-naphthyl butyrate esterase. On the other hand none of the esters affected the human activity's kinetics, indicating that these compounds are not metabolized by the human a-naphthyl butyrate esterase. To begin to see whether the toxicologically important esters are metabolized in human nasal mucosa we tested the ability of human nasal homogenate to hydrolyze dimethylsuccinate, essentially according to the method of Bogdanffy (32). Figure 9 shows that dimethylsuccinate is hydrolyzed by human nasal homogenate in a time- and protein concentration-dependent manner. In an experiment to measure the kinetics of dimethylsuccinate hydrolysis by human nasal homogenate the Km was 9.2 mM and the Vmax was 410 nmol/min/mg protein. Thus it appears that human nasal homogenate contains separate esterase activities for α-naphthyl butyrate and dimethylsuccinate.

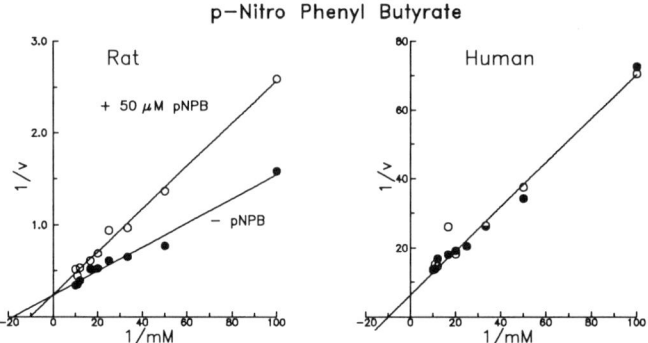

Figure 5. Kinetics of rat and human nasal α-naphthyl butyrate esterase in the presence and absence of 50 μM p-nitrophenylbutyrate.

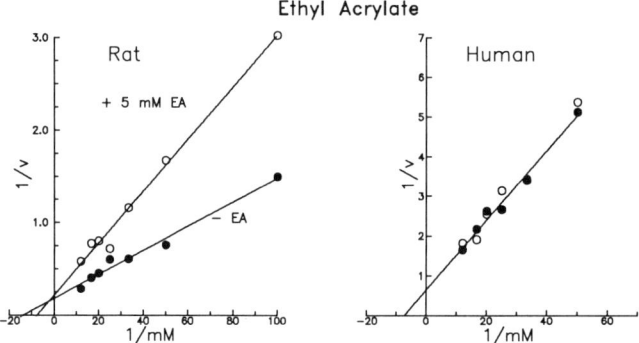

Figure 6. Kinetics of rat and human nasal α-naphthyl butyrate esterase in the presence and absence of 5 mM ethyl acrylate.

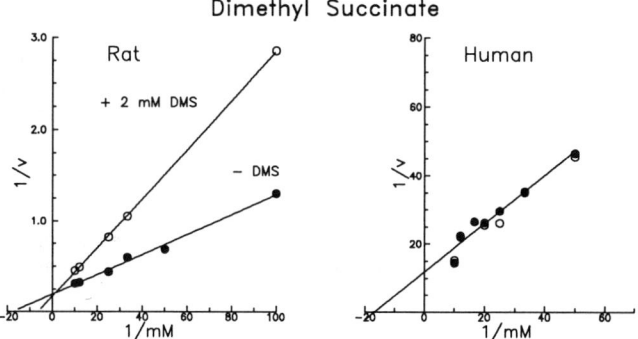

Figure 7. Kinetics of rat and human nasal α-naphthyl butyrate esterase in the presence and absence of 5 mM dimethyl succinate.

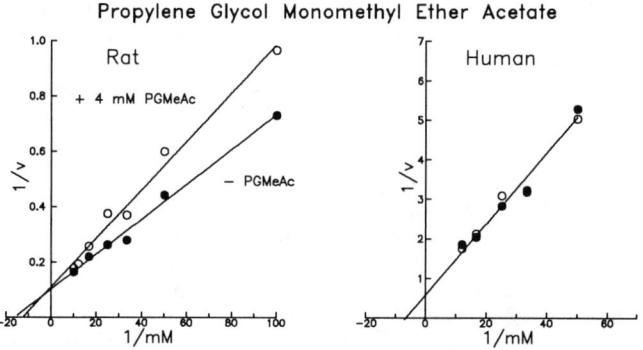

Figure 8. Kinetics of rat and human nasal α-naphthyl butyrate esterase in the presence and absence of 5 mM propylene glycol monomethyl ether acetate.

In conclusion, these data suggest that rat nasal α-naphthyl butyrate esterase has a very broad substrate specificity, and measurement of its activity in rat cells is expected to be a useful indicator of the ability of rodent nasal cultures to metabolize the industrial esters. On the other hand, the human activity apparently has a more narrow substrate specificity, necessitating further studies to determine the minimum number of esterase substrates needed to screen cultured human nasal cells for toxic carboxylester-activating activity.

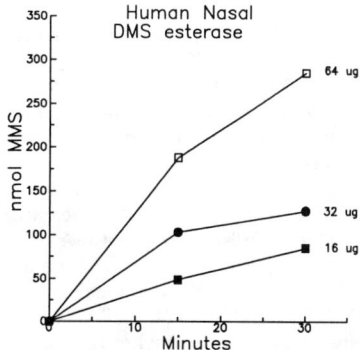

Figure 9. Time course of hydrolysis of dimethylsuccinate (8mM) to monomethylsuccinate by human nasal homogenate.

Acknowledgments

We thank Dr. John Morris for performing the HPLC analyses for the dimethylsuccinate esterase assays. This work was supported in part by a grant from the Johns Hopkins Center for Animal Testing (P.M.M.) and by PHS grant HL28669-10 (Dr. Michelle Cloutier, University of Connecticut Health Center).

References
1. CAMERON, G.R., et al. (1946) J. Pathol. 58: 449-456.
2. TORJUUSSEN, W. (1983), Nasal cancer in nickel workers. Histopathological findings and nickel concentrations in the nasal mucosa of nickel workers, and a short review of chromium and arsenic, Nasal Tumors in Animals and Man, Vol 2, G. Reznik and S.F. Stinson, (Eds.), CRC Press, Boca Raton, 33-53.
3. KOENIG, J.Q. and PIERSON, W.E. (1984) Nasal responses to air pollutants. (1984) Clin. Rev. Allergy 2: 255-261.
4. PRASAD, U. (1983) Nasopharangeal carcinoma in man. Nasal Tumors in Animals and Man, Vol. 1, G. Reznik and S. F. Stinson (Eds.), CRC Press, Boca Raton, 151-186.
5. BUIATTI, E., GEDDES, M., CARNEVALE, F., and MERLER, E. (1983) Nasal cavity and paranasal sinus tumors in woodworkers and shoemakers in Italy compared to other countries. Nasal Tumors in Animals and Man, Vol 1, G. Reznik and S.F. Stinson (Eds.), CRC Press, Boca Raton, 111-136.
6. BUCKLEY, L.A., JIANG, X.Z., JAMES, R.A., MORGAN, K.T., and BARROW, C.S. (1984) Respiratory tract lesions induced by sensory irritants at the RD50 concentration. Toxicol. Appl. Pharmacol. 74: 417-429.
7. SCHREIDER, J.P. (1986), Comparative anatomy of the nasal passages. Toxicology of the Nasal Passages, C.S. Barrow, (Ed.), Hemisphere, Washington, D.C., 1-23.
8. STOTT, W.T., RAMSEY, J.C., and MCKENNA, M.J. (1986), Absorption of chemical vapors by the upper respiratory tract of rats, Toxicology of the Nasal Passages, C.S. Barrow (Ed.), Hemisphere, Washington, D.C., 191-210.
9. DAHL, A.R., and HADLEY, W.M. (1991), Nasal cavity enzymes involved in xenobiotic metabolism: Effects on the toxicity of inhalants, Crit. Rev. Toxicol. 21: 345-372.
10. DAHL, A.R., HADLEY, W.M., HAHN, F.F., BENSON, J.M., and MCCLELLAN, R.O. (1982), Cytochrome P-450-dependent monooxygenases in olfactory epithelium of dogs: Possible role in tumorigenicity, Science 216: 57-59.5.
11. DAHL, A.R. (1986), Possible consequences of cytochrome P-450-dependent monooxygenases in nasal tissues, Toxicology of the Nasal Passages, C.S. Barrow (Ed.) Hemisphere, Washington, D.C., 263-273.
12. CASANOVA-SCHMITZ, M., DAVID, R.M., and HECK, H.D. (1984), Oxidation of formaldehyde and acetaldehyde by NAD+-dependent dehydrogenases in rat nasal mucosal homogenates, Biochem. Pharmacol. 33: 1137-1142.
13. DAHL, A.R., and WARUSZEWSKI, B.A. (1989), Metabolism of organonitriles to cyanide by rat nasal tissue enzymes, Xenobiotica 19: 1201-1205.
14. BOND, J.A. (1983) Some biotransformation enzymes responsible for polycyclic aromatic hydrocarbon metabolism in rat nasal turbinates: effects on enzyme activities of in vitro modifiers and intraperitoneal and inhalation exposure of rats to inducing agents, Cancer Research 43: 4804-4811.
15. STOTT, W.J., and MCKENNA, M.J. (1985), Hydrolysis of several glycol ether acetates and acrylic esters by nasal mucosal carboxylesterase in vitro, Fundam. Appl. Toxicol. 5: 399-404.
16. MILLER, R.R., YOUNG, J.T., KOCIBA, R.J., KEYES, D.G., BODNER, K.M., CALHOUN, L.L., and AYERS, J.A. (1985), Chronic toxicity and oncogenicity bioassay of inhaled ethyl acrylate in Fischer-344 rats and B6C3F1 mice, Drug Chem. Toxicol. 8: 1-42.
17. MILLER, R.R., HERMANN, E.A., YOUNG, J.T., CALHOUN, L.L., and KASTL, P.E. (1984), Propylene glycol monomethyl ether acetate (PGMEA) metabolism, disposition, and short-term vapor inhalation toxicity studies, Toxicol. Appl. Pharmacol. 75: 521-530.
18. KEENAN, C.M., KELLY, D.P., and BOGDANFFY, M.S. (1990), Degeneration and recovery of rat olfactory epithelium following inhalation of dibasic esters, Fundam. Appl. Toxicol. 15: 381-393.
19. MILLER, R.R., et al. (1981) Fundam. Appl. Toxicol. 1: 271-277.
20. TRELA, B.A., and BOGDANFFY, M.S. (1990), Carboxylesterase-dependent cytotoxicity of dibasic esters (DBE) in rat nasal explants, Toxicol. Appl. Pharmacol. 107: 285-301.

21. BOGDANFFY, M.S., RANDALL, H.W., and MORGAN, K.T. (1987), Biochemical quantitation and histochemical localization of carboxylesterase in the nasal passages of the Fischer-344 rat and B6C3F1 mouse, Toxicol Appl. Pharmacol. 88: 183-194.
22. MATTES, P.M., and MATTES, W.B. (1992), a-Naphthyl butyrate carboxylesterase activity in human and rat nasal tissue. Toxicol. Appl. Pharmacol. 114: 71-76.
23. VAN DOREN, K., and GLUZMAN, Y. (1984) Efficient transformation of human fibroblasts by Adenovirus-Simian Virus 40 recombinants. Mol. Cell. Biol. 4: 1653-1656.
24. MATTES, P.M., and GUGGINO, W.B. (1986), Derivation of virally transformed CF and non-CF nasal epithelial cultures and characterization of electrophysiological properties. Am. J. Hum. Genet. 39: A16.
25. WU, R., YANKASKAS, J, CHENG, E., KNOWLES, M.R., and BOUCHER, R.C. (1985), Growth and differentiation of human nasal epithelial cells in culture, Am. Rev. Resp. Dis. 132: 311-320.
26. LECHNER, J.F., and LAVECK, M.A. (1985), A serum-free method for culturing normal human bronchial epithelial cells at clonal density. J. Tissue Cult. Methods 9: 43-48.
27. MATTES, P.M., MATTES, W.B., and MORRIS, J.B. (1991), Rat nasal epithelial cell lines for *in vitro* toxicity testing: derivation and partial characterization. In Vitro Toxicology: Mechanisms and New Technology, Alternative Methods in Toxicology, Book 8, A. Goldberg (Ed.) Mary Ann Liebert,Inc., New York, pp.425-434.
28. STEELE, V.E., and ARNOLD, J.T. (1985). Isolation and long term culture of rat, rabbit, and human nasal turbinate cells. In Vitro Cell. Devel. Biol. 21: 681-687.
29. SUN, T.T., and GREENE, H. (1978), Immunofluorescent staining of keratin fibers in cultured cells. Cell 14: 469-476.
30. STEELE, R.E., PRESTON, A.S., JOHNSON, J.P., and HANDLER, J.S. (1986) Porous bottom dishes for culture of polarized cells. Am. J. Physiol. 251: C136-C139.
31. HANDLER, J.S., PERKINS, F.M., and JOHNSON, J.P. (1980) Studies of renal cell function using cell culture techniques. Am. J. Physiol. 238: F1-F9.
32. BOGDANFFY, M.S., KEE, C.R., HINCHMAN, C.A., and TRELA, B.A. (1990), Metabolism of dibasic esters by rat nasal mucosal carboxylesterase. Drug Metab. Disp. 19: 124-129.
33. SEGEL, I. (1976), Biochemical Calculations, 2nd edition, Wiley, New York, 234.
34. KRAJINA, Z., and ZIRDUM, A. (1987), Histochemical analysis of nasal polyps. Acta Oto Laryngol. 103: 435-440.
35. BONNEFOI, M.S., RANDALL, H.W., LEVINE, R., KENAN, P.D., MORGAN, K.T. (1992), Metabolism of aldehydes and esters in human respiratory nasal mucosa: a biochemical and histochemical study. The Toxicologist 12: 399.
36. MATTES, P.M., MATTES, W.B., and MORRIS, J.B. (1992), Human and rat nasal alpha-naphthyl butyrate esterase activity: kinetics and substrate specificity. The Toxicologist 12: 398.

ABO# Development of a Characterized Human Renal Proximal Tubule Cell Line

LORRAINE RACUSEN[1] and JOHNG S. RHIM[2]

[1]Department of Pathology
The Johns Hopkins University School of Medicine
720 Rutland Avenue
Baltimore, MD 21205

[2]Laboratory of Cellular and Molecular Biology
National Cancer Institute
Bethesda, MD 20894

An Adeno-12-SV_{40} hybrid vector has been used to develop continually proliferating clones of human renal proximal tubular cells. While non-immortalized cells from the human nephrectomy specimen used for tubular cell harvesting grew in vitro for less than 6 passages, cells from the same kidney exposed to the immortalizing agent have been grown in vitro for over 40 passages. At passage 21, 15 clones were developed using dilution cloning. Of these clones, 3 clones with typical epithelial cell morphology, monolayer growth pattern, and expression of the proximal tubular brush border enzyme gamma-glutamyl transpeptidase were selected for further characterization. All 3 clones were found to be non-producers of the immortalizing vector in a Vero cell assay. Monitoring of cells over subsequent passages revealed a subgroup of cells within each of the selected clones which had strong cell surface expression of brush border enzymes, in contrast to weaker expression in the majority of cells. We are currently using an immunodissection technique utilizing antibody to one of these enzymes, alkaline phosphatase, to develop a subclone or subclones which strongly express this differentiated property. These differentiated clones will then be exposed to a panel of compounds we have found to enhance differentiation in non-immortalized cells, including phorbol esters and agents which elevate intracellular c-AMP, and further characterized by ultrastructural, biochemical, and electrophysiologic techniques. An optimal clone grown under conditions producing maximal differentiation will then be utilized for toxicity testing using the known tubular toxin mercuric chloride, to validate its usefulness as a model system for the human renal proximal tubule.

The renal proximal tubule is sensitive to a variety of environmental and chemotherapeutic toxic agents, and is an important site of toxic injury (1-3). In humans, however, this epithelium is inaccessible to direct study, and harvesting of fresh renal tissue from humans for in vitro studies is also difficult. The kidneys of other mammals can be directly studied in vivo, and tissue and cells harvested for in vitro studies, but this requires, of course, the sacrifice of the animals. My laboratory and a few others have harvested and cultured tubular cells from normal cortex of human kidneys surgically removed for trauma or tumor for study with some success (4-7), but many laboratories do not have access to such tissue, and cells are generally utilized in primary culture or early passages, requiring a steady supply of human kidney tissues.

Previous studies have demonstrated that non-transformed human proximal tubular cells can be isolated and grown readily in culture and express differentiated properties in vitro. Inability to propagate these cells beyond 6-7 passages, however, and the need to constantly control for isolate-to-isolate variation, in addition to difficulty in obtaining suitable human tissue, makes it highly desirable to develop a cell line or cell line from such isolates. Well-differentiated human renal tubular cell lines have not been developed, (probably in part due to difficulty in obtaining suitable human kidney tissue). There have been reports of transformation of human kidney cells by transfection (8, 9), but these cells have not been well characterized.

Human epithelial cells have historically proven relatively difficult to transform and immortalize. Strategies such as manipulation of growth conditions or exposure to chemical transforming agents which have been used to transform rodent cells have rarely been successful with human cells (10). However, there are now viral antigens which have been developed and used to immortalize human epithelial cells from skin (11, 12), respiratory epithelium (12-14), and salivary gland (15). Human cells can now be transformed via transfection with plasmids or infection with hybrid viruses. Using these agents, human epithelial cell lines have been developed which retain differentiated features, and are non-oncogenic. A differentiated proximal tubular cell line of human origin should be possible to develop and characterize.

The long-range goals of these studies, then, are: a) to develop immortal human proximal tubule cell line(s) which will propagate indefinitely in vitro; b) to characterize immortal clones morphologically and physiologically to define level of differentiation and allow selection of optimally differentiated clones; and c) to utilize selected cell lines for toxicity testing, comparing cytopathic effects of mercuric chloride, a known proximal tubule toxin, on non-transformed isolates of human proximal tubule cells and selected immortal cell lines. The ultimate aim is to develop a human renal proximal tubule cell line or cell lines which can be used in lieu of kidney tissue and cells from experimental animals for detection and study of toxic effects on the renal tubule.

Research Plan and Methods

Normal renal proximal tubular cells were harvested for these studies from normal cortex of a surgical nephrectomy specimen removed for tumor. The capsule overlying uninvolved normal cortex was removed and strips of outer cortex harvested using sterile techniques. Cortical tissue was then minced in Joklik's modification of Eagle's minimum essential medium (JMEM, GIBCO) plus 10mM Hepes, 1.2mM $CaCl_2$ and freshly added collagenase, 100 units/ml (Sigma) at 37° in a laminar flow hood and transferred to Spinner flasks. Tissue was then further digested for 15-minute spins x3 at 37°C, with the supernatant collected after each spin and fresh collagenase solution added. Cells and tissue fragments in the supernatant were pelleted by gentle centrifugation (72g x 5 min) and resuspended in JMEM with 15 units/ml DNAase, to prevent cell clumping. Tubular fragments and glomeruli were removed by filtering the suspension through 160u and then 40u nylon mesh, following which 5% heat-inactivated fetal calf serum was added. Cell viability was assessed using a hemocytometer and Trypan blue exclusion. For culture, cells from primary isolates were plated in precoated plastic culture plates at $1x10^6$ viable cells/ml.

Cultures were maintained at 37°C in a 95% CO_2;95% air atmosphere, and refed every 2-3 days with Hams F12:DMEM with 10mM Hepes and tapering amounts of fetal calf serum (10%/5%/2.5%). At 5% and below, medium was supplemented with 5ug/ml insulin, 5 ug/ml transferrin, 5×10^{-8}M Na selenite, 5×10^{-8}M hydrocortisone, and 3×10^{-8}M triiodothyrone. This medium has been shown to promote growth and differentiation of cultured renal proximal tubular cells.

For initial transformation studies, we used an SV40 antigen-containing plasmid, pSV_3-neo, which has been used successfully to transform human epithelial cells (12). Briefly, the cells were transfected with the SV40T-bearing plasmid while in exponential growth phase, using polybrene (10ug/ml) exposure for 6 hours in conjunction with dimethyl sulfoxide shock (30% DMSO for 4 minutes) (16). This agent, however, was not successful in prolonging cell survival in vitro beyond the usual period of senescence of these cells in culture.

In additional studies, we used an agent which had proven successful in transforming a range of human cells in culture (11-15), an Adeno 12:SV40 hybrid virus which carries SV40 viral genomic material into the cell by infection via the adenovirus 12. The virus was introduced into the culture medium while the human renal proximal tubular cells were in exponential growth phase in the first passage from primary culture. The cells were then maintained in culture and monitored. Cells from the same isolate which had not been exposed to the viral agent were cultured in parallel. Growth of culture cells was monitored by phase contrast microscopy. Once monolayers reached confluence, cells were harvested by trypsin digestion and passaged. Monolayers were monitored serially for expression at the proximal tubular brush border enzyme gamma-glutamyl-transpeptidase (GGTP).

For <u>GGTP staining</u>, cells were fixed for 30 seconds in cold citrate-acetone fixative, rinsed well, and allowed to air-dry. Assays for GGTP were performed using a histochemical method based on measurement of the 4-methy-2-naphthylanine liberated from the artificial substrate gamma-glutamyl-p-nitroaniline (17). Briefly, air-dried specimens were incubated in a substrate solution containing gamma-glutamyl-4-methoxy naphthylamide in Tris-buffered saline (pH 7.4) with glycylglycine and fast Blue BB for 5 minutes. Specimens were then rinsed in saline, transferred to .1M cupric sulfate for 2 minutes, rinsed again with saline and then distilled H_2O, dried and mounted. A red reaction product forms in the presence of the enzyme. Negative controls were run in adjacent chambers of the chambered slide, and positive and negative controls were done on frozen sections of human kidney as well.

After cloning, alkaline phosphatase activity was also determined using a standard histochemical method (18).

<u>Results</u>

The non-transformed cells quickly lost proliferative capacity and become senescent. In contrast, populations of cells exposed to the adeno 12:SV40 virus continued to grow, forming monolayers of epithelial-appearing cells through successive passages. At passage 19, cells in confluent monolayers were stained for the brush border enzyme gamma-glutamyl transpeptidase, an enzyme localized to the proximal tubule of the nephron. Most cells in the monolayer expressed enzyme activity, demonstrating that they retained this differentiated feature of the renal proximal tubule. At passage 21, cells from confluent monolayers were harvested, diluted to cloning density, and seeded into two 24-well plates. Growth was carefully monitored, and only wells containing a single clone of cells were maintained. Eighteen separate clones have been isolated by this technique.

A range of growth characteristics were seen in the propagated clones. A few attached and grew in a net-like pattern without forming confluent monolayers.

Others grew as monolayer but began proliferating and mounding above the monolayer while still only partially confluent. Some, however, grew to confluent flat monolayers of epithelial-appearing cells. At passage 27, as the cells from the clones were being passaged, cytospin preparations were prepared and stained for gamma-glutamyl transpeptidase as above. Three clones that expressed moderate enzyme activity, had appropriate cell morphology and a monolayer growth pattern were then evaluated for viral shedding.

To test for evidence of viral shedding, media from confluent monolayers of the selected clones were placed on cultures of Vero cells, a cell line highly sensitive to viropathic effects. All three of the selected clones appear to be non-producers, with no evidence of viropathic effects in the Vero cells.

The three selected clones are being propagated in vitro for studies of morphologic and functional properties. They have now maintained excellent in vitro growth capacity to 40 passages. At passage 37 of the three selected clones, it was noted that while cells maintained epithelial morphology, a subpopulation of cells in each clone were larger and showed stronger expression of brush border enzymes GGTP and alkaline phosphatase than the remaining cells. One of these clones was selected and a subclone has been developed using an immunodissection technique (18). Briefly, a plastic culture plate was coated with human monoclonal IgG antibody to human kidney-type alkaline phosphatase, and cells from the clone were layered briefly onto this coated plate. Non-adherent cells were removed and the growth surface washed repeatedly. Cells which remained adherent to the antibody-coated plate are currently being propagated in vitro for further characterization.

Discussion

These studies are designed to develop an immortal human renal proximal tubule cell line which retains differentiated features, and can be used as an in vitro model system to study injury to this epithelial cell system. An understanding of the mechanisms of human tubular cell injury would lead to better strategies for prevention and treatment of such toxicity. The availability of human cells for study would also reduce the need to use tissues and cells from other small mammals for such studies. The overall aim is to develop a cell line which could be utilized by many investigators for studies of proximal tubular cell injury.

In vitro cell culture systems, and especially cell lines, in addition to providing an alternative to live animal experimentation, actually offer several advantages over in vivo animal studies for the detection and analysis of mechanisms of action of toxic chemicals on a give target cell. These include: absence of in vivo factors such as hemodynamic, hormonal and neural influences which may modify cellular response to the toxin; precise definition and control of cellular milieu; rapid cellular response to a potential toxin and equally rapid detection of that cellular response; and ability to replicate observations in a uniform population of cells. Human cell culture systems are desirable as they are probably most applicable to in vivo toxicity in humans. Even a partially differentiated cell line, provided it is well-characterized, would be a useful tool in defining toxic effects on the human proximal tubule.

The next phase of development of this cell line is currently underway. The newly derived subclone will be tested for ploidy using fluorescence activated cell sorting. A variety of differentiating growth factors and matrix components will be screened for effects on growth and expression of differentiated structural and ultrastructural properties, biochemical properties, and electrical resistance and transport properties characteristic of human proximal tubule.

To validate the cell line for suitability for a model system for toxic injury to the human proximal tubule, in vitro toxicity testing is planned using normal human proximal tubule cells as controls. The known proximal tubular toxin mercuric chloride will be used (19-22). Dose response studies of effects on morphology, lactate dehydrogenase releases, vital dye exclusion, and electrical and transport properties will be carried out. Demonstration that the immortalized cell line shows pathologic and pathophysiologic changes the same or similar to those seen in wild-type cells would support the usefulness of the cell line as a model system for this important and vulnerable human epithelial cell system.

References

1. Solez, K. (1983), Acute renal failure, Pathology of the Kidney, R.H. Heptinstall (Ed.) Little, Brown and Co., 1069.

2. Bennett W.M., Elzinga, L.W., Porter, G.A. (1991). Tubulointerstitial disease and toxic nephropathy, The Kidney, B. Brenner and F. Rector (Eds.) W.B. Saunders Co., 1491.

3. Olsen, S. (1989), Acute tubular necrosis and toxic renal injury, Renal Pathology, C.G. Tisher, and B.M. Brenner (Eds.) Lippincott, 656.

4. Trifillis, A.L., Regec, A.L., and Trump, B.F., (1985). Isolation, culture, and charterization of human renal tubular cells. J. Urol. 133:324.

5. Detrisac, C.J., Sens, M.A., Garvin, A.J., Spicer, S.S., and Sens, D.A. (1984), Tissue culture of human kidney epithelial cells of proximal tubule origin. Kidney Int. 25:383.

6. Wilson, P.D., Dillingham, M.A., Breckon, R., and Anderson, R. J., (1985). Defined human renal tubular epithelia in culture: growth, characterization, and hormonal response. Am. J. Physiol. 248:F436.

7. Kempson, S.A., McAteer, J.A., Al-Mahrouq, H.A., Dousa, T.P., Dougherty, G.S., and Evan, A.P., (1989). Proximal tubule characteristics of cultured human renal cortex epithelium. J. Lab. Clin. Med. 113:285.

8. Graham, F.L., Smiley, J., Russell, W.C., Nairn, R., (1977). Characteristics of a human cell line transformed by DNA from human adenovirus type 5. J. Gen. Virol. 36:59.

9. Whittaker, J.L., Byrd, J., Grand, R.J., and Gallimore, P.H., (1984). Isolation and characterization of 4 adenovirus type-12 transformed human embryo kidney cell lines. Mol. Cell Biol. 4:110.

10. Rhim, J.S., (1989). Neoplastic transformation of human epithelial cells in vitro. Anticancer Res. 9:1345.

11. Rhim, J.S., Jay, G., Arnstein, P., Price, F.M., Sanford, K.K., and Aaronson, S.A., (1985). Neoplastic transformation of human epidermal keratinocytes by Ad12-SV_{40} and Kirsten Sarcoma virus. Science 227:1250.

12. Rhim, J.S., Park, J.B., and Kawakami, T., (1988). Techniques for establishing human epithelial cell cultures: sensitivity of cell lines for propagation of herpesviruses. J. Virol. Methods 21:209.

13. Zeitlin, P.L., Lu, L., Rhim, J.S., Cutting, G., Stetten, G., Kieffer, K.A., Craig, R. and Guzzino, W.B., (1991). A cystic fibrosis bronchial epithelial cell line: immortalization by Ad12-SV$_{40}$ infection. Am. J. Resp. Cell and Mol. Biol. 4:313.

14. Scholte, B.J., Bijman, J., Hoogeveen, A.T., Willemse, R., Rhim, J.S. and Van der Kamp, W.M., (1989). **Immortalization of nasal polyp epithelial cells** from cystic fibrosis patients. Exp. Cell. Res. 182:559.

15. Rhim, J.S., Rhim, J.S., Fox, R.I., Ablashi, D.V., Salahuddin, S.Z., Buchbinder, A., and Joseph, S.F. (1988). Establishment of salivary gland epithelial cell lines from patients with Sjogrens Syndrome and normal individuals, Epstein-Barr Virus and Human Disease, Alblashi, Fag-Faggin\oni, Krueger, Pagano, Pearson (Eds.) Humana Press, 155-161.

16. Rhim, J.S., Park, J.B. and Jay, G., (1989). Neoplastic transformation of human keratinocytes by polybrene-induced DNA-mediated transfer of an activated oncogene. Oncogen 4:1403.

17. Rutenberger, A.M., Kim, N., Fischbein, J.W., Hasker, J.S., Wasserkrug, H.L., and Seligman, A.M., (1981). Histochemical and ultrastrucutral demonstration of gamma glutamyl transpeptidase activity in serum and plasma. Clin. Chem. 27:1190.

18. Ackerman, G.A., (1962). Substituted naphthol AS phosphate derivatives for the localization of leukocyte alkaline phosphatase activity. Lab. Invest. 11:563.

19. Flamenbaum, W., McDonald, F.D., DiBona, G.F., Oken, D.E., (1971). Micropuncture study of renal tubular factors in low dose mercury poisoning. Nephron 8:221.

20. McDowell, E.M., Nagle, R.B., Zalme, R.C., McNeil, J.S., Flamenbaum, W., and Trump, B.F., (1976). Studies on the pathophysiology of acute renal failure. I. Correlation of ultrastructure and function in the proximal tubule of the rat following administration of mercuric chloride. Virchows Arch. [Cell Pathol.] 22:173.

21. Weinberg, J.M., Harding, P.G., and Humes, H.D., (1982). Mitochondrial bioenergetics during the initiation of Mercuric chloride-induced renal injury. J. Biol. Chem. 257:60.

22. Troyer, D.A., Kreisberg, J.I., and Venkatachalam, M.A., (1986). Lipid alterations in LLC-PK$_1$ cells exposed to mercuric chloride. Kidney Int. 29:530.

D. Draize Eye Testing Alternatives

Draize Eye Testing Alternatives—A Perspective

JAMES P. McCULLEY[1] and THOMAS J. STEPHENS[2]

[1]*Department of Ophthalmology*
University of Texas Southwestern Medical School
Dallas, TX 75235

[2]*Thomas J. Stephens & Associates, Inc.*
Carrollton, TX 75006

ABSTRACT

There has been considerable public and scientific interest in the Draize ocular test in recent years; consequently, there have been major efforts to develop *in vitro* alternatives to this test which has traditionally been carried out in rabbits. Realization that the Draize test is used for different purposes by different industries has allowed adjustments to be made in animal testing even without regulatory agency acceptance. For instance, the pharmaceutical industry can use *in vitro* methods to screen products for non-toxicity and take only those products that appear to be non-toxic onto animal and human testing.

Progress has been made in identifying *in vitro* tests to replace the Draize eye test; however, a universally accepted test or battery of tests have yet been identified. Most likely, the test battery will consist of test(s) that will predict cytotoxicity, non-cytotoxicity induced inflammation, and, possibly, effects on nutrition and metabolism of cells. Problems related to *in vitro* testing of non-water soluble preparations in tissue culture must also be addressed. It is anticipated that with continued research, it will be possible to develop a battery of endpoints or tests that will allow testing in animals only of substances that are thought to be non-toxic.

BACKGROUND

All consumers want safe products; however, there is no consensus among interested parties on how to achieve this goal. For over forty years, the Draize eye test has been the accepted standard for substantiating the safety of consumer products, ocular medications and chemicals that might accidently be splashed into the eyes of workers (1).

Prior to the 1930's, the manufacturers of products were not required to substantiate the safety of their products, including drugs. In 1937, 107 Americans tragically died when Elixir of Sulfanilamide was marketed without safety testing. The company that manufactured the product used a toxin, diethylene glycol, as the solvent (2).

****
Dedicated to the Memory of Dale R. Meyer, Ph.D.
****

The development of Draize eye test has its origin in cosmetics usage. In the early 1930's, an untested eyelash product containing a synthetic aniline was marketed under the name of Lure-Lash. Usage of the product by the public was catastrophic. Recorded adverse effects included allergic contact dermatitis of periocular tissue, loss of vision, and death. Congress responded with the promulgation of the the Food, Drug, and Cosmetic (FDC) Act of 1938 (3). This law was rapidly followed by the development of animal testing methods designed to protect the American public. A pharmacologist named John Draize was hired by the FDA to develop animal tests to predict eye and skin irritation (2). In spite of the criticism of animal activists, John Draize should be considered an American pioneer in product safety assessment.

The FDC Act of 1938 established the concept that the cosmetic manufacturer must substantiate the safety of ingredients and finished products prior to marketing the product. Under the law, any ingredient or product whose safety is not adequately substantiated prior to marketing is inadequately labelled (i.e. misbranded) unless it is labelled with the statement "**The safety of this product has not been determined**"(4).

Interestingly, the authors of the act did not specify the types of tests required to substantiate the safety of products. This wording was not an accident. They undoubtedly expected the methods of testing to improve with time and did not want the law to specify outdated test methods.

During the last decade, the cosmetic industry became the target of the animal rights movement (5). The early goal of the movement was to reduce and refine animal tests and, when possible, replace them with *in vitro* tests. The cosmetic industry responded by having their trade group, the Cosmetic, Toiletry, and Fragrance Association (CTFA), provide seed money to help establish the Johns Hopkins Center for Alternatives to Animal Testing (CAAT). The major focus of research was the replacement of the Draize eye test with a suitable *in vitro* test. Many of the early tests were simple, cytotoxicity assays with monolayer cultures and *in vitro* measurements of inflammation using fertilized chick eggs (6).

In 1991, the CTFA, as well as over one hundred corporations, government agencies and individuals, provided contributions to support the mission of CAAT. CAAT provides financial support to individual and group scientists in order to foster the development of scientifically acceptable *in vitro* tests and other alternative methods. The Humane Society of the United States presented its first Russel and Burch Award to Dr. Alan Goldberg, Ph.D., Director of CAAT, in order to honor his contributions to the advancement of alternatives to the use of animals in research, testing, and education (7).

The FDA, as well as other regulatory agencies, remains skeptical about the possibility of *in vitro* tests rapidly replacing the Draize eye test. This skepticism is based in inherent over-simplification of the physiology and response of the whole animal system (8). This does not mean that FDA is not concerned with animal testing. Their goal is to assure the safety of the American public using the best available test methods. At present, this includes animal testing. Many other professional organizations including the Society of Toxicology (SOT), the American College of Toxicology (ACT), the American Medical Association (AMA), and the European Chemical Industry Ecology and Toxicology Centre (ECETOC) stress the continued need for using animals in research and testing (9).

In our quest to eliminate animal suffering, we should not become discouraged. It is likely that pressure from the public and scientific community, as well as the expense associated with animal testing, will continue to drive the development of *in vitro* tests to replace the Draize eye test. The cost of safety testing on animals has been estimated to range from $20,000 to over $1,000,000 for a comprehensive safety work-up (10). The use of *in vitro* tests could substantially reduce this cost.

Additionally, public opinion polls continue to show that the American public would prefer to purchase products from companies that have not been tested on animals (11). This is reflected by the public's pressuring for laws attempting to limit animal testing. In 1990 alone, ten bills were pending in eight states that would eliminate cosmetic testing on animals. A major focus of these bills was to eliminate the Draize eye and skin test. Although none of the bills became law, the bill introduced in California passed both Houses only to be vetoed by by the Governor. It is likely that such bills will be reintroduced in the future.

Recently, the European Community Parliament voted 202 to 60 to accept a total ban on animal testing of cosmetics and cosmetic ingredients. Under the ban a committee on alternative non-animal testing methods would, in cooperation with the Parliament's Scientific Committee on Cosmetology, evaluate the safety of non-animal testing methods proposed by the Commission or member states. The ban is scheduled to go into effect in 1994 (12).

The intent of this article is to give the reader a new perspective on alternative tests to the Draize eye test. An alterative test can be either an *in vitro* test or a human clinical procedure that reduces the dependency on the Draize eye test. In this article we will review recent progress in Draize alternative test development as well as discuss how alternatives tests fit into the safety decision process.

TERMINOLOGY

In vitro Test - Any test procedure that is not conducted in animals or humans. *In vitro* tests are placed into the categories of "predictive" or "diagnostic," based on their use. These tests typically involve measuring changes, or endpoints, such as chemical reactions or alterations in cellular functions in eukaryotes or prokaryotes. Depending on the level of confidence, *in vitro* tests may be used as screening tests or as replacement tests.

Alternative Test - Any procedure that refines, reduces or replaces (i.e. the three R's of alternatives) the use of whole animals. Unlike an *in vitro* test, an alternative test may include a human test procedures as well as alternative *in vivo* procedures.

Draize Eye Test - A whole animal test method developed by Friedenwald and refined by Draize to assess the ocular irritation potential of products. The test is based on instilling either 0.1 ml (liquids) or 0.1 g (powder) onto one eye of each of three to six rabbits for a specified, short period of time (usually one second). The contralateral eye serves as an untreated control. Using no instrumentation, eyes are graded at 24, 48, and 72 hours and sometimes up to 21 days after instillation and assigned a numerical score based on ocular damage. The grading scale is weighted so that 73% of the scoring assesses gross changes in the cornea, 9.0% of the score assess the iris and 18% of the score assess damage to the conjunctivae. The Draize test has the ability to assess ocular damage as well as recovery of ocular tissues. At present, there are separate applications of the Draize eye test in the chemical industry, biomedical research, consumer product testing, and the ophthalmic pharmaceutical industry (1).

Ocular Irritant - Any material intentionally instilled or accidently spilled into the eyes that produces undesirable changes in vision or deleterious effects on ocular tissues, either immediately or at a later time.

Cytotoxin - Any agent that has the ability to damage or kill cells, *in vivo* or *in vitro*. Ocular irritants may or may not be cytotoxic depending on their mechanism of toxicity.

Inflammation - A reproducible change in a tissue or organ characterized by redness (erythema), edema (chemosis), warmth, pain, and an influx of immune cells. Inflammation is associated with the synthesis and release of active agents and hormones from cells. These agents include vasoactive amines, eicosanoids, complement components, and cytokines.

Validation - The process by which the credibility of a candidate test is established for a specific purpose. Scientific criteria for the validation of *in vitro* toxicity tests have been developed by Dr. John Frazier. The factors which are considered essential to validation include a standard protocol, intra-laboratory and inter-laboratory studies on standardized chemicals representing the category of interest, and the derivation of the sensitivity and specificity of the assay (13, 14).

Mechanistic Test - An *in vitro* test that measures an endpoint that has clear biological or pathophysiological relevance to the effects that would be detected *in vivo*. *In vitro* cell culture systems which measure cytotoxicity and inflammation are examples of mechanistic tests for dermal and ocular irritation. It is anticipated that only mechanistic based *in vitro* tests will receive regulatory and scientific acceptance as Draize eye and skin test replacements.

Phenomenological Test - An *in vitro* test that measures an endpoint that does not show a clear relevance to the effects that would be detected *in vivo*. Phenomenological tests may be correlative tests in that a mathematical relation may exist between the non-mechanistic endpoint measured *in vitro* and the toxicological endpoint observed *in vivo*. In some circumstances, phenomenological tests may have value as simple toxicity screening tests, although they are not good candidates for regulatory or scientific community acceptance. Examples of phenomenological test are protein matrix tests for eye and skin irritation.

MECHANISMS OF OCULAR INJURY (PATHOPHYSIOLOGY)

While there are undoubtedly numerous biological pathways for tissue or organ injury to occur, the prediction of some events seem more fundamental than others. This is especially true for many ocular and skin irritants. Clues for understanding the events of ocular irritation can be found by studying the gross responses of various ocular tissues after instillation of an irritant.

Ocular irritants simultaneously produce change in multiple ocular tissues of the anterior segment of the eye. The severity of the damage to each of the tissues is related to the strength of the irritant. Many ocular irritants affect the vascular beds of the conjunctiva and lids, directly producing symptoms of redness, vascular injection, and edema. These reactions are the result of cytotoxic effects on surface epithelial cells and deeper lymphoid tissue or by directly effecting mast cells that release histamine and other vasoactive substances.

The cornea of primates and birds is composed of five layers including epithelium, Bowman's membrane, stroma, Descemet's membrane and endothelium. Other animals have only four layers since they lack Bowman's membrane. Damage to any of these layers as well as alterations in the tear film that bathes the cornea may affect visual acuity. Mild irritants that disrupt the tear film of the eye eye can alter the wettability of the corneal epithelium resulting in corneal erosions or ulcers (15). This can occur independent of changes in transparency. Fluorescein or rose bengal staining will detect damage to the corneal epithelium.

The cornea is transparent because of the regular arrangement of uniform collagen fibers in the stroma. Table A lists the frequent causes for corneal opacification. Toxic events such as the disruption of the stroma, the presence of stromal edema and the influx of inflammatory cells have the potential to produce corneal opacity. These events often produce opacity by disturbing the arrangement of the collagen in the stroma so that the distance between the fibers exceeds one-half the wavelength of light or by altering the collagen fibrils themselves..

TABLE A
CAUSES FOR CORNEAL OPACIFICATION
Disruption of Stroma
Stromal Edema
Inflammatory Infiltrate
Epithelial Coagulation
Deposition of Opaque Material in Cornea

Coagulation of epithelial cells occurs when external contact agents such as strong acids or bases are instilled into the eyes. The degree of damage due to acids is related to the pH and the capacity of the anion or cation to bind to the epithelial protein or penetrate more deeply into the cornea (16). In general, the coagulation of the protein in the anterior segment of the eye by an acid often provides a barrier that limits the amount of damage to the endothelium of the cornea. The damage observed in the first few hours often reflects the extent of the long term damage. In contrast, alkali burns are often produced by such compounds as household ammonia and sodium hydroxide which disrupt epithelium and pass rapidly through the cornea disrupting both stromal and endothelial cells. Later events such as infiltration, ulceration and perforation are often observed up to one to four weeks after the initial contact (16).

The deposition of opaque material in the cornea can produce opacity. Hydroquinone is a colorless dust that when oxidized produces a brown benzoquinone. Exposure to the eye to this material results in the formation of brown lines. This brown band keratopathy is the result of storage of this opaque material in or near the basal layer of the epithelium (16).

The determinants of ocular recovery are the degree and extent of cell death. Cells with reversible changes have a better chance of recovering compared to disrupted cells or cells with latent toxic effects. Damage to critical epithelial stem cells located at the corneal limbus and corneal endothelium cells as well as diffuse surface damage will impede or prevent recovery. Corneal endothelium has little to no regenerative capability. A healthy endothelial layer is critical to corneal clarity as it constantly pumps fluid out of the stroma (i.e. prevents stromal edema) which has an innate tendency to swell.

Eyes dosed with a test material that does not penetrate into Bowman's membrane and the stroma have a greater potential to recover than eyes dosed with test materials that do penetrate these layers. Clearing or reversing of changes in opacity are associated with the movement of fluid and inflammatory cells out of the stromal layers and wound healing of the epithelial layer.

Irreversible opacity occurs when irritants produce significant cell death, especially of the corneal endothelium and epithelial stem cells, disruption of stromal proteins or induce severe inflammation. Strong acids and alkalies are examples of chemicals that frequently produce irreversible effects.

Direct injury to the iris is characterized by engorged leaky blood vessels with aqueous cell and flare and thickening of the stromal layer (edema). Aqueous flare is caused by the presence of plasma proteinaceous material in the anterior chamber. When light is shown into healthy eyes it passes through unimpeded. When protein is present in the aqueous humor as a result of ocular injury, the light will refract and the beam will be seen in the anterior chamber. This is called the the "Tydall Phenomenon." Anterior chamber cell and flare may also occur secondarily if there is sufficient ocular surface damage which in a short period of tome will cause iris vessels to become leaky, probably via the influence of released inflammatory mediators. A secondary iridocyclitis with resultant vascular leakage will lead to cell and flare in the aqueous humor.

The development of an alterative test battery must be based on mechanisms of injury depending on the nature of the test materials and the need of the investigator. While it may be impossible to have a battery that will account for all mechanisms, we can strive to select a basic test battery that will sufficiently predict acute toxicity. In establishing a battery of Draize alternative tests, it is essential that we have tests that, at a minimum, detect cytotoxicity and non-cytotoxic induced inflammation produced by vasoactive amines and eicosanoids. The ideal test battery will also include tests for predicting ocular recovery.

NEW *IN VITRO* ALTERNATIVE TESTS SINCE 1987

In 1987 Bausch & Lomb provided funding to CAAT for the development of a monograph entitled, *A Critical Evaluation of Alternatives to Acute Ocular Irritation Testing* (1). The book provided readers with a comprehensive review of the *in vitro* methods identified as potential replacements for Draize eye irritancy test and/or acute ocular irritancy testing. *In vitro* tests were classified into six different groups based on the type of endpoint measured (see Table B). Of the thirty plus assays reviewed by the authors, only a limited number of tests in the categories of cell metabolism (i.e. neutral red uptake and MTT reduction in mammalian tissue culture), cell and tissue physiology

TABLE B
CATEGORIES OF *IN VITRO* ALTERNATIVES
Morphologic
Cytotoxic
Cell and Tissue Physiology
Inflammation / Immunity
Mathematical Modeling
Phenomenologic (other)

(i.e. bovine corneal/corneal opacity), inflammation /immunity (i.e. HET-CAM, CAMVA and bovine corneal cup model), mediator release (i.e. PGE_2 synthesis in mammalian cell models), and phenomenological tests (i.e. protein matrix assays, computer based structure-activity relationships, and the Tetrahymena motility assay) were thought to show promise as first generation *in vitro* tests for ocular irritation. While none of the tests alone have the potential to replace the Draize eye test, they appear to have some potential as screening assays depending on the type of test materials.

The authors also identified the Draize alternative needs in the categories of research and validation (see Table C). Their recommendations were to hold a series of highly structured workshops to address technical and logistical issues of conducting *in vitro* tests, initiate micro- and macro-validation programs, standardize the Draize eye test and to educate scientists about the uses of *in vitro* tests.

TABLE C
SUMMARY OF 1987 DRAIZE ALTERNATIVE NEEDS
Development of improved methodology (especially for recovery and repair)
Understand toxico- and pharmaco- kinetics of materials *in vitro* and relationship to *in vivo*
Method to evaluate pain
Methods to assess complex mixtures, solids, and water insoluble materials
Relate QSAR to mechanisms
More clearly define specific aspects of validation

Several of these recommendations have been initiated, and in some circumstances, completed. With sponsorship from several companies, CAAT has published reports from two workshops to address the issues of technical problems associated with *in vitro* toxicity testing systems and structure-activity relationships (17, 18). Tufts University has held a series of workshops which developed a plan for the development, evaluation, validation, and implementation of alternative methods in the safety evaluation process (19).

Several organizations and trade groups have initiated either evaluation or validation programs of *in vitro* tests. The list includes Frame, the Soap and Detergent Association, the Cosmetic, Toiletries and Fragrance Association, The Commission of European Communities, Oeuvre pour l'Assistance aux Animaux de Laboratoire (OPAL), and the Bundesgesundheitsamt (BGA) (20). Many companies have begun private evaluation and validation programs of *in vitro* tests. These companies are in a unique position in that they have well define test formulations that have often been evaluated in both animal and human testing programs. While several of these programs have been made publicly available, the information from many other in-house programs are likely to remain proprietary. In June, 1991, the CAAT and the cellular toxicology committee of the Tissue Culture Association held a joint workshop to discuss current efforts of validation and the need to facilitate future validation. The conclusions of the meeting will be published as the CAAT Technical Report Number 5 (21).

In September, 1991, a workshop was held to update or harmonize the Draize eye test and the application of methods for assessing ocular safety. The workshop was the output of an as *ad hoc* group of scientists from the Consumer Product Safety Commission, Environmental Protection Agency, and the Food and Drug Administration. The topics discussed at the workshop included the use of various procedures to screen test materials for ocular irritation, the use of topical ocular anesthetics, the volume of test material instilled into a rabbit's eye, the number of test animals, scoring methods, sequential testing approaches, and the evaluation and classification of unknown test materials (14). Although the output of the workshop did not represent official positions of the regulatory agencies, it did represent an important step in standardization of the Draize eye test.

Education institutions such as the University of Texas, Johns Hopkins University, University of California, and others have begun educational efforts aimed at teaching students about the use of *in vitro* tests in product safety assessment. These efforts include classroom and laboratory training as well as site visits to corporate R&D and toxicology testing facilities. In addition, scientists can read about new *in vitro* tests and information gained through research in a number of new journals dedicated to *in vitro* technology.

In 1990, members of the drug safety subsection of the Pharmaceutical Manufacturers Association reviewed alternatives to the Draize test using volume 4 of *Alternative Methods in Toxicology* as a guide. The committee identified four tests (i.e. the enucleated superfused rabbit eye system, the corneal cup model, the corneal opacity test and the mouse eye permeability test) that, in their opinion, have the potential to serve as alternatives to the current Draize eye procedure. It is not in our opinion that these necessarily hold the greatest potential. The committee acknowledged that these tests fit into the category of refinement as opposed to replacement. Nineteen of the thirty-three *in vitro* tests, although not mechanistically relevant to eye injury, were classified as possibly useful for general acute irritation screens (see Table D). A third group of test systems, also not mechanistically relevant to eye injury, were designated inadequate. These tests are listed in Table E.

TABLE D
ACUTE IRRITATION SCREENING TESTS
Balb / c 3T3 Cells / Morphological Assays (HTD)
BHK Cells / Growth Inhibition
BHK Cells / Colony Formation Efficiency
BHK Cells / Cell Detachment
SIRC Cells / Colony Forming Assay
Balb / c 3T3 Cells / Total Protein
BCL-D1 Cells / Total Protein
LS Cells / Dual Dye Staining
Thymocytes / Dual Fluorescent Dye Staining
RCE-SIRC-P815-YAC-1 / Cr Release
L929 Cells / Cell Viability
Bovine Red Blood Cell / Hemolysis
Rabbit Corneal Cell Cultures / Plasminogen Activator
LS Cells / ATP Assay
Balb / c 3T3 Cells / Uridine Uptake Inhibition Assay
Balb / c 3T3 Cells / Neutral Red Uptake
HeLa Cells / Metabolic Inhibition Test (MIT-24)
Bovine Eye Cup / Histamine (Hm) and Leukotriene C4 (LT-C4) Release

TABLE E INADEQUATE TESTS	
Test	Reason Inadequate
Epidermal Slice / Electrical Conductivity	Irrelevant to eye
Rabbit Ileum / Contraction Inhibition	Irrelevant to eye; pharmacological model
Chorioallantoic Membrane (CAM)	Irrelevant to eye; *in vivo* test; correlations poor
Rat Peritoneal Cells / Histamine or Serotonin Release	Irrelevant to eye
Rat Vaginal Explant / Prostaglandin Release	Irrelevant to eye
Rabbit Corneal Epithelial Cells / Wound Healing	Potentially relevant to repair studies, but not injury
Protein Matrix Assay	Physiochemical reaction irrelevant to eye
Computer Based Structure Activity Relationship (SAR)	Output limited to database inputted; inadequate for novel structures / mixtures
Tetrahymena / Motility	Irrelevant to eye; questionable relevance to mammals

In 1992, a report of a double blind study was published in ATLA in which 465 cosmetic product formulations and raw ingredients were evaluated in Eytex™ (protein matrix assay) using one of four protocols. Data from these tests were correlated with historical eye tests provided by Avon.

The ability of Eytex to detect ocular irritants varied with the type of test and product class. The Eytex system is designated to provide data which approximates the maximum acute ocular irritant response and does not provide direct/mechanistic information on cytotoxicity or inflammation (22).

Diverse product types may require retesting in multiple versions of a protein matrix assay in order to obtain meaningful results. This can off-set the cost advantage of routine use of protein matrix systems. Eytex is classified as a phenomenological test.

The application of tissue isoelectric focusing (TIF) techniques to human and rabbit corneal specimens have been proposed as a useful screen for detecting chemicals that produce irreversible effects by denaturing ocular proteins (23). The *in vitro* exposure of corneal sections to acetic acid (1% and 4%) and ammonium hydroxide (0.25% and 2%) resulted in selective modifications of tissue protein profiles which could be evaluated by scanning densitometry. Modification of certain protein bands were selective. The author states that using this refinement procedure, a single rabbit corneal donor would replace approximately 50 rabbits undergoing *in vivo* ocular irritation. Although the test has not been shown to detect classes of ocular irritants other than acids and bases,.it does have the potential of improving the performance of protein matrix assays.

Monolayer tissue culture techniques continue to provide a cost effective approach to assessing ocular irritation. The development of serum-free medium has eliminated many of the technical difficulties of non-specific binding of test materials and interferences with measuring inflammatory mediators. A disadvantage of monolayer culture as an *in vitro* ocular irritation test is the disproportional relationship between the concentration of a test material required to produce cytotoxicity and the non-reactiveness of the same concentration in a rabbit's eye. Additionally, the testing of powders and anhydrous systems can be difficult, if not impossible, with monolayer culture. Meyer and McCulley reported pH and osmotic tolerance limits for rabbit corneal epithelium and endothelium in tissue culture. These data may prove useful for screening in drug development programs including epithelial and endothelial tolerances (24, 25).

Three dimensional skin models provide a new category of *in vitro* tests which allow the measurement of multiple endpoints on the same tissue. These models are composed of dermal keratinocytes and fibroblasts surrounded by a supporting natural or artificial matrix (26, 27). Test materials are often dosed directly onto the surface of the tissues for a specified period of time. Some commercially available tissue models are bathed in culture media, while other models have air interfaces. Damage to the tissue can be assessed by measuring changes in tissue morphology, cytotoxicity (MTT conversion, neutral red uptake, and LDH release) and the release of eicosanoids and cytokines in spent media. Damage is assessed by measuring either concentration dependent changes (exposure time remains constant) or time dependent changes (concentration remains constant).

Although these models are best suited for evaluating the dermal irritancy of test materials, they do provide useful information about the ocular irritation potential of certain classes of test materials such as cosmetics (28, 29). These models are limited in studying all pathways of inflammation in that mast cells, Langerhan cells, and other immune cells are removed in order to make the skin acceptable for transplantation. Some of the newer models are incorporating murine mast cells in order to study the release of vasoactive amines. Additionally, these models do not mimic the mucous membrane-like structure of the eye. Dosing the test materials directly onto the surface of the tissue eliminates some of the confounding factors affecting cells in submerged culture. These include osmotic effects, difficulty with dosing insoluble test materials, reactions between test materials and culture medium, protein binding, and chromatic effects from test materials. They do not address the unique character of the ocular surface which is bathed in a complex aqueous solution.

The adaptation of LAPS (Light Addressable Potentiometric Sensor) technology to a flow chamber offers an exciting advancement in studying intercellular recovery after pulse exposure of test material. Good statistical correlations have been reported between the Draize low volume test and LAPS data (30). The disadvantage of this technology is the cost and the questionable relevance of acidification measurements and ocular injury and recovery.

The use of corneal epithelial fluorescein staining in conjunction with bovine corneal opacity test has made this a promising refinement technique. The test system requires an electronic device to measure light transmittance through fresh bovine corneas treated with test materials. The test has an advantage over existing *in vitro* tests in that it is relatively inexpensive, it can evaluate both insoluble and soluble materials, and it measures both opacity and the destruction of the corneal epithelium (31). For opacity alone, values obtained for 44 common chemicals showed an excellent correlation with *in vivo* data. (32). In a ten company collaborative evaluation of alternatives to the eye irritation test, the bovine cornea opacity and permeability test (BCOP) showed the most promise in predicting the ocular irritation of the test materials. In addition to the BCOP, the evaluation included Eytex, the neutral red uptake assay, Testskin™ LDM™, and Microtox™ Bioassay.

The Microtox™ Bioassay has been shown to be a useful test for screening for ocular irritation (33). The test is conducted by exposing the bacterium, Photobacterium phosphoreum to varying dilutions of a test material. Toxicity is determined by measuring a ratio of light reduced to light remaining (gamma value). Using a threshold of 50 ppm, the test separated irritants and non-irritants for hair care products, anionic surfactants, and cosmetics (33, 34, 35). The test cannot always discriminate the degree of irritation.

HUMAN *IN VIVO* ALTERNATIVE TESTS

The use of human clinical studies can often reduce the need for animals and, in some cases, provide additional information about the ocular safety of certain types of formulations. While the Draize test assesses the objective signs, human clinical studies can provide valuable symptomatic information about subjective irritation such as burning, itching, and tearing which cannot be measured by standard eye safety tests (36). Products that produce mild subjective symptoms will have a difficult time being successful in the market place.

A test that has become popular in Europe and in the US is the human eye instillation test. The test is conducted on healthy volunteer subjects that are free of ocular pathology. A board certified ophthalmologist serves as the principle investigator in these studies. Prior to instilling the test material into the eye, each subject receives a slit lamp examination confined to the anterior segment. A presumed to be non-irritating concentration of the test material is instilled into the subject's eye while the other eye serves as a control. Subjects are examined at one and 24 hours after instillation, and subjective symptoms are recorded (36). Products which are candidates for this type of testing include baby shampoos, cosmetics, eye care products, and eye makeup removers.

Occasionally, the Draize eye test.cannot detect human eye area symptoms. Localized eye area sensitivity syndrome (LEASS) is a collection of subjective and objective signs and symptoms that has occurred when susceptible individuals have applied moisturizers to the periocular area. Symptoms range from itchy, burning, stinging, and watery eyes to foreign body sensations. Ophthalmological examinations reveal bulbar conjunctival chemosis and injection consistent with the release of vasoactive amines. Test materials that produce LEASS do not produce these signs and symptoms when instilled into the eyes of rabbits. It should not be assumed that products that pass the Draize eye test will not cause symptoms in humans (37).

CAVEATS ON THE DRAIZE ALTERNATIVE TESTS

There are several caveats that we should be aware of in our development of alternative tests to predict human ocular irritation. *In vitro* tests that use animal tissue, including those from rabbits, may not totally reflect the Draize eye test. Likewise, the use of human tissue, even from the eye area, may never predict human response one hundred percent of the time.

Does this mean that we should stop the development and use of *in vitro* tests because of the magnitude of the uncertainty? The answer is no! Just as the Draize eye test has its limitation in predicting the human response, so will a battery of *in vitro* tests. The use of *in vitro* tests in conjunction with animal tests is likely to strengthen the safety decision process by providing a mechanistic basis for understanding ocular injury.

Researchers need to be careful in verifying their successes. A successful *in vitro* test should not only correlate to Draize eye data, but also to the human response. We must continue to demand that good science be an integral part of the verification process; otherwise, we run a risk much greater than simply failing to replace the Draize eye test. Success can only be assured by understanding the strengths and weakness of the *in vitro* test and by standardizing each level of testing.

Each of us has a role to play in this process. Educators must play the role of facilitator. Too often we think our responsibilities stop with publication of our research in a peer reviewed journal. We have a responsibility to develop training programs and internships in industry for scientists so that they better understand the safety decision process and can intelligently interpret *in vitro* test results.

Industry, not federal agencies, has the responsibility of validating and implementing *in vitro* tests. Only industry has a complete understanding of the complexity of assessing the safety of products. Regulatory agencies can provide clear direction to interested parties on the role of *in vitro* tests in the safety evaluation process. The safety of a product cannot be justified based solely on the results of an *in vitro* test. Clinical results and exposure conditions must be used in conjunction with *in vitro* data before deciding whether a product is safe. The *in vitro* test is but one tool in the safety decision process. *In vitro* testing for many industries will allow only apparently non-toxic products to be tested in animals, and those found to be non-toxic to either be tested in humans or to be marketed without further testing.

In vitro tests that are found to be reliable in predicting severe eye irritants may be used in conjunction with physical measurements such as pH, structure-activity relationships (SAR), and

TABLE F
MATRIX OF *IN VITRO* TEST OBJECTIVES AND OPERATIONS

Objective	User	Type of Use	Goal / Purpose	Barrier to Acceptance	Value
Evaluation of the irritation / corrosion potential of chemicals not intended to come into contact with the eye and unlikely to do so	Petrochemical industry	Screen	Worker's safety (MSDS) Labeling (DOT)	Toxicity cut-offs Education of toxicologists	Reduces animal usage
Understanding mechanism(s) of injury and as therapeutic screens	Biomedical / pharmaceutical industry	Research and development	To develop animal models to elucidate disease and formulate therapy for humans and animals	Data extrapolation to animals and humans	Mechanistic basis for treatment
Determination of the ocular irritation potential of new and reformulated consumer products	Cosmetic, personal care, and household product industries	Screen	Formulate products Substantiate product claims Labeling Quality Assurance	Regulatory acceptance Added cost Data interpretation Problems with testing formulations	Improves safety decisions Shortens R&D time Reduces and eliminates animal usage

clinical data to make a judgment about the safety of the product. This approach will help reduce our dependency on Draize eye testing.

CONCLUSION

The need for conducting an alternative test is as varied as the need for the Draize eye test. Table F shows the matrix of test objectives, users, applications, goals, barriers to acceptance, and value of *in vitro* tests.

The first step in managing *in vitro* testing is to set realistic goals for their application and use. *In vitro* tests cannot be used as stand alone technology for predicting ocular irritation; however, when used in conjunction with physical measurements, pre-clinical safety data, and clinical data, they can strengthen the safety assessment process. *In vitro* methods are especially useful in screening for severe eye irritants. This level of validation is less extensive than for replacement tests and can be conducted internally by individual companies.

There is consensus on the need for having a battery of Draize alternative tests for ocular irritation testing. A test battery should stress multiple endpoints, not necessarily multiple tests. The battery should, at a minimum, measure cytotoxicity, non-cytotoxic induced inflammation (eicosanoids, vasoactive amines), and, ideally, recovery. It is likely that only mechanistically based tests will achieve this goal. It is anticipated that both public and economic pressures will continue to drive the development and implementation of *in vitro* tests.

REFERENCES

1. FRAZIER, J.M., GAD, S.C., GOLDBERG, A.L., and McCULLEY, J.P., (1982), Historical perspective in eye irritation testing, Alternative Methods in Toxicology, A Critical Evaluation of Alternatives to Acute Ocular Irritation Testing, Vol. 4, Mary Ann Liebert, Inc., New York.

2. PARASCANDOLA, J., (1991), Historical perspectives on *in vitro* toxicology, Alternative Methods in Toxicology, *In Vitro* Toxicology: Mechanisms, and New Technology, Vol. 8, Mary Ann Liebert, Inc., New York.

3. JACKSON, C.O., (1970), Food, and Drug Legislation in the New Deal, Princeton University Press, Princeton, NJ.

4. 21 CFR 740, 10(a).

5. STEPHENS, T.J. and SPENCE, E.T., (1992), The Rule of *In Vitro* Tests in Assessing the Safety of Cosmetics and Consumer Products, presented at a symposium on current concepts and approaches on animal test alternatives, Feb. 4-6.

6. GOLDBERG, A.M. and FRAZIER, J.M., (1989), Alternatives to Animals in Toxicity Testing, Scientific American, 261: 2.

7. BARLOW, A., (1992), The Johns Hopkins Center for Alternatives to Animal Testing, CAAT Newsletter, 9: 3.

8. Statement to the Maryland Governor's Task Force to Study Animal Testing, April 17, 1989, The U.S. Food and Drug Administration.

9. European Chemical Industry Ecology and Toxicology Centre, 1988, Monograph II.

10. ROWAN, A.N., (1981), Alternatives and Laboratory Animals, Animals in Research: New Perspective in Animal Experimentation, D. Sperlinger (Ed.), John Wiley and Sons, Chechester.

11. McGILL, D.C., Cosmetic Companies Quietly Ending Animal Tests, The New York Times, August 2, 1987.

12. EC Cosmetics Directive Modified Animal Testing Ban Passed, 1992, The Rose Sheet.

13. FRAZIER, J.M., (1990), Validation of *In Vitro* Models, Journal of American College of Toxicology, Vol. 9: No. 3.

14. Workshop on Updating Eye Irritation Test Methods, Proposals for Regulatory Consensus, September, 1991.

15. McDONALD, T.O., SEABAUGH, V., SHADDUTS, J.A., and EDELHAUSER, H.F., (1987), Eye Irritation on Dermatotoxicology, 3rd Edition.

16. POTTS, A.M. and GONASUN, L.M., (1980), Toxic Responses of the Eye in Toxicology, The Basic Science of Poisons, MacMillian Publishing, New York.

17. FRAZIER, J.M. and BRADLAW, J.A., (1989), Technical Problems Associated with *In Vitro* Toxicity Testing Systems, A Report of the CAAT Technical Workshop of May 17-18, CAAT Technical Report No.1.

18. SEHNERT, S.S., (1990), Structure-Activity Relationships in Predictive Toxicology, A Report of the CAAT Technical Workshops of June 21-22, CAAT Technical Report No. 2.

19. ROWAN, A.N., (1990), Tufts Alternatives Program National Agenda Project: The Alternatives Report, 2: 6.

20. FRAZIER, J.M., (1990), Scientific Criteria for Validation of *In Vitro* Toxicity Tests, document prepared for the Organization for Economic Co-Operation and Development, Environmental Monograph No. 36.

21. FRAZIER, J.M., (1992), Report on the CAAT/TCA Workshop on the International Status of Validation of *In Vitro* Toxicity Tests, CAAT Draft Technical Report No. 5.

22. KRUSZEWSKI, F.H., HEARN, L.H., SMITH, K.T., TEAL, J.J., GORDON, V.C., and DICKENS, M.S., (1992) Applications of the Eyetex™ System to the Evaluation of Cosmetic Products and Their Ingredients, ATLA 20: 146.

23. EURELL, T.E., SINN, J.M., GERDING, P.A., and ALDEN, C.L., (1991), *In Vitro* Evaluation of Ocular Irritants Using Corneal Protein Profiles, Toxicol. Appl. Pharmacol., 108: 374.

24. MEYER, D.R. and McCULLEY, J. P., (1992), pH Tolerance of Rabbit Corneal Endothelium in Tissue Culture, J. Toxicol.-Cut. and Ocular Toxicol., 11 (1): 15.

25. MEYER, D.R. and McCULLEY, J. P., (1992), Osmotic Tolerance of Rabbit Corneal Endothelium in Tissue Culture, J. Toxicol.-Cut. and Ocular Toxicol., 11 (1): 31.

26. BELL, E., IVARISON, B., and MERRILL, C., (1979), Production of a Tissue-Like Structure by Contraction of Collagen Lattices by Human Fibroblasts of Different Proliferative Potential *In Vitro*, Proc. Natl. Acad. Sci. U.S.A., 76 (3): 1274.

27. TRIGLIA, D., SHERARD BRAA, S., DONNELLY, T., KIDD, I., and NAUGHTON, G.K., (1991), A 3-Dimensional Human Dermal Model Substrate for *In Vitro* Toxicological Studies, Alternative Methods in Toxicology, Vol. 8, A.M. Goldberg (ed.), Mary Ann Liebert,Inc., New York.

28. SHERARD BRAA, S. and TRIGLIA, D., Predicting Ocular Irritation Using 3-Dimensional Human Fibroblast Cultures, Cosmetics and Toiletries, Vol. 106, No. 12.

29. GAY, R.J., SWIDERELS, M., NELSON, D., and STEPHENS, T.J., (1992), The Living Dermal Equivalent as an *In Vitro* Model for Predicting Ocular Irritation, J. Toxicol.-Cut. and Ocular Toxicol., 11 (1): 47.

30. PARCE, J.W., OWICKI, J.C., WADA, H.G., and KERCSO, K.M., (1991), Cells on Silicon: the Microphysiometer, <u>Alternative Methods in Toxicology, Mechanisms and New Technology</u>, A. M. Goldberg (Ed.), Mary Ann Leibert, Inc., New York.

31. GAUTHERON, P., DUKIC, M., ALIX, D., and SINA, J.F., (1992), Bovine Corneal Opacity and Permeability Test: An *In Vitro* Assay of Ocular Irritancy, <u>Fundamental and Applied Toxicology</u>, 18: 442.

32. GALLER, D.M., CURREN, R., GAD, S.C., GAUTHERON, P., LEONG, B., MILLER, K., SARGENT, E., SHAH, P.V., SINA, J., and SUSSMAN, R.G., (1992), ATO-Company Collaborative Evaluatin of Alternatives to the Eye Irritation Test Using Chemical Intermediates, Poster A12, *In Vitro* Toxicology: 10th Anniversary Symposium of CAAT, April 14.

33. SANDERS, C., SWEDLUND, T.D., STEPHENS, T.J., and SILBER, P.M., (1990), Evaluation of Six *In Vitro* Toxicity Assays; Comparison with *In Vivo* Ocular and Dermal Irritation Potential of Prototype Cosmetics Formulations, <u>The Toxicologist</u>, 11(1): poster 1085.

34. HEINZE, J.E., STEPHENS, T.J., SWEDLUND, T.D., and SILBER, P.M., (1990), Assessing the Mildness of Anionic Surfactant Systems with the Microtox Luminescent Bacteria Test (LBT), The Tetrahymena Motility Assay, and Testskin™ Living Dermal Equivalent (LDE™) Multiple Endpoint Tests, <u>The Toxicologist</u>, 11(1): poster 1083.

35. LAKE, L.K., STEPHENS, T.J., and SPENCE, E.T., (1992), Use of Four *In Vitro* Assays to Evaluate the Ocular Irritation Potential of Hair Care Products, Poster C1, *In Vitro* Toxicology: 10th Anniversary Symposium of CAAT, April 16.

36. DROTMAN, R.B., McCULLEY, J.P., STEPHENS, T.J., MATOBA, A., and GUNST, R.F., (1985), Assessing the Irritation Potential of Eye Area Products in the Human Eye, <u>J. Toxicol.-Cut. and Ocular Toxicol.</u>, 4 (1): 3-11.

37. STEPHENS, T.J., McCULLEY, J.P., THARPE, M., MARBACH, H.I., PATRICK, E., SILBER, P.M., DRAKE, K., and FLOYD, A., (1989-1990), Localized Eye Area Sensitivity Syndrome, <u>J. Toxicol.-Cut. and Ocular Toxicol.</u>, 8 (4): 569.

E. A Ten-Year Progress Report of the Center

E1

Pride and Prejudice: Ten Years of CAAT—An Industry Perspective

STEPHEN D. GETTINGS

The Cosmetic, Toiletry and Fragrance Association
Washington, DC 20036

INTRODUCTION

During the past two decades the general public has become increasingly aware of the potential of chemicals to cause toxic effects. As a consequence there are increasing demands for more stringent safety evaluation of new chemicals, drugs and consumer products. At the same time there has been growing public concern with respect to the use of animals in toxicity testing. Industry is in the business of providing society with a wide choice of commodities and finished products but also has a responsibility to ensure the safety of its employees, consumers and the environment. Consistent with this responsibility, industry also shares the concern of those persons committed to supporting animal welfare initiatives to reduce and, wherever possible, to replace the use of animals in safety testing. To this end, industry has committed substantial resources toward the search for reliable and scientifically valid alternative methods to the use of animals for purposes of safety substantiation. The Johns Hopkins Center for Alternatives to Animal Testing (CAAT), founded on the initiative of the cosmetic and personal-care industry in 1981, is a happy product of such commitment.

HISTORY

At the beginning of the 1980's, both the private and the public sector were under some pressure from the animal rights movement. In 1980, the General Accounting Office (GAO) prepared a report on "Alternatives to Use of Animals in Research" in response to a request from Congress to investigate whether or not research would benefit from the allocation of funds specifically to the development of alternatives (1). The report cited the National Institutes of Health (NIH) as acknowledging the existence of some non-animal testing alternatives. In February 1981, NIH conducted a conference, in part, to discuss with other government agencies the use of *in vitro* techniques in bioassay methodology (2). The conference was held at the suggestion of the Chairman of the House Science, Research and Technology Subcommittee, Rep. George Brown, Jr. (D-Calif.), who saw the conference as an appropriate forum to develop technical background data for legislation conceived in the 96th Congress to encourage non-animal testing.

GOVERNMENT

By early 1981, there were several proposals pending in the 97th Congress whose goal was to promote alternative, non-animal test methods in research (for a brief review of U.S. and European animal rights-influenced legislation in the 1970's and early 1980's, see [3]). Two of these proposals (Senate Resolution 65 and House Concurrent Resolution 27) focused on the Draize rabbit eye irritancy test (requiring that the Consumer Product Safety Commission (CPSC), the Environmental Protection agency (EPA) and the Food and Drug Administration (FDA) develop alternative non-animal testing procedures to replace currently used ophthalmic testing procedures), and two (H.R. 556 and House Concurrent Resolution 38) called for funding to develop and validate alternative ophthalmic testing procedures that did not require animals. In particular, H.R. 556 called for the establishment of a National Center for Alternative Research, funded by a percentage of the money then currently available to the federal agencies involved in animal testing.

FEDERAL REGULATORY AGENCIES

In response to pressure from Congress, the federal agencies were beginning to re-evaluate their use of testing procedures which utilized experimental animals. In May 1980, the Executive Director of the CPSC ordered agency scientists to suspend routine testing of products for eye irritation for three months (the purpose of this directive was to allow staff scientists to evaluate the use of topical anesthetics administered directly to the eyes of rabbits immediately prior to instillation of test substance. CPSC concluded that although there was some evidence that use of topical anesthetics reduced the discomfort of the rabbits, there was also evidence that in some instances anesthetics actually increased discomfort and increased the time treated eyes took to recover from test substance-related injury). Press reports at the time suggested that the EPA was also questioning conduct of rabbit eye irritancy testing, and whether anesthetics might be used. The Food and Drug Administration was reportedly approached by animal rights groups who requested that the agency institute a moratorium on its in-house use of the Draize rabbit eye irritation test. FDA declined to do so. Although at that time FDA had not apparently earmarked any funds to develop alternatives to animal tests, the agency was of the opinion that non-animal tests might appropriately be developed. In a May 1980 "Talk Paper" affirming the Draize rabbit eye irritation test as the best test available to assure the safety of substances that may enter the human eye, it was noted that FDA "encourages research toward finding a better and more humane method for testing and safety of products"; in addition, it was noted that FDA would review carefully the outcome of the CPSC anesthetics program because of FDA's concern "with the safety and well-being of all animals used to test products for human use."

INDUSTRY

The cosmetic industry was also beginning to respond to the issues raised by animal rights advocates, in the federal agencies, and in Congress (Table 1). In December 1980, Revlon announced a $750,000 grant to Rockefeller University for work on alternatives to animal testing, and the Cosmetic, Toiletry and Fragrance Association (CTFA) formed a working group (Test Systems Review Task Force) which was charged with the exploration of alternative testing procedures which might ultimately eliminate the need for animals in product safety testing. In the first instance, the working group was directed to address the issue of the possible modification or replacement of the acute eye irritation test commonly referred to as the Draize procedure. As a first step, CTFA organized and sponsored the CTFA Ocular Safety Testing Workshop in October 1980 (4). Participants in the workshop included scientific experts representing government, industry, academia, and animal rights groups. Given (i) an appreciation of the immensity and complexity of the task of replacing animal tests with scientifically-viable alternatives which arose from the workshop; (ii) the prevailing legislative climate; and (iii) the results of several meetings between CTFA and animal rights groups (including Beauty Without Cruelty, United Action for Animals, the American Fund for Alternatives to Animal Research, the Humane Society of the United States, and with Henry Spira of the Coalition to Abolish the Draize Test), in March 1981, CTFA's Board of Directors agreed in principle to establish a National Center for Alternatives. In an internal memo written at the time it was noted, "It is prudent and responsible for the cosmetic industry to take affirmative action. We too are interested in the welfare of animals used in testing and research, and the advancement of scientific methods to reduce the need for testing." CTFA further concluded that "establishment of a fund for a National Center would accomplish the goal of commencing a coordinated program that no one has yet been able to start - research to develop animal testing alternatives. Establishing and contributing to a Center would assure that duplicative testing is avoided. Selection of a highly respected individual or group to manage the Center would assure that CTFA members are getting high quality, credible scientific research for their investment".

CTFA proceeded on two fronts: (i) the CTFA Test Systems Review Task Force evolved into the Modified Ocular Safety Testing Task Force that had as its goal the development of interim modifications to the Draize eye test that could be adopted by the cosmetic industry to lessen the discomfort of test animals used in safety testing, and to decrease the number of animals that were used; and (ii) establish the feasibility of creating and funding a "National Center for Alternatives". It was perceived that the work of the Task Force would result in short-term benefits (the Task Force went on to conduct a collaborative program, involving 9 industry laboratories, which evaluated the effects of (i) decreased dose volume; (ii) application to the cornea *vs*. the conjunctiva; and (iii) treatment of rabbit eyes with topical anaesthetic prior to test substance administration [5]), whereas establishing a National Center would result in long-term benefits (e.g., the elimination of some animal tests altogether). At a March 25, 1981, meeting of the CTFA Board of Directors Subcommittee on Research, approval of the Center approach was reaffirmed and it was decided that once the Center was established, CTFA should adopt a "hands off" policy (i.e., would not be involved in the actual selection of grant proposals other than to assure that funding be applied to the development of appropriate alternative methods). CTFA envisioned that the institution receiving these funds would have the sole responsibility of administering the research program, of reviewing research proposals, of performing appropriate research, and of selecting others to perform research where necessary. It was further envisaged that, once established, CTFA (and the Center itself) would encourage additional funding from other industries, from government agencies, from individuals, and from foundations. Based upon these guidelines, proposals were solicited from several organizations and institutions, including Johns Hopkins. By early summer of 1981, a selection had been made and negotiations completed; by September, CAAT was in place. Commitment of additional funding was made by Bristol-Myers Co. in November 1981, and in December the Geraldine R. Dodge Foundation agreed to support publication of the CAAT Newsletter. Corporate funding for the Centre has increased steadily ever since (Figure 1).

TABLE 1.

SIGNIFICANT EVENTS IN CAAT HISTORY
1980 - 1992

1980
October — 1st CTFA Ocular Safety Testing Workshop.
December — Revlon announces $750,000 grant to Rockefeller University for work on alternatives to animal testing.

1981
March — CTFA Board of Directors agrees in principle to establish funding for a "National Center".
September — CAAT funded with $1 million grant from CTFA over 3 yrs.
November — Commitment of additional funding by Bristol-Myers, Co.
December — Geraldine R. Dodge Foundation supports publication of CAAT Newsletter.

1982
May — 1st CAAT Symposium. "Product Safety Evaluation: Development of New Methodological Approaches".
CAAT solicits first research proposals.
November — CAAT funds first 16 grants.

1983
May — 2nd CAAT Symposium. "Acute Toxicity Testing: Alternative Approaches".

1984
January — Commitment of funding by Exxon Corp. signifies first corporate funding of CAAT outside cosmetic/personal-care industry.
October — 3rd CAAT Symposium. "*In Vitro* Toxicology: A Progress Report".

1985
January — SDA initiates *In Vitro* Alternatives Program.
June — CAAT *In Vitro* Toxicology Laboratory established.
September — Bausch & Lomb, Inc. award CAAT grant to conduct and publish critical review of **Draize eye test and potential alternatives**.

1986
April — 4th CAAT Symposium. "*In Vitro* Toxicology: Approaches to Validation".
CAAT/Bausch & Lomb, Inc. sponsored workshop "A Critical Evaluation of Alternatives to Acute Ocular Irritation Testing".

1987
November — 5th CAAT Symposium. "Progress in *In Vitro* Toxicology".

1988
February — Colgate-Palmolive Co. awards first SOT Post-Doctoral Fellowship in In Vitro Toxicology.
The Procter & Gamble Co. awarded Corporate Conscience Award for long-time leadership in search for alternatives.

TABLE 1 (continued).

SIGNIFICANT EVENTS IN CAAT HISTORY
1980 - 1992

1988
- March — *CTFA announces Evaluation of Alternatives Program.*
- April — **Avon Products, Inc. funds CAAT program of directed research (Program Project) in alternatives to contact allergy testing.**
- September — *Joint Government - Industry Workshop on Progress Towards Non-Animal Alternatives to the Draize Test sponsored by CPSC, EPA, FDA, SDA, CTFA, CSMA, CMA.*
- December — *First meeting of Industrial In Vitro Toxicology Group (IIVTG).*

1989
- January — *Noxell Corp. announces implementation of Agarose Diffusion Method.*
- February — **First meeting of CAAT Subcommittee on Validation and Technology Transfer.**
- March — **Mary Kay Cosmetics, Inc. funds two-year project in CAAT *In Vitro* Toxicology Laboratory.**
- April — **6th CAAT Symposium. "*In Vitro* Toxicology: New Directions".**
  Avon Products, Inc. announces that it will no longer use the Draize eye test.
- May — **NIH/NIEHS grant signifies first federal funding of CAAT.**
  CAAT Technical Workshop on problems involved in *in vitro* testing sponsored by Procter & Gamble, Mary Kay Cosmetics, Hoffmann-LaRoche and EPA.
  The Procter & Gamble Co. announces University Animal Alternatives Research Program.
- June — **First meeting of CAAT Government Exchange Group.**

1990
- January — **CAAT/ERGATT Workshop on Validation.**
- June — **CAAT/Ciba-Geigy Technical Workshop on Structure - Activity Relationships in Predictive Toxicology.**
  1st CAAT/TCA Workshop: Cell Culture and *In Vitro* Toxicity Tests.
- September — *2nd CTFA Ocular Safety Testing Workshop.*
  OECD Monograph No. 36 "Scientific Criteria for Validation of In Vitro Toxicity Tests" published by Fraizer.
- November — **7th CAAT Symposium. "*In Vitro* Toxicology: Mechanisms and New Technology".**

1991
- June — **2nd CAAT/TCA Workshop: The International Status of Validation of *In Vitro* Toxicology Tests.**
- September — *IRAG Regulatory Consensus Workshop on Eye Irritation Methodology.*
- November — **Goldberg presented with Russell and Burch Award by HSUS.**
  OECD accepts Fixed Dose Procedure as alternative to classical LD_{50}.

1992
- January — **EPA funds CAAT program of directed research (Program Project) in *in vitro* neurotoxicology.**
  CAAT launches *In Vitro* Toxicology Program at Johns Hopkins School of Public Health.
- April — **In Vitro Toxicology: 10th Anniversary Symposium of CAAT.**

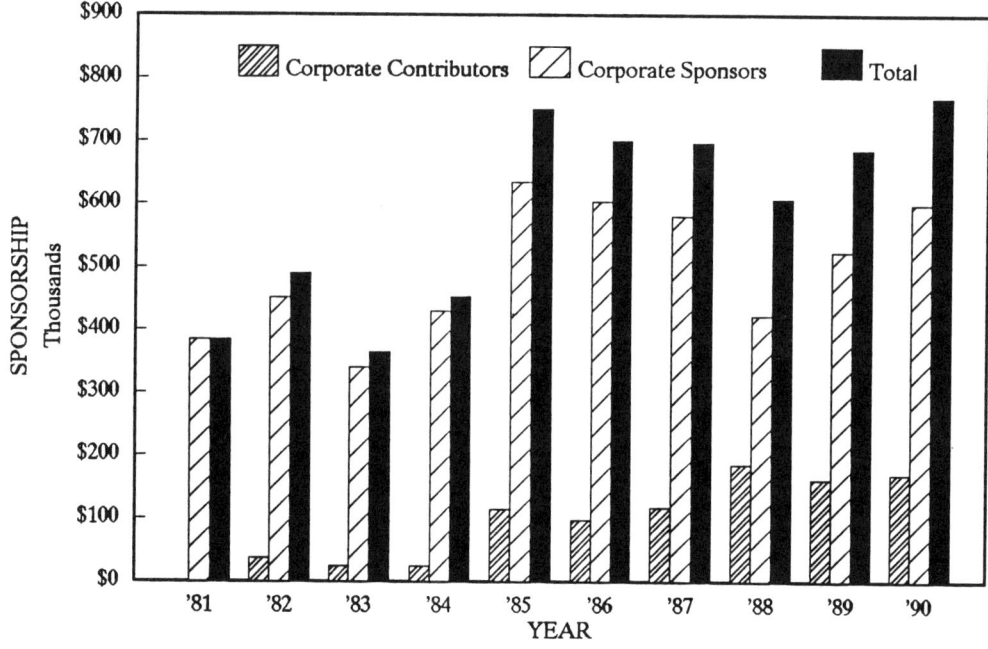

Figure 1. Corporate Funding 1981-1991.

MISSION

The mission of the Center is to develop and disseminate appropriate basic scientific knowledge pertaining to the use of innovative non-whole animal methods for safety substantiation of commercial and/or therapeutic products. CAAT recognizes that non-whole-animal (alternative) methods act in concert with whole animal and clinical studies to advance science, develop new products and drugs, and to prevent, treat and cure disease. Specifically, CAAT's goals are to (*i*) encourage basic research that will provide the foundation for *in vitro* and other non-animal test procedures designed to evaluate the safety of chemicals and/or commercial products; (*ii*) develop specific methodology that will provide alternative approaches to whole animal studies for the evaluation of safety; (*iii*) disseminate research progress through symposia, publications and workshops; and (*iv*) encourage and promote the *acceptance* of applicable methods (technology transfer) of non-whole-animal safety testing in the industrial and regulatory arenas (6,7). To attain these goals, CAAT has engaged in a variety of activities organized under three major areas: (*i*) Research; (*ii*) Validation and Technology Transfer; and (*iii*) Education and Communication.

RESEARCH

Research Grants Program. CAAT's primary goal is achieved through an intramural and extramural grants program. Proposals submitted by investigators from within the institution (i.e., at Johns Hopkins) must undergo the same selection procedure as those submitted by investigators from outside institutions. Grants are funded through an investigator-initiated peer review process culminating in a final decision by the Center's Advisory Board in November of each year. The scope of the research program is international: The first 9 grants were funded in November 1982, and the first grantees included two investigators from overseas (P.H.Bach, University of Surrey; T.J.B. Gray, BIBRA) as well as from institutions in the United States. In the last 10 years, over 160 research projects have been funded in the United States, Canada and Europe. In the 1992 grant period over 100 proposals were received and 16 grants funded in the areas of neurotoxicity, phototoxicity, dermatotoxicity, teratology, renal toxicity and hepatotoxicity. CAAT grants are funded in the range of $15-20,000 (to be increased to $30,000, beginning in 1993). Although not a large figure by today's standards, CAAT grants often serve as a springboard for further funding (*CAAT Newsletter (1988) 6 (1), 9-10*) or support from industry (*CAAT Newsletter (1989) 7 (1), 1-2*). In many cases a CAAT grant funds work to evaluate the application of a promising test methodology based upon an investigator's basic research (so-called "piggy-back" approach); in other cases, a CAAT grant is the only likely means of supporting research which has the potential to reduce animal use. Research proposals are funded by CAAT for a maximum of three years; beginning in 1992, CAAT will actively review currently funded grants for potential commercial interest as a means of securing support for research projects after CAAT-funding is terminated.

Directed Research Grants. In 1988, CAAT initiated a program of *directed* research ("Program Projects") designed to hasten the development of animal test alternatives in *specific* areas targeted by corporate sponsors, and to spur technology transfer *(CAAT Newsletter (1988) 6 (2), 1-2)*. On the basis of recent advances in immunology, Avon Products, Inc., concluded that (if harnessed appropriately) a program of directed research in the area of contact allergy testing could lead rapidly to alternative testing procedures and thus impact animal use in the cosmetic, pharmaceutical, food additive, household product and industrial chemical industries. In April 1988, Avon sponsored the first of a series of semi-annual workshops at Hopkins as the first step in bringing together company scientists and interested outside investigators. As a result of the workshop, grant proposals were solicited and presented to the CAAT Advisory Board at its November meeting. Subject to the same peer-review procedure as all CAAT proposals, projects were selected for funding from among the proposals with high priority scores. The Program Project approach provides a mechanism for bridging research and development, allowing the Center to participate directly with sponsors in areas of mutual interest. Corporate sponsors must agree to a minimum annual commitment of $100,000 for three years (each grant is awarded for three years, and each project is reviewed annually). The approach incorporates peer review and maintenance of intellectual independence for academic researchers, whilst providing sponsors with a focused research program (8). Preliminary findings from the Avon Contact Allergy Program Project were presented at the 7th CAAT Symposium, *"In Vitro Toxicology: Mechanisms and New Technology"* (9). The success of the Avon Program Project has led to the implementation of a similar program of directed research (EPA Neurotoxicology Program Project) funded by the Environmental Protection Agency (*CAAT Newsletter (1992) 9 (3),8*); similarly, in June 1992, CAAT sponsored a Cell Immortalization Workshop at Johns Hopkins as part of its first attempt to initiate a "Program Project" involving five current grantees. The scientists who presented at the workshop had all been funded by CAAT to investigate the utility of developing differentiated cell lines for toxicity testing. Four of the five were using viral vectors to immortalize cells; three of the five were working with kidney cells. As noted by the coordinator of the workshop, Dr. Joanne Zurlo (Assistant to the CAAT Director), "The success of the Cell Immortalization Workshop - measured by the collaborative interaction it inspired - provides the impetus for CAAT to put together other working groups in the future. We hope CAAT's "informal" Program Projects will cultivate joint publications and cross-pollenization of research, in addition to creating a grants program in which the whole is greater than the sum of its parts" *(CAAT Newsletter (1991) 9 (2), 5)*.

In Vitro Toxicology Laboratory/In Vitro Toxicology Program. To supplement the research program, CAAT established its own *in vitro* toxicology laboratory at Johns Hopkins in June 1985. Initial funding was supplied by Allied Corp., American Hospital Supply Corp., the Shell Companies Foundation and private donors. Envisioned as a means of facilitating technology transfer by offering short training programs in *in vitro* techniques, the laboratory also conducts basic research on identifying mechanisms of cellular toxicity. In March 1989, Mary Kay Cosmetics Inc., committed $110,000 over two years in support of research on evaluating *in vitro* methods for determining phototoxicity and photoallergic responses. Recently CAAT has established an *In Vitro* Toxicology Program in the Johns Hopkins Division of Toxicological Sciences *(CAAT Newsletter (1992) 9 (3), 4)*. The goal of this program is to facilitate interaction among Johns Hopkins faculty with expertise and interest in the use of *in vitro* systems and the study of mechanisms of toxicity to (*i*) foster the development of new cell systems, (*ii*) develop novel strategies for the detection of toxicity; and (*iii*) assess cellular toxicity and *in vitro* parameters for extrapolation of risk. It is expected to serve as a focal point for intra- and inter-institutional program projects in the areas judged to be important and fruitful for the development of new *in vitro* test systems.

VALIDATION AND TECHNOLOGY TRANSFER

CAAT has played a key role in the debate over validation. Staff from the Center (most prominently Dr. John Frazier, CAAT Associate Director) have participated in (or organized) every major workshop, conference or symposium addressing validation since 1981. In September 1988, representatives of government, industry, academia and the general public gathered to participate in the Joint Government-Industry Workshop on Progress Towards Non-Animal Alternatives to the Draize Test. The workshop was sponsored by CPSC, EPA, FDA, SDA, CTFA, CSMA, CMA. The objective of the workshop was to provide a forum for interested parties to present data and discuss policy regarding the development and validation of alternatives to *in vivo* ocular irritation testing procedures. Several important areas of consensus were developed and reported by CAAT *(CAAT Newsletter (1989) 6 (3), 9)*. In particular, it was agreed that (*i*) development and validation of *batteries* of tests for *specific classifications* of chemicals would lead to a more rapid acceptance and implementation of *in vitro* tests than would occur if *universal* validation of *in vitro* tests were required; and (*ii*) in the absence of an extensive quantitative human data-base, rabbit ocular irritation data (using the Draize scale) should be used in the assessment of *in vitro* performance (although what limited human data exists should be used to confirm irritancy classification based on the Draize score). Both of these consensus findings were incorporated in two industry-sponsored programs (10,11) which were conceived and first initiated in the mid-1980's (Table 1). As was noted at the workshop, development and validation of test methods for specific classifications of materials will, in all likelihood lead to a more rapid acceptance and implementation of *in vitro* tests than would occur if universal validation were required (for example, the detergent industry must evaluate granular, alkaline solids while these substances do not concern the paint or cosmetics industries). Each industry will identify unique aspects about their spectrum of chemicals and products that will lead to a unique validation program for that industry *(CAAT Newsletter (1988) 6 (2), 4-5)*.

In addition to producing one of the most comprehensive treatises on the scientific criteria for the validation of *in vitro* toxicity tests, *OECD Environment Monographs, No. 36* (12), CAAT is actively trying to promote practical moves toward the acceptance of validated test methods by the regulatory agencies. In a *CAAT Newsletter* feature article in 1986, Dr. Salvatore De Salva (Colgate-Palmolive Co.) noted, "Industry's role in the drive to find alternative methods is as an equal partner with academia and governmental agencies. Industry has provided financial support to academic institutions and some companies have undertaken studies within their own research facilities. Industry should not have the sole responsibility of supporting these efforts. The federal government... ...must assume part of the financial and technical burden for validation of alternative methods" *(CAAT Newsletter (1986) 4 (2), 1-4)*. In the same issue Dr. W. Gary Flamm (then Director of Toxicological Sciences, Center for Food Safety and Applied Nutrition, FDA) further noted, "The best contribution regulatory agencies can make (to furthering acceptance of alternative methodology) is to become participants in the validation process. Both the agencies and industry must gain hands-on experience with a new method before they can accept it". CAAT is endeavoring to play a unique role in fostering the validation process by acting as mediator between industry and the regulatory agencies. Specifically, CAAT has encouraged dialogue. In 1989, CAAT instituted the first of a series of meetings between the staff of the Center and representatives of several regulatory agencies including CPSC, EPA and FDA. At the second CAAT-Government Information Exchange meeting in June 1990, CAAT discussed the feasibility of a proposal designed to facilitate validation. Dr's. Frazier and Goldberg presented the outline of a plan (which aims to combine the best of government, corporate and academic expertise) that might best be used to establish an *administrative framework* for facilitating validation of *in vitro* methodologies *(CAAT Newsletter (1990) 8 (1), 3)*. In a presentation entitled "Diffusion of a New Methodology" presented at the 4th CAAT Symposium *"In Vitro Toxicology: Approaches to Validation"* in 1986, several predictions were made about the likely course of the spread and acceptance of alternatives *(CAAT Newsletter 4 (3), 5)*; in particular it was noted that *(i)* even after a new methodology is developed and validated, it may take some considerable time before adoption of a new test; and *(ii)* specific communication strategies designed to promote the widespread adoption of a new testing methodology can affect the rate and course of this diffusion process. CAAT's growing recognition of the validity of these predictions led to the formation of the Subcommittee on Validation and Technology Transfer which first met in February 1989. The objective of the committee is to promote the transfer of new testing technology from the research laboratory to practical application in toxicity assessment. The committee maintains strong links with the academic, industrial and regulatory research communities, and has formed a network of organizations for the exchange of information on validation activities. Long-range plans include developing a data bank to identify and catalog validation activities and *in vitro* methodologies in the United States. The primary short-term goal of the committee is to develop the administrative framework, proposed by CAAT, establishing a scientific structure for validation.

EDUCATION AND COMMUNICATION

Symposia. In order to provide impetus and focus for the research program, CAAT has conducted a series of symposia designed to bring together participants from academia, government, industry and the animal welfare movement (Table 1). The first symposium, *"Product

Safety Evaluation: Development of New Methodological Approaches", in May 1982, surveyed existing knowledge about alternatives to animal testing and outlined problems impeding the search for alternatives. A major focus was potential *in vitro* alternatives to tests for irritation and inflammation, such as the Draize eye test. In May 1983, the second symposium, *"Acute Toxicity Testing: Alternative Approaches,"* produced a scientific consensus on short-term measures that could be taken to reduce animal use in acute toxicity testing and led to actions by FDA and EPA that encouraged industry to re-examine use of the classical LD_{50} test. In April 1986, in conjunction with the 4th CAAT Symposium, *"In Vitro Toxicology: Approaches to Validation"*, Bausch & Lomb, Inc. sponsored a workshop specifically for the purpose of identifying promising *in vitro* alternative tests for eye irritation. It was concluded that a battery of alternative tests would be needed to replace the Draize test and that different batteries of tests, dependent upon product type, would probably be required. It was also apparent that a number of cosmetic and personal care companies were at the forefront of research on *in vitro* alternatives, and that many of them were sponsoring the development of *in vitro* tests. Based upon these findings, CTFA initiated planning for an industry-wide program that could be focused to fit the needs of the cosmetic and personal care industry, and that could be initiated (and result in useful information on the application of *in vitro* test methodologies) as expeditiously as possible. The CTFA Evaluation of Alternatives Program was publicly announced in March 1988 and preliminary results presented at a meeting of the Industrial *In Vitro* Toxicology Group in May 1990 (13). More definitive analyses of the data arising from Phase I of the CTFA Program have been published subsequently (14,15). A similar program, focused on the needs of the soap and detergent industry, has been instituted and reported on by the Soap and Detergent Association (10,16).

Workshops. Workshops are also a mechanism by which CAAT has focused attention on validation and promoted technology transfer. In June 1989, CAAT held the first in a series of technical workshops. Entitled *Technical Problems Associated with In Vitro Toxicity Testing Systems*, and sponsored by Procter and Gamble, Mary Kay Cosmetics, Hoffman-LaRoche and EPA, the workshop addressed two problem areas (*i*) identification of artifacts that adversely affect *in vitro* test results; and (*ii*) techniques to handle insoluble test chemicals in *in vitro* test systems. Representatives from the regulatory and corporate communities participated in a two-day workshop and collaborated in writing a technical report of the workshop (17). Topics for future workshops include such subjects as (*i*) chemical selection for validation; (*ii*) interpretation, extrapolation, and relevance of *in vitro* data; (*iii*) good laboratory practices for *in vitro* testing; (*iv*) culture conditions and how they affect toxicity testing; (*v*) validation; and (*vi*) information transfer. A second technical workshop on *Structure-Activity Relationships in Predictive Toxicology* was held in June 1990. The goal of the workshop was to discuss state-of-the-art approaches concerned with reducing the number of animals used in testing, minimizing stress and discomfort to laboratory animals and maximizing the scientific data obtained from whole animal and *in vitro* studies. The workshop, supported by the Ciba-Geigy Corporation, focused on two aspects: computational chemical modeling to predict toxicity, and alternative techniques that permit bioeffects to be predicted accurately *in vitro* (18). CAAT has also co-organized a workshop (*1st CAAT/TCA Workshop: Cell Culture and In Vitro Toxicity Tests*) in conjunction with the Tissue Culture Association which addressed the effects of cell culture conditions on the toxic responses of cells to test chemicals (19). Recognition that validation is a truly international issue is evidenced by CAAT's organization and participation in the joint *CAAT/ERGATT Workshop on the Validation of Toxicity Test Procedures* held in Amden in January 1990 (20), and the *2nd CAAT/TCA Workshop: The International Status of Validation of In Vitro Toxicology Tests* held in Anaheim, California, in June 1991 (21).

Information Program. The CAAT Newsletter is an obvious example of the success of CAAT's information program. The book series, *Alternative Methods in Toxicology,* which presents the proceedings of the Center's annual symposia, is also an important vehicle for disseminating the results of the CAAT grant program. Goldberg and Fraizer's publication of an article on alternatives to animal testing in *Scientific American* (22) has made a significant contribution to educating the general public and increasing awareness of the issue. In an early edition of the *CAAT Newsletter* it was noted that "Public attention, scientific awareness and monetary support will contribute to an accelerated production of information" and "As new alternatives and support research are developed, there will be an obvious need to disseminate this information to scientists who can put it to use" *(CAAT Newsletter (1982) 1 (1), 1-2).* As the result of a collaboration with the CAAT, the National Library of Medicine introduced "animal testing alternatives" as a new subject heading in all its new catalogs, periodicals and computer data bases *(CAAT Newsletter (1985) 3 (2), 2-3).* The new heading has improved communication on alternatives amongst scientists worldwide.

Educational Outreach Program. CAAT is very aware of the lack of knowledge on the part of the public with regard to animal testing and alternatives issues. In particular, in the past several years the number of students at the elementary, secondary and college levels calling the Center to request information on alternatives to animal testing has increased significantly. Students at all levels are more aware of animal issues and are conducting research for class projects. During 1991 over 1500 requests were received. In response to this overwhelming need for information, CAAT (under the direction of Assistant to the Director, Dr. Joanne Zurlo) has developed an Educational Outreach Program sponsored by Mary Kay Cosmetics, Inc., with additional funding from Merck, Sharp & Dohme Research Laboratories and the Geraldine R. Dodge Foundation. The goal is to develop an informational package addressing the use of alternatives and animals in scientific research and testing, and is designed to promote interaction between the scientific and lay communities.

CAAT IN PERSPECTIVE

By increasing scientific and public awareness of the advantages and limitations of *in vitro* toxicology, CAAT has legitimized the study and implementation of alternatives. CAAT has had an impact. The Center endorses the concept of alternatives (reduction, refinement, replacement) first proposed with publication of Russell and Burch's *"Principles of Humane Experimental Technique"* (23). CAAT defines alternatives as new methods that refine existing procedures by minimizing animal distress, reducing animal usage, or replacing whole animal tests; thus, progress may be viewed as (*i*) any modification of currently accepted testing strategy which results in decreased animal use; and (*ii*) any modification in societal perceptions which result in increased awareness and realistic expectations from both animal and non-animal tests.

REDUCTION, REFINEMENT, REPLACEMENT

Industry has a legal and moral responsibility to provide safe products and to ensure the safety of workers engaged in the manufacture of such products. As part of this responsibility, industry tests its raw materials and finished products using current state-of-the-art methods. Industry is willing to use non-animal alternatives when and if they are developed and accepted by the regulatory and scientific communities. In the interim, industry has demonstrated a willingness to develop and adopt modifications to current testing procedures which may produce some short-term benefits, e.g., use of fewer animals, reduced discomfort, etc. As a result of these efforts, the number of animals used in safety testing has been dramatically reduced. As an example, during the period from 1980 to 1989, CTFA estimates that the number of rabbits used in eye irritancy evaluations for cosmetic products was reduced by 87 percent; the number of animals required for all other cosmetic product safety testing was reduced by an estimated 73 percent. In addition to a commitment to research on alternatives, other measures supported by the cosmetic industry have made such progress possible. The CTFA Cosmetic Ingredient Review (CIR) program has played a key role in minimizing the use of animals in safety testing. The program's mission is to collect, evaluate, and publicize all available published and unpublished safety data on cosmetic ingredients (24). By making publicly available the data maintained in an ingredient data bank, the CIR plays an important role in reducing duplicative animal testing.

Although definitive statistics are not available in the United States, figures on the numbers of scientific procedures performed in the U.K. are available on an annual basis. The latest year for which figures are available is 1990 (25). The *total* number of project license holders on which the 1990 statistics are based was 4,500 (i.e., an increase of just over 300 more than in 1989). Even so, the number of scientific procedures (or experiments) performed on animals in 1990 fell by 100,000 (3%) compared to the previous year, thus marking the fourteenth successive fall in the annual number of scientific procedures started in any one year (Figure 2).

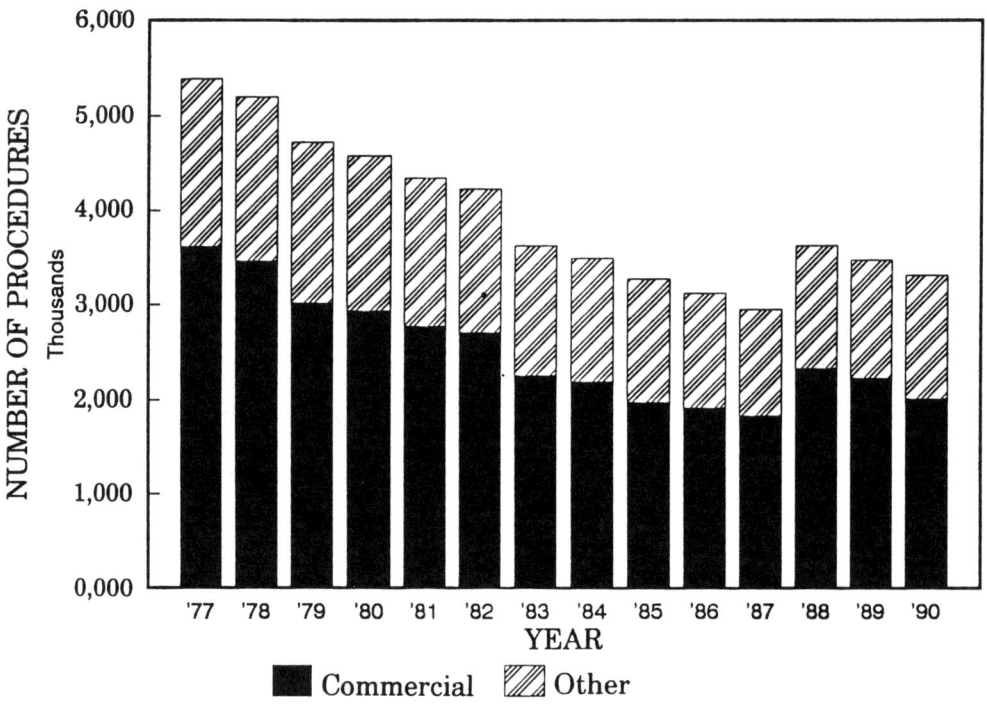

Figure 2. Number of Scientific Procedures Performed on Animals in Great Britain 1977-90.

As noted in a recent review of the Home Office's figures *(FRAME News (1991) 28, 20-21)*, the data indicate a sharp fall in the number of animals used in cosmetic testing from 12,090 in 1989 to 4,365 (64%) in 1991. However (perhaps not surprisingly, given consumer pressure for a safer environment), there appears to have been an increase in the number of animals used for safety evaluation concerned with environmental pollution (24%), agricultural substances (35%) and industrial chemicals (7%), and also more safety evaluation procedures for food additives (90%), tobacco (70%) and alcohol (28%). Interestingly, the major increases in numbers of procedures appear to have come from government departments and non-profit making organizations, rather than from commercial organizations.

As has been pointed out by FRAME, many well-intentioned people apparently believe that they are being consistent in both supporting organizations concerned with so-called "cruelty-free" living, and those which aim to force government and industry to give greater protection to workers, consumers and the environment *(FRAME News (1991) 28, 20-21)*. Ironically, increased assurance of human and environmental "safety" may currently rely upon extensive testing in animals. Examination of Table 2, showing trends in the use of animal procedures since the *Animals (Scientific Procedures) Act* came into effect in 1987, reveals that the quest for "environmentally-safe" products has resulted in a marked increase in the number of animal tests

Table 2.   Number of Scientific Procedures Perfomed on Animals in Great Britain Classified by Commercial Category (1987 vs. 1990).

Category	Procedures (thousands)		
	1987	1990	% Change
Agricultural chemicals	77.5	108.9	+40.5
Industrial chemicals	70.3	92.0	+30.9
Environmental pollution	28.2	43.2	+53.2
Cosmetics and toiletries	14.5	4.4	-69.7
Household materials	6.9	1.5	-78.3
Alcohol	3.7	1.4	-62.2
Food additives	3.3	10.8	+227.3
Tobacco	1.3	0.7	-46.2
Other	37.9	13.8	-63.4
Total	243.6	276.7	+13.6
(Total - all procedures)	3,631.4	3,207.1	-11.7

Due to changes in reporting requirements, it is likely that some testing listed in Table 2 in the "other" category for 1987, has since been re-allocated to the specific subjects listed. (Reproduced, by permission from FRAME News (1991) 28, 20-21).

undertaken to evaluate their toxicity (a 13.6% increase *vs.* an overall decrease of 11.7% for all procedures). This increase cannot be blamed on the cosmetics and household products industries (combined 72.4% decrease), but rather is due to significant increases in tests on agricultural chemicals (fertilizers and pesticides), industrial chemicals and food additives, and in ecotoxicity testing.

PUBLIC PERCEPTION

Scientists are not the only audience interested in the development of alternatives. Through its publications and presentations, CAAT has successfully drawn attention to alternative testing methods and provided essential information to scientists, industry executives, government officials, animal protection advocates, and (through the news media) the general public. The *CAAT Newsletter* has grown from an initial circulation of 1,000 to more than 20,000, and reaches an international audience in 62 countries. CAAT has reached millions of people through coverage in the news media. The Center's activities have been covered by newspapers, magazines, radio and television stations, and scientific, industry and animal-protection publications throughout the United States and in several other countries. Publicity has appeared in many large-circulation periodicals, including *The Wall Street Journal, The New York Times, The Los Angeles Times, The Chicago Tribune, USA Today, Newsweek* and *Business Week*.

Even in its infancy, it was recognized that the Center would occupy a pivotal societal position. While it's own role would be a strictly scientific one, other questions - of ethics, law and policy - all turned on a scientific base *(CAAT Newsletter (1982) 1 (1), 3)*. At the first CAAT Government Exchange Group meeting in June 1989 (attended by representatives from EPA, USDA, NIH, FDA, U.S. Fish and Wildlife Service, National Institute of Standards and Technology, Association of American Veterinary Medicine Colleges, American Veterinary Medical Association and Tufts Center for Animals and Public Policy), it was noted that "The public often has unreasonable expectations about the complete substitution of *in vitro* tests for all product testing" *(CAAT Newsletter (1989) 7 (2), 5)*, and that this misunderstanding may pose a danger to science if the public pressures (federal) legislators and regulatory agencies to place more restrictions on biomedical research". Although attendees at the first CAAT Government Exchange Group meeting identified *Congressional* staff members as being a key constituency in terms of educating non-scientists with regard to progress and the limits of *in vitro* toxicology tests, it has been at the *State* legislative level where the greatest dangers to the maintenance of responsible biomedical and scientific regulation lie. As a specific example, since the creation of the Center in 1981, CTFA has contested legislation which would outlaw or restrict the use of animal testing procedures in at least 12 states (Arizona, California, Connecticut, Hawaii, Illinois, Maryland, Massachusetts, Michigan, New York, New Jersey, Pennsylvania, and Vermont).

Overestimation and overpromotion of the usefulness and validity of non-animal techniques benefit no one. The assistance of CAAT has been invaluable in helping to dispel the, sometimes false and often misleading, statements made by misinformed individuals concerning the availability of alternatives capable of totally replacing animal testing methods. There is some evidence, however, that the public is *beginning* to understand the issues involved, and that CAAT's message is finding at least some receptive audiences: A Consumer Federation of America (CFA) Policy Resolution, adopted in February 1988, affirmed that CFA opposes efforts to outlaw the use of animals for the purpose of testing the safety of consumer products such as household substances, drugs and cosmetics. Whilst supporting laboratory guidelines/standards to promote the humane treatment of animals, and believing that alternative non-animal tests should be developed, the resolution further states that "Outlawing animal testing would have a chilling effect on biomedical research and would make it impossible to determine the adverse effects of many chemical ingredients used in thousands of consumer products".

PRIDE AND PREJUDICE

During its first ten years, the CAAT has been influential in two important areas. Through its research program, the Center has demonstrated to the scientific community that a directed effort to find and develop alternatives can succeed. Through its information program, the Center has improved the public's understanding of animal testing and the potential value of alternatives. The Center has legitimized worldwide the scientific pursuit of alternatives to animal testing. Its procedures have achieved international recognition and have served as the model for similar programs established in Europe. Industry is proud to have played a part in CAAT's success. Why *"Pride and Prejudice"?* Industry is proud of CAAT's achievements, but our opinion is prejudiced by the fact that industry feels a measure of responsibility for CAAT's success. Industry has been a partner with CAAT. Industry had the foresight to found the Center in 1981, and to continue to fund it's activities (Figure 1). The *number* of corporate contributors, and the

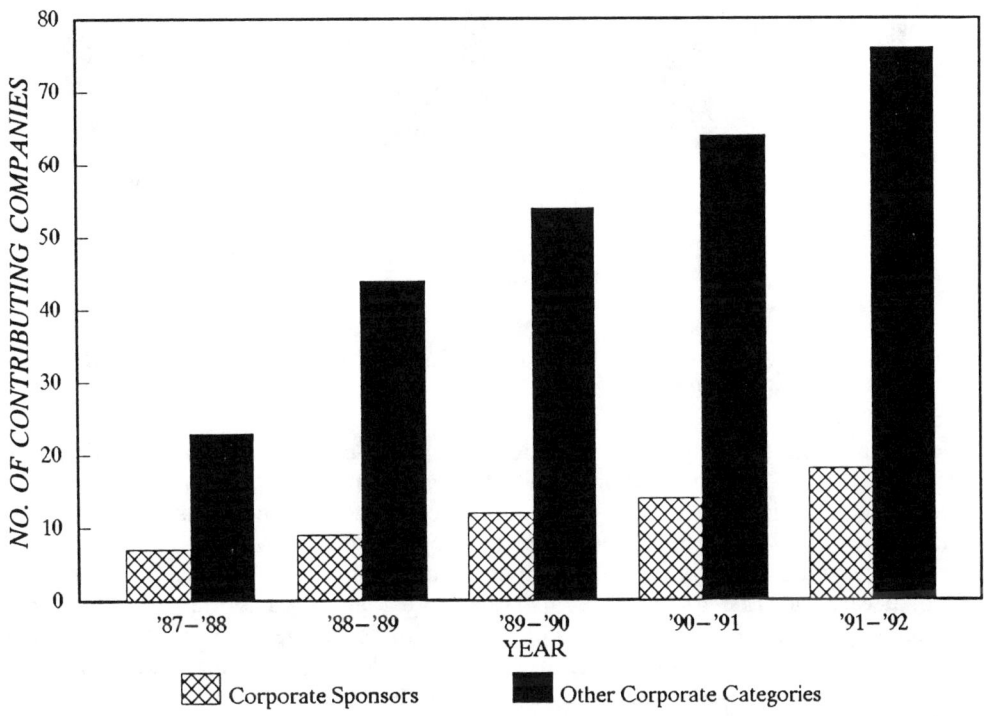

Figure 3. Level of Participation by Corporate Sponsors 1987-1991.

level of participation by CAAT's supporters have been increasing over the past ten years (Figure 3). Core support for CAAT remains within the cosmetic and personal-care industry (Figure 4). Commitment of funding by Exxon Corp., in January of 1984, signified the first corporate funding of CAAT outside the cosmetic and personal-care industry (Table 1); May 1989 signalled the first Federal funding of the Center when CAAT was awarded a five-year grant by the U.S. Public Health Service (funding of the grant was provided through the National Institutes of Health, Division of Research Resources, and the National Institute of Environmental Health Sciences). From 1981-92, over 140 corporations (Appendix) have contributed approximately $5.9 million to the Center. Industry has committed *significant* resources and millions of dollars in the search for alternatives, particularly with regard to finding replacements to the Draize test. Given their current state of development, reliance by industry on alternative tests is limited. Although

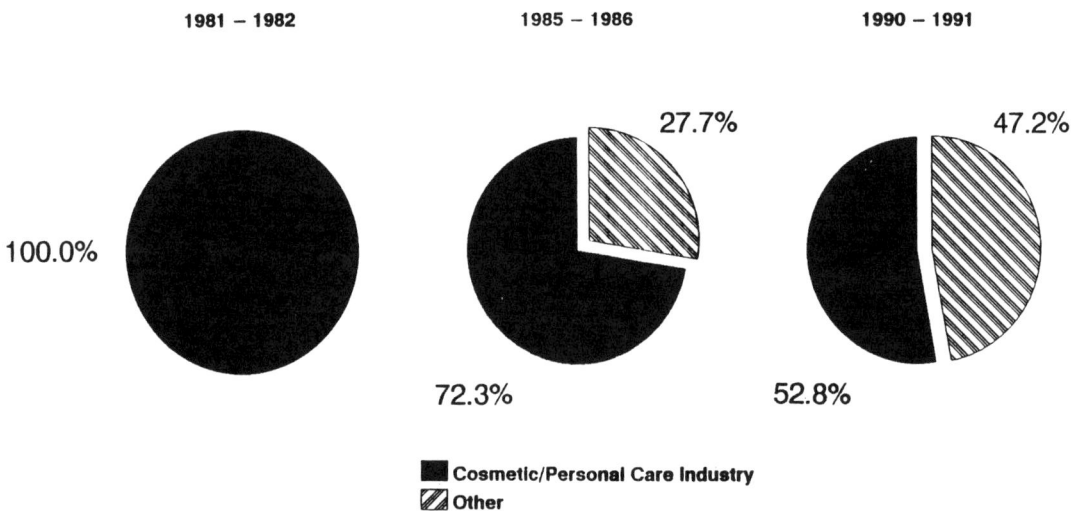

Figure 4. Percentage Funding by Cosmetic/Personal-Care Industry (i) 1981-1982; (ii) 1985-1986; (iii) 1991-1992.

several companies (notably in the cosmetic and personal-care industry) have publicly announced their ability to use (to a greater or lesser extent) alternatives to substantiate the safety of their products, others maintain that they have no choice but to test on animals. *Diversity should not be confused with division.* Industry is *united* in its opposition to any measure which would restrict the use of animals in safety substantiation and is also united in the search for alternatives. The personal care industry, for example, markets more than 80 categories and more than 5,000 individual products. For certain types of products there is, at present, *no* demonstrated viable non-animal alternative to *any* type of toxicity test which currently utilizes animals, and industry must continue to rely on animal data to substantiate the safety of raw materials and finished products.

At the 6th CAAT Symposium *"In Vitro* Toxicology: New Directions", Dr. John Yam (The Procter & Gamble Co.) presented a paper entitled *Development of Alternatives in a Consumer Product Company* (26), in which he notes "This paper outlines one company's approach to alternatives development. Obviously, a different approach may be more suitable for another company. The key is no one company can do it on its own. To be successful, alternatives development needs the cooperation of industry, the scientific community, regulatory agencies, and the animal rights community." The Johns Hopkins Center for Alternatives to Animal Testing (CAAT) provides a forum which fosters such cooperation. May CAAT be as successful in the next ten years as it has been in the last.

Acknowledgments -- The author wishes to thank the following individuals for their advice and contributions to the preparation of this paper: Dr. Alan Goldberg, Dr. John Fraizer, Marilyn Principe, and Richelle Lewis (CAAT); Louis DiPasquale (Gillette Medical Evaluation Labs.); Dr. G.N. McEwen, Jr., Jane Cavins, Pandora Dennis and Krista Merker (CTFA).

REFERENCES

(1) U.S. General Accounting Office (1980). Report #HRD8070, *Alternatives to Use of Animals in Research,* Washington DC: U.S. Government Printing Office.

(2) National Institues of Health (1981). *Trends in Bioassay Methodology: In Vivo, In Vitro and Mathematical Approaches,* pp. 371. Washington, DC: U.S. Government Printing Office.

(3) Rowan, A.N. & Andrutis, K.A. (1990). Alternatives: A socio-political commentary from the USA. *ATLA* 18, 3-10.

(4) CTFA (1980). Proceedings of the CTFA Ocular Safety Testing Workshop: *In Vivo and In Vitro Approaches.* Washington DC: The Cosmetic, Toiletry and Fragrance Association.

(5) Arthur, B.H., Pennisi, S.C., DiPasquale, L.C., Re, T., Dindardo, J., Kennedy, G.L., North-Root, H., Penney, D.A. & Sekerke, H.J. (1986). Effects of anesthetic pretreatment and low volume dosage on ocular irritancy potential of cosmetics: A collaborative study. *Journal of Toxicology-Cutaneous and Ocular Toxicology,* 5, 215-227.

(6) Goldberg, A.M. (1983). The Johns Hopkins Center for Alternatives to Animal Testing. In *Product Safety Evaluation* (Alternative Methods in Toxicology Vol. 1, ed. A.M. Goldberg), pp. 297-305. New York: Mary Ann Liebert, Inc.

(7) Frazier, J.M. & Goldberg, A.M. (1990). Alternatives to and reduction of animal use in biomedical research education and testing. *The Cancer Bulletin* 42, 238-245.

(8) Teal, J.J. (1991). Introduction to Avon Program Project. In *In Vitro Toxicology: Mechanisms and New Technology* (Alternative Methods in Toxicology Vol. 8, ed. A.M. Goldberg), pp. 23-25. New York: Mary Ann Liebert, Inc.

(9) Sauder, D.N. & Feliciani (1991). The skin as an immunologic organ: Role of epidermal cytokines. In *In Vitro Toxicology: Mechanisms and New Technology* (Alternative Methods in Toxicology Vol. 8, ed. A.M. Goldberg), pp. 27-36. New York: Mary Ann Liebert, Inc.

(10) Booman, K.A., Cascieri, T.M., Demetrulias, J., Driedger, A., Griffith, J.F., Grochoski, G.T., Kong, B., McCormick, W.C. III., North-Root, H., Rozen, M.G. & Sedlak, R.I. (1988). in vitro methods for evaluating eye irritancy of cleaning products Phase I: preliminary assessment. *Journal of Toxicology - Cutaneous and Ocular Toxicology* 7 (3), 173-185.

(11) Gettings, S.D. & McEwen, G.N. (1990). Development of potential alternatives to the Draize eye test: The CTFA Evaluation of Alternatives Program. *ALTA* 17, 317-324.

(12) Frazier, J.M. (1990). Scientific criteria for validation of *in vitro* toxicity tests. *OECD Environment Monographs, No. 36.*

(13) Gettings, S.D., DiPasquale, L.C., Bagley, D.M., Chudkowski, M., Demetrulias, J.L., Feder, P.I., Hintze, K.L., Marenus, K.D., Pape, W.W.W., Roddy, M., Schnetzinger, R., Silber, P.M., Teal, J.J., & Weise, S.L. (1990). The CTFA Evaluation of Alternatives Program. An evaluation of *in vitro* alternatives to the Draize primary eye irritation test. (Phase I) Hydroalcoholic formulations; a preliminary communication. *In Vitro Toxicology* 3, 293-302.

(14) Feder, P.I., Lordo, R.A., DiPasquale, L.C., Bagley, D.M., Chudkowski, M., Demetrulias, J.L., Hintze, K.L., Marenus, K.D., Pape, W.J.W., Roddy, M.T., Schnetzinger, R., Silber, P.M., Teal, J.J., Weise, S.L., & Gettings, S.D. (1991). The CTFA Evaluation of Alternatives Program. An evaluation of *in vitro* alternatives to the Draize primary eye irritation test. (Phase I) Hydroalcoholic formulations; (Part 1) Statistical methods. *In Vitro Toxicology* 4, 231-246.

(15) Gettings, S.D., Bagley, D.M., Demetrulias, J.L., DiPasquale, L.C., Hintze, K.L., Rozen, M.G., Teal, J.J., Weise, S.L., Chudkowski, M., Marenus, K.D., Pape, E.J.W., Roddy, M.T., Schnetizinger, R., Silber, P.M., Glaza, S.M., & Kurtz, P.J. (1991). The CTFA Evaluation of Alternatives Program. An evaluation of *in vitro* alternatives to the Draize primary eye irritation test. (Phase I) Hydroalcoholic formulations; (Part 2) Data analysis and biological significance. *In Vitro Toxicology* 4, 247-288.

(16) Booman, K.A., De Prospo, J., Demetrulias, J., Driedger, A., Griffith, J.F., Grochoski, G.T., Kong, B., McCormick, W.C. III, North-Root, H., Rozen, M.G., & Sedlak, R.I. (1988). The SDA alternatives program: comparison of *in vitro* data with Draize test data, *Journal of Toxicology - Cutaneous and Ocular Toxicology* 8 (1), 35-49.

(17) Frazier, J.M. (1989). *Technical Report No. 1*. Technical Problems Associated with In Vitro Toxicology Testing Systems. (June 1989).

(18) Sehneit, S.S. (1990). *Technical Report No. 2*. Structure-Activity Relationships in Predictive Toxicology. (November 1990).

(19) Bradlaw, J., Flint, O.P., & Frazier, J.M. (1992). *Technical Report No. 4*. Cell Culture Systems and *In Vitro* Toxicity Testing. *Cytotechnology* (In Press).

(20) Balls, M., Blaauboer, B., Brusick, D., Frazier, J., Lamb, D., Pemberton, M., Reinhardt, C., Roberfroid, M., Rosenkranz, H., Schmid, B., Spielman, H., Stammat, A-L., & Walum, E. (1990). Report and recommendations of the CAAT/ERGATT Workshop on the validation of toxicity test procedures. *ATLA* 18, 313-338.

(21) Frazier, J.M. (1992). *Technical Report No. 5*. International Status of Validation of *In Vitro* Toxicity Tests. (In preparation).

(22) Goldberg, A.M. & Frazier, J.M. (1989). Alternatives to animals in toxicity testing. *Scientific American* 261 (2), 24-30.

(23) Russell, W.M.S & Burch, R.L. (1959). *The Principles of Humane Experimental Technique*, pp238, London: Methuen.

(24) Elder, R.L. (1984). The Cosmetic Ingredient Review - a safety evaluation program. *J.Am. Acad. Dermatol.* 11, 1168-1174.

(25) Home Office (1990). *Statistics of Scientific Procedures on Living Animals in Great Britain 1990,* London: HMSO.

(26) Yam, J. & Winters, R. (1989). Devlopment of alternatives in a consumer product company. In *In Vitro Toxicology: New Directions* (Alternative Methods in Toxicology Vol. 7, ed. A.M. Goldberg), pp. 23-32. New York: Mary Ann Liebert, Inc.

APPENDIX

The Johns Hopkins Center for Alternatives to Animal Testing
A History of Corporate Contributions 1981-1992

Corporate Sponsors

3M
Abbott Laboratories
Amoco Corporation
ARCO
Avon Products, Inc.
BP America, Inc.
Bausch & Lomb
Bernice Barbour Foundation, Inc.
Bristol-Myers Squibb Company
Charles River Laboratories, Inc.
CIBA-GEIGY Corporation
The Cosmetic, Toiletry & Fragrance Association, Inc.
The Geraldine R. Dodge Foundation
The Estee Lauder Companies
Exxon Corporation
Hoffmann-La Roche
IBM Corporation
Johnson & Johnson
L'Arome (U.S.A.) Inc.
L'Oreal
Mary Kay Cosmetics, Inc.

Federal Sponsors

Environmental Protection Agency
  Health Effects Research Laboratory
National Institutes of Health

Corporate Patrons

Alberto-Culver Company
Benetton Cosmetics Inc.
The Clorox Company
Cosmair Inc.
E.I. du Pont de Nemours & Company
Eli Lilly & Co.
Gilette Medical Evaluation Laboratories

Corporate Patrons (continued)

Glaxo Inc.
Hoffmann-LaRoche
ICI Pharmaceuticals Group
S.C. Johnson Wax
Miles, Inc.
The Procter & Gamble Company
Unilever (UK)
Xerox Corporation

Corporate Benefactors

Abbott Laboratories
Allied-Signal, Inc.
American Hospital Supply Fdn.
Amoco Foundation, Inc.
Baxter American Fdn.
BeautiControl Cosmetics
Best Foods (a division of CPC International Inc.)
The Body Shop Inc.
Colgate-Palmolive Company
Elizabeth Arden
Hoechst Celanese Corporation
Gulf Oil Fdn.
Kimberly-Clark Corporation
Maybelline
The Mennen Co.
Merck Sharp & Dohme
Neutrogena Corporatrion
Parfums Christian Dior
Pfizer Inc.
The Upjohn Company

Corporate Contributors

Louis & Ann Abrons Foundation, Inc.
Allergan

The Johns Hopkins Center for Alternatives to Animal Testing
A History of Corporate Contributions 1981-1992

Corporate Contributors (continued)

Block Drug Company Inc.
Boyle-Midway Household Products, Inc.
Chanel, Inc.
Chesebrough-Pond's Inc.
The Coca-Cola Company
The Dow Chemical Company
Dow Corning Corporation
Guerlain Inc.
Helene Curtis, Inc.
Hershey Foods Corporation
L & F Products
Microbiological Associates, Inc.
Monsanto Company
Parfums Nina Ricci, U.S.A. Limited
Rickett & Colman Household Products
Shaklee Corp.
Shell Oil Company Foundation
Society of Cosmetic Chemists
Sterling Drug Inc.

Corporate Friends

A.K.A. Saunders Inc. DBA TerraNova DBA Nectarine
Allergan
AMA Laboratories Inc.
Airwick Industries
Alcon Laboratories, Inc.
Alza Corporation
American Cyanamid
The Andrew Jergens Company
Arbonne Manufacturing/North America, Inc.
Australian Society of Cosmetic Chemists
BF Goodrich Co. Specialty Polymers
 & Chemicals Division
BDF Beiersdorf Inc.
Bayer/AG Miles
Beatrice Fdn.
Beecham Products
Benetton Cosmetics Inc.
Blistex Inc.
Bonne Bell Inc.
Bradford
Bundesverband
Carme, Inc.
Carson Products Company
Charles of the Ritz
Church & Dwight Co., Inc.

Corporate Friends (continued)

Clarins U.S.A., Inc.
Concept Now Cosmetics
The Dial Corp.
Evyan Perfumes, Inc.
Fred Hayman Beverly Hills
Georgette Klinger Labs
Gryphon Development, L.P.
H_2O Plus
Hawaiian Tropic Tanning Research Laboratories, Inc.
Hazelton Labs Corp.
Health Designs Inc.
Health Industry Manufacturers Association (HIMA)
Houbigant, Inc.
J&J Baby Products
Key West Fragrance & Cosmetic Factory
L&F Products
Lever Bros Co. Fnd.
Life Technologies, Inc.
Lion Corporation Biological Science Laboratories
MEM Company, Inc.
M&M/Mars
M.A.C. Cosmetics (Make-Up Art Cosmetics Limited)
Mary Ann Liebert Inc.
Merle Norman Cosmetics
Mibelle AG
Miranol Inc.
The Pennsylvania SPCA
Presperse, Inc.
ROC, S.A.
Rakuma Labs
Redken Laboratories, Inc.
Richardson-Vicks
Shell Oil Company Foundation
Sherex Chemical Co.
Shiseido Cosmetics (America) Ltd.
SmithKline Beecham Consumer Brands
Soundscape
St. Ives Laboratories, Inc.
Taconic Farms
Tevco Inc.
Walgreens
Warner-Lambert Foundation
The Wella Corporation
West Coast Cosmetics Associates
Whittaker Bioproducts Inc.
Yves Rocher, Inc.

E2

Alternatives in the 90's: What's Next?

HENRY SPIRA

Animal Rights Coalitions
Box 214, Planetarium Station
New York, NY 10024

ABSTRACT

The 80's was a decade of remarkable and innovative research and development of alternatives. We see the 90's as the decade of validation and implementation.

From an activist's perspective, the 80's was very encouraging,-- alternatives gained acceptance, legitimacy and credibility within the toxicology, corporate and regulatory communities. And The Center for Alternatives to Animal Testing (CAAT) at Johns Hopkins University played a significant role in making this acceptance possible.

But these new technologies have yet to realize their full potential; the focus to date has been on development more than on bringing these technologies into routine usage. And the public, including the more forward-looking sectors of the science community, is eager for results.

One way that activists in the 90's may promote alternatives is the development of a new "chic" in research, testing and education, in much the same way that anti-smoking groups have successfully turned around the image of smoking. With the support of pioneering groups, including the CAAT community, a trickle-down phenomenon can change the outlook and mind-set of future scientists. Starting with teenagers, we can turn around the tradition that sees animals as test tubes with whiskers towards the "chic" of Replacement, Reduction and Refinement as well as zero-based animal usage.

ALTERNATIVES IN THE 90's:
WHAT'S NEXT?

A sure sign of success in any movement is that it becomes self-sustaining. The size and diversity of this meeting testifies to the fact that the "Three R's" -- Reduction, Replacement and Refinement -- have a life of their own. Clearly, the concept of alternatives has gained legitimacy, become institutionalized and is moving into the scientific mainstream. But the pace needs to be accelerated.

There's a growing recognition that our treatment of animals merits serious consideration. Animal rights is recognized as a rapidly growing movement, with support across the entire spectrum, from young to old, from Right to Left, from rich to poor. It's one of three issues generating the largest amount of Congressional mail. It has made the covers of major publications and been the focus of national TV programs. It has rapidly gained credibility and legitimacy as a movement which has a rational foundation, has political clout, and is making real progress. The term animal rights is no longer belittled with quotation marks.

I believe that much of the movement's recent success can be traced to Peter Singer's 1975 manifesto, _Animal Liberation_. Singer provides a rational foundation for animal rights by framing it as a logical extension of earlier movements for human rights. He made it possible for social activists and professionals to rally to the cause. This new influx of talent has helped the movement gain widespread acceptance over the past decade.

DO PEOPLE CARE?

Polls show that the public increasingly feels that the suffering of animals does matter. Doyle Dane Bernbach reported that nine out of ten people are concerned with protecting animals. To place this in a larger context, we need to remember that only fairly recently has it become generally accepted that all humans, regardless of sex, race, nationality, religious or political beliefs, abilities or popularity are entitled to equal consideration -- that they have the right to not be harmed. The next reasonable step, once all humans have been included in this "circle of concern," is to expand the circle to include non-human animals. In our view, animal rights will continue to gain public support, not as the latest fad vying for media attention, but as a natural progression, an additional ethical consideration, a matter of consistency, justice and fair play.

Still, many people perceive the movement for animal protection as negative and anti-science. To counteract this perception, we have continually accentuated the fact that members of the science community are part of the nine out of ten people concerned with protecting animals. We have attempted to turn walls into bridges by promoting the shared goals of better science, efficiency, economy and humanity.

Our role has been largely that of catalyst and amplifier. Members of the science community have been the first to note that humane science can also be better science. The "Three R's" had for some time been a quiet, pioneering enterprise; we encouraged proliferation of the concept within the corporate, regulatory, scientific, and educational sectors.

What is particularly encouraging is that within the past decade a whole new discipline of in-vitro toxicology has begun to enter the mainstream. There are now university centers, data bases, scientific journals, newsletters, books and professional associations devoted to alternatives. And the subject is routinely included in major scientific conferences, seminars, symposia and data bases.

HOW DID THESE EFFORTS GET UNDERWAY?

In the old days, biological scientists and animal protectionists were usually to be found at each other's throats,-- each screaming that the other was immoral. This deplorable state of affairs, dependent on a black-and-white, saints-and-sinners way of looking at the issues, ruled the past century and did no good to anyone, including the animals.

Fortunately, early in the century, a small but rapidly growing cadre of visionary philosopher/scientists emerged. They conceived the possibility that the goals of science and of the animal protection movement need not be contradictory, that difficult as the idea might at first appear, humane science would be better science.

Individuals working within this framework produced a series of suggestions as to what was doable. In 1959, W.M. Russell and R.L. Burch published their ground-breaking study, <u>The Principles of Humane Technique</u>, which suggested that humane science can also be better science. They developed the concept of alternatives through the "Three R's" -- methods which (1) Replace the use of animals, (2) Reduce the number of animals used, or which (3) Refine existing procedures so that animals are subject to less pain and suffering.

Then, in 1978, David Smyth, the late head of the British Research Defense Society, published <u>Alternatives to Animal Experiments</u>, which explored potential alternatives in biology. As Russell and Burch had done, Smyth attempted the difficult task of defining where alternatives were possible versus areas in which animal use, at the time, appeared essential. In 1984, Andrew Rowan's thoughtful assessment of the use of animals in research, <u>Of Mice, Models, & Men</u>, was, among other things, instrumental in changing the attitude within the science community from "<u>if</u> an alternative can be developed" to "<u>when</u> we develop an alternative."

And the movement toward alternatives gained energy from the traditional practise in science of questioning the usual ways of doing things and attempting to think through what is really necessary and sufficient for solving any problem.

HOW WE CAN "KICK THE HABIT"

Since 1980, this theme was also promoted by our animal protection coalitions. We maintained that much unnecessary animal suffering is due to "creeping routinism," and suggested that this be countered by clear goals and questioning of methods. I use "we" rather than "I" to indicate that both the actions and the ideas described are the product of a loose network of organizations and individuals with a variety of expertise, meeting informally to develop and implement programs and campaigns.

One method of challenging "creeping routinism" is through the concept of "zero-based" animal use. This calls for an institution to examine its entire animal research program as if it had just begun, from ground zero, so that people do not mindlessly repeat what was done in previous years.

People and institutions tend to do tomorrow what they did yesterday. To counter this, we have suggested that before any laboratory animals are used, the review process must question: "Is this research/data really necessary?" "Can this information be obtained without using animals?" "With fewer animals?" "With less pain?" We feel that such a program can rapidly eliminate zeros from the more than 20,000,000 laboratory animals currently being used in the USA every year.

STARTING WITH THE DRAIZE

Smyth was a pioneer of this concept and proposed replacing the Draize test. The Draize presumes to measure the potential for chemicals to damage the human eye based on the damage inflicted in the eyes of conscious rabbits. It clearly causes suffering and Smyth felt that the development of alternatives should not present any major scientific problems. We therefore decided to approach corporations involved in Draize testing, hoping to gain their collaboration in seeking alternatives. We began by attempting dialog with cosmetics industry leader, Revlon.

At first, Revlon refused to consider the potential of alternatives, perhaps "considering the source". But after more than two years of protests, Revlon responded with an historic initiative: multi-year funding of research at Rockefeller University to seek cell biological and other humane alternatives to the Draize test. Revlon launched a program that led to institutionalizing and carrying forward the seminal suggestions of Smyth and others.

This momentum and our negotiations with Avon, Bristol-Myers, Estee Lauder and other major corporations, all of whom were concerned with the image they were projecting, led to the creation of the Johns Hopkins Center for Alternatives to Animal Testing. CAAT distributed many small grants, piggybacking the search for alternatives onto massive research projects already in progress. This resulted in established researchers becoming sensitized to emerging opportunities in new methods, and thereby expanding the alternatives loop. In addition, symposia and publications under the aegis of CAAT Director Alan Goldberg did much to promote networking among scientists developing new methods, as well as to legitimize the concept of alternatives.

As part of this initial thrust, the idea of giving alternatives a fair shake was furthered significantly by the trailblazing activities of a number of corporate toxicologists, including Ted Brenner, John Corbett, Pam Danneman, Yale Gressel, Jack Griffith, Myron Mehlman, Emil Pfitzer, Jim Russo, Bob Scala, Janice Teal, Alex Vongries, and John Yam; the initiatives of government scientists, including June Bradlaw, Gary Ellis, Ted Farber, Sid Green, Dick Hill, Kailash Gupta, John Moore, Gary Flamm, Victor Morgenroth and David Rall; and the work of science writers Jeannie Blake, Mary Brevnik, Ron Dagani, Barnaby Feder, Susan Fowler, Jane Gregory, Cathy Heinze, Constance Holden, Rex Rhein, Helen Smith, Nicholas Wade, and Jonathan Weiner, among others.

These initiatives were the "big bang,"-- an immense leap forward in establishing the legitimacy and promise of alternatives. They have generated new ideas and findings and spawned similar major programs elsewhere.

Meanwhile visionary high-tech entrepreneurs have begun to realize the great promise in alternatives. In addition to R&D they are aggressively marketing new methods: setting up laboratories, organizing workshops to familiarize technicians with the state of the art, and, most excitingly, joining forces with major multinational corporations.

ON TO THE LD50

Similar progress has taken place in phasing down the 65-year-old classic LD50 test. The LD50 (Lethal Dose 50% Test) measures death slowly, painfully and badly. It generates, with meaningless precision, a number indicating how much of every product, per body weight, is needed to kill half of a group of lab animals.

Just ten years ago, the LD50 was considered the foundation of safety testing. Now, there's almost unanimous agreement that the LD50 is wasteful and unnecessary. And this change is due in large part to our amplifying the criticisms made by leading toxicologists, including Gerhard Zbinden, who in 1982 asserted that "clinical experience shows that the LD50 value determined in animals rarely bears a meaningful relation with the lethal dose in man." Zbinden suggested regulatory change from the LD50 to range-finding tests using one-tenth the number of animals with careful observation. Furthermore, Smyth had noted the incongruity of mortality being used as a test for morbidity, a lethal dose providing assurances about non-lethal toxicity.

A turning point in the campaign to phase out the LD50 was a letter from David P. Rall, then Director of the National Toxicology Program, who called the LD50 "an anachronism... I do not think the LD50 test provides much useful information about the health hazards to humans from chemicals, the NTP does not use the LD50..."

THE EXPANDING LOOP

Progress toward phasing out the LD50 and the Draize tests has been rapid. Ten years ago, replacing these tests appeared overwhelmingly difficult. But as events developed, it was the scientific objections to these tests, plus growing support for alternatives from sectors of the toxicology, corporate, and governmental communities that led to encouraging results.

Over the past decade, major corporations such as Avon, Bristol-Myers, Colgate, Hoffmann-La Roche, Johnson & Johnson, L'Oreal, Mobil, Procter & Gamble, Revlon, and Unilever, among others, have instituted structural changes to promote alternatives. Here are some examples:

Hoffmann-La Roche has decreased its use of animals by 67% over a seven-year period. One of the techniques that made this possible is computer-assisted molecular modeling, which allows the shape and structure of an experimental compound to be visualized in a three-dimensional image on a computer screen; predictions of biological effects can then be made on the basis of similarities between the structure of molecules.

In 1991 alone, Procter & Gamble spent over $4.6 million on alternatives research and they are sharing these results with others to help advance scientific and governmental acceptance of alternative methods. P&G also publishes "Alternatives Alert," the first corporate newsletter devoted specifically to promoting alternatives. P&G researchers have published and presented more than one hundred papers on alternatives.

Colgate-Palmolive has publicly committed itself to the long-term goal of completely replacing the use of animals with alternative methods. They have developed the CAM Test, which uses the membrane of a fertilized chicken egg to predict the potential of materials to cause eye irritation, and they are sharing the results.

One of the most dramatic examples of a science-driven move toward alternatives is happening at the National Cancer Institute. NCI has developed a new in-vitro screen for testing potential anti-cancer compounds which has reduced their animal use from 6,000,000 to less than 300,000 annually, while improving the quality of research.

WHERE DO WE GO FROM HERE?

Now that the concept of alternatives has been legitimized and even institutionalized, the question becomes: Where do we go from here? Despite all the progress, energy and creativity, it's not clear where things are now, nor where it's all going. There are no timetables, no benchmarks and nobody has yet attempted to pull it all together. While each research project may well be brilliant and well organized, it's not necessarily linked to what others may be doing, nor to any overarching plan. If we keep pursuing the current trajectory, it's not at all clear what will be nailed down in any of our lifetimes. The potential is there to keep developing more and more candidates for alternatives when we need to focus serious energies on assessing, validating and implementing the most promising tests already developed.

It seems to us that we now need to shift gears,-- that what is now needed, in the common interest, is a blueprint.

To illustrate this concept, consider an orchestra. An orchestra can consist of brilliant, accomplished musicians, but if these musicians are not playing the same piece, if there is no agreed musical score nor even a conductor, then the many random sounds will not likely produce the coherent, harmonious music you are aiming for.

As another example, consider space exploration. Regardless of one's own sense of social priorities, NASA could never have met the challenge of putting people on the moon in the relatively short period of less than ten years without strong central direction, an absolute commitment to planning and coordination, and, above all, a strong conviction in their ability to succeed.

HOW DO WE GO ABOUT CONSTRUCTING A BLUEPRINT?

The European community already recognizes that validation of potential alternatives is a key stumbling block in the application and use of alternatives. Accordingly, they are establishing the European Center for the Validation of Alternative Methods (ECVAM) in Ispra, Italy, whose primary focus will be to coordinate the validation of alternatives within the European Community. ECVAM will also serve as an information exchange on alternatives and promote dialogue among legislators, industry, biomedical scientists, consumer organizations and animal welfare groups.

Unlike the European Community, the USA has yet to establish a national center for the validation and implementation of alternatives.

Clearly, leadership is one of the first issues which will need to be addressed in the construction of a center and a plan. It has been suggested in several quarters that the National Toxicology Program/National Institute of Environmental Health Sciences (NTP/NIEHS) represents a natural setting for this initiative, and that its Director, Kenneth Olden, may well be the ideal person to pull it all together and set up a steering group.

It would be important that this steering group have representation from all the relevant sectors including industry, members of the Interagency Regulatory Alternatives Group (IRAG), academia, animal protectionists and consumer advocates such as perhaps the Council on Economic Priorities (CEP).

One of the first tasks that would need to be undertaken by this group is a "situation analysis" to summarize and assess where we are now, what's happened to date, the successes and obstacles to step by step implementation.

Upon completion, this "situation analysis" would form the basis for setting clear objectives, strategies and time-tables. In developing such a plan, it is crucial that there be guidance, input and participation from as many sectors as possible who will be affected by the outcome. And in the process of preparing the blueprint, additional ideas may well be generated.

We're not proposing a straitjacket, but rather a living, breathing, flexible plan, that is fine tuned as it progresses, a program that is modified and adapted on the basis of real world experience.

To ensure optimal progress, the Center's steering group should meet regularly to update progress and monitor implementation.

A PRACTICAL PLAN FOR CHANGE

We're talking about a plan that leads to meaningful change. This is not wishful thinking since there are many initiatives that can be acted on immediately.

For example, the "zero-based" concept of animal use, while currently accepted by forward-looking researchers, needs to become the norm throughout the corporate, academic and governmental sectors.

In tandem with the "zero-based concept," corporate and government agencies need to adopt the "Three R's." The "Three R's" are methods which, as stated earlier, (1) Replace the use of animals, (2) Reduce the number of animals used, or (3) which Refine existing procedures so that animals are subject to less pain and suffering.

Practical application of these policies will lead to scrapping those animal tests that have no significant value in protecting the public or the environment and whose only justification appears to be "this is the way we've always done it." Testing requirements should be science-driven, not based on historical baggage and check-lists.

Another thing a blueprint can do is to help avoid unnecessary and costly duplication by providing for a system of data sharing which also addresses concerns such as proprietary interests and compensation. A possible prototype: the FIFRA provisions used by the Registration Division of the EPA's Office of Pesticide Programs. This Office actively encourages data sharing, with the result that the majority of data submitted come from existing EPA files, not from needless duplication. Fair compensation is worked out between the submittor and user; if they cannot agree, the final determination is made by US Department of Labor arbitrators.

There's also the need to promote international regulatory acceptance of the most modern, most reliable and most humane methods. With commerce being global, international harmonization is crucial. Recently, there have been some encouraging agreements among officials from the FDA, the European Community and Japan to end the classic LD50, and to accept reproductive toxicology data that meet USA, EC or Japanese standards rather than duplicating the testing.

Finally, we need to address the issue of who will pay for this proposed undertaking which will be, in effect, a center for the validation and implementation of alternatives. One possibility is that this initiative be jointly funded by the corporate sector, government and the animal protection community.

THE NEED TO MONITOR PROGRESS

It will be difficult to assess or quantify progress without a benchmark and tracking mechanism. It has been suggested that this can only be done with an Animal Utilization Survey, a basic tool which is used overseas but not yet in the USA. Such surveys provide a baseline against which to measure progress; they make it possible to prioritize goals and allocate resources on the basis of the numbers of animals, the opportunities for change and the pain involved.

Such a survey should be sufficiently detailed to make it possible to track animal usage in relation to objectives. Categories could include: drug discovery and development; data for regulatory purposes; education; production of biological products, etc.

Not least, an animal utilization survey can increase sensitivity. The research community and the public at large may well have the impression that nobody counts the numbers because the numbers don't count.

GETTING THE BALL ROLLING

It has been suggested that closure for one specific animal test in one specific product category however narrow and specific, can provide a prototype to get the ball rolling. In this connection, the Draize eye irritancy test is most frequently mentioned.

The movement for new methods could be enormously energized were there a prototype for bringing a predetermined line of products to market without using traditional testing methods and without compromising consumer safety.

The first steps toward such a prototype are already underway: some of the largest household products companies are now working together to establish guidelines to identify shampoo formulations that would no longer require the traditional routine

Draize animal tests. While developing a shampoo matrix might not appear of historic import, the matrix could in fact open the door to a revolution in toxicology. If carried to fruition, it could serve as a possible prototype for defining regulatory needs for other product lines.

But, in replacing the Draize test, as would be true for replacing other traditional tests, the point is not to daydream or "ivory tower" to the point of abstract perfection. Rather, let us seek methods that have practical application. And this is the audience that can make it happen.

To summarize, we've had a decade of brilliant development. What's needed now is a decade of aggressive implementation. As an engineering friend of mine told me, "there comes a point when you have to stop designing and start shipping."

E3

A Ten-Year Progress Report of The Center for Alternatives to Animal Testing: A Governmental Perspective

GERALD B. GUEST

Center for Veterinary Medicine
Food & Drug Administration
Rockville, MD 20857

It is a real pleasure for me to meet with you today to celebrate the 10th Anniversary of the Johns Hopkins Center for Alternatives to Animal Testing (CAAT) and to present "A Government Perspective" on the progress of the CAAT and issues concerning animal testing. My view of the CAAT comes largely from an awareness of its activities since the beginning, ten (10) years ago, and more recently as a member of the CAAT Advisory Board. Although I communicate frequently with other parts of the Federal Government on animal issues, my perspective is largely from my position in the Food and Drug Administration (FDA).

The Food and Drug Administration is a public health agency. Our job is to promote the public health as well as to protect the public health. The National Institutes of Health (NIH), the Centers for Disease Control (CDC), the Environmental Protection Agency (EPA), and the Consumer Product Safety Commission (CPSC) each have a purpose similar to the FDA, but each occupies a unique niche in the government's framework. FDA as it now exists and as it evolved geneologically, is a scientific organization. It dates from at least 1862 when the U.S. Department of Agriculture (USDA) established laboratories for the Bureau of Chemistry to investigate food-related issues.

We have tended to dramatize the development of food, drug and cosmetic regulation by highlighting crises such as the embalmed beef scandal of the Spanish-American War of 1989, the disgusting packing house conditions so graphically depicted in Upton Sinclair's The Jungle, the elixir of the sulfanilamide disaster, and the thalidomide tragedy, to name but a few. These provided impetus and helped marshal public support for stronger food and drug laws. But, in a less public way, food and drug regulation has quietly developed in parallel with scientific progress, particularly in chemistry and toxicology. Research with laboratory animals and toxicological evaluation of compounds in laboratory animals is a very major part of food and drug regulation.

As scientific knowledge progressed the Federal laws became more complex and more demanding. Passage of the 1906 Pure Food and Drugs Act was followed by the 1938 Food, Drug, and Cosmetic Act. In 1949, Representative James T. Delaney of New York began 2 years of legislative hearings which produced several amendments. Most notable is a proviso in the food and color additives laws which says that the FDA can not approve an additive as safe if found to cause cancer in man or experimental animals. The evaluation of drugs and food additives by conducting feeding studies in rats and mice took on new importance.

The march of science and regulation continued with the 1962 drug amendments requiring that drugs be both safe and effective, followed by the 1976 amendments covering medical devices and the 1980 Infant Formula Act.

Through the late 1970's and into the late 1980's, the FDA and the scientific community have struggled with the large societal issues of risk assessment, risk management, risk benefit evaluations, and what is meant by zero when one thinks of indirect or inadvertent chemical additives that may be carcinogenic at some level. In general we, you and I, try to determine how safe must a product or a process be. As sophisticated as our science and scientists have become, these kinds of issues are still debated as particular issues concerning particular products as they arise. Notable among these are saccharin, aspartame, and the color additives.

As scientists evolved the mechanisms and models for risk assessment, animals became an important surrogate for man, and in laboratories all over the world, important advances in public health are linked closely with the use of animals in biomedical research and in toxicological testing. All the while, of course, a very small part of the world's population were asking whether animal research was necessary. A feeling began to evolve among some that scientists were perhaps too comfortable with animal use or said another way, unconcerned about animal welfare. Some would abolish animal use in product testing, others would restrict the use of animals in research of any kind and still others are opposed to the confinement rearing of livestock as is practiced in many parts of the world today. It would be easy for us to think that this is a new issue and that our generation of scientists is being particularly singled out and our jobs made harder because of these outside forces. I will speak for a moment on the historical perspective of the antivivisection movement. Much of what I say historically on this issue is borrowed from a paper by Dr. Lester M. Crawford presented to the French Academy of Veterinary Medicine in Paris on June 21, 1984. Dr. Crawford preceded me at the FDA as Director of the Center for Veterinary Medicine.

Perhaps the most formidable antivivisection debate of all times occurred in Washington, D.C. in the 1890's. In 1898, Senate Bill 1063 which would have severely restricted animal experimentation in the District of Columbia by a system of stringent regulation, and periodic inspection of laboratories was reported unanimously by the relevant committee, the Committee of the District of Columbia. The proposed legislation was titled "A Bill for the Further Prevention of Cruelty to Animals in the District of Columbia." The Bill was defeated on the floor of the Senate primarily because of the debate and argument offered at the time by William Henry Welch, the great pathologist and Dean of the Johns Hopkins Medical School. An earlier version of the same Bill had failed in 1896. When the same legislation was introduced in 1900, as Senate Bill 34, Welch and his supporters resolved to lay the matter to rest once and for all.

There is a long list of scientific and medical societies that opposed the 1896, 1898, and 1900 proposals. Most of these organizations exist today. Among those supporting Welch were the National Academy of Sciences, the American Association for the Advancement of Science, the Society for Promotion of Aricultural Science, the American Medical Association, the

American Public Health Association, the American Veterinary Medical Association, and the Association of American Medical Colleges.

The proponents of the Bill were the Washington Humane Society. The record shows that the Washington Humane Society actually drafted the legislation and by the time it had been introduced for the third time both sides obviously saw the D.C. Bill as a harbinger of things to come for the rest of the nation. The list of scientists and leaders in the medical field who spoke out against this proposed law reads very much like a list of who's who of that day. Notable among the witnesses who spoke to the Congress at that time was Joseph Lister, the English surgeon who founded antiseptic surgery.

The Bill was ultimately defeated. Welch and his colleagues prevailed and prevailed so well that it was not until 1966 that similar legislation again surfaced in the Congress. This Bill as finally passed was called the Animal Welfare Act and is now administered by the U.S. Department of Agriculture.

Ten years ago when the Johns Hopkins Center for Alternatives to Animal Testing came into being, clearly the animal issue needed such an institution. By 1980, some of the public were focusing on the morality of animal experimentation and others on the three R's of animal welfare --- replacement, reduction, and refinement. (The three R's were presented by Russell and Bertch in Principles of Human Experimental Techniques.) In 1975 the Food and Drug Administration had published regulations on safety testing of cosmetics. The regulations generally stated that cosmetic manufacture must provide a product that is safe for the consumer, but no pre-market approval by the FDA is required. The implication, of course is that the cosmetic sponsor will develop convincing documentation of safety through testing in animals, or if appropriate in man. The Draize eye and skin irritation test were very much a part of the routine expected testing for cosmetic ingredients. Testing of cosmetics was and is a logical target for critics of animal use. The thought by some, of course, is that animals should not be used for testing products that could easily be eliminated from personal use. Divergent views on how to show safety of cosmetics in large part assisted in the birth of the CAAT and the Cosmetic, Toiletries, and Fragrance Association (CTFA) was responsible for the early funding of the Center.

Dr. Gary Flamm, a toxicologist and the FDA representative to the CAAT Advisory Board until 1988, has said that the Center was the first to enter into the unprecedented activity of getting toxicologists and other biologists from academia, industry, and government to discuss replacement alternatives to animal testing. Dr. Flamm told me in a recent conversation that he credits CAAT with finding a "formalized and dignified way" to cause us to face-up to an issue that had been largely ignored, because it was not the "politically correct" thing to talk about. Dr. Flamm said that CAAT, in the early years did a good job laying out problems and issues, for example the Draize Tests, and developing a strategy to deal with alternatives. He also offered that the Center then approached research in a very different way -- that of one university granting money to other universities.

Dr. Richard Hill an M.D., Ph.D. toxicologist with the Environmental Protection Agency and a member of the CAAT Advisory Board since the mid-eighties at my request offered his perspective on CAAT. Dr. Hill said that for the beginning CAAT has served as a focal point for the U.S. considerations for alternatives to animal testing. He credits Dr. Goldberg and others in CAAT for finding just the "right way to kick-off" the thinking on alternatives. The right way, according to Dr. Hill, was to approach alternatives in a deliberative way through scientific research and the funding of research.

Dr. Hill believes that, the CAAT moved quietly and efficiently into what was then a scientific void. Government at the time had no strategic programs which focused on alternatives to animal testing. In fact, it is only recently that some Government funding was extended to the CAAT. Today there are research grants coming to CAAT from the EPA and NIH.

In addition, Government scientists are actively involved in the peer review process for grant applications received by CAAT and Dr. Goldberg, Dr. Frazier, Dr. Zurlo and others on the CAAT staff meet regularly with Government staffers from a wide variety of agencies in Washington to discuss issues of mutual interest. The CAAT has also formed the Government Information Exchange Committee to facilitate increased communication.

I personally see the CAAT as an important entity for a number of reasons:

- CAAT conducts and funds research in search of alternatives to animal testing.

- Serves as important source of scientifically correct information.

- Provides an important bridge between academia, industry, government, and the animal welfare activists.

- Provides leadership in the U.S. and internationally as we move toward harmonization of requirements of regulatory agencies for product testing.

- Provides a vehicle for scientific consensus in the alternatives arena.

The Center continues to plan and set goals for the future. At the most recent planning retreat by the Center, in June 1991, the question of validation and the coming to closure on the acceptance of alternative was a much discussed topic. The feeling that the scientific community both within and outside government need to come to consensus and agree on replacement for at least the Draize tests is on everyone's mind. When researching this paper, I noted that Alan Goldberg in his column in the Fall 1984 issue of the CAAT Newsletter said:

"The next step is to begin to develop the mechanics for 'validation,' establishing the accuracy of those methods that have the greatest potential for replacing animals. There now are several methods ready for validation. These methods are possible Draize eye test replacements that correlate well with Draize scores, used to rank the effects of eye irritants."

Dr. Goldberg was correct then and what he wrote is true today. We simply must find the way to accomplish what Alan has suggested. Those of us in government are recognizing that government needs to become involved in this process, because in the end, it's the regulatory agencies on a global basis which must accept these alternatives and acceptance comes through scientific consensus and validation procedures. This is our challenge for the future.

This is a rather brief review of the ten years of CAAT from a government perspective. I would like to close this paper by acknowledging what an enormous contribution the Johns Hopkins University and the people at the CAAT have made to the science of alternatives to animal testing and the thinking that has come out of these activities as we all strive for more humane care and use of animals in biomedical research. I would like to congratulate Alan M. Goldberg, John M. Frazier, Joanne Zurlo, Marilyn Principe, and the remaining staff at the Johns Hopkins Center for Alternatives to Animal Testing for the fine job and the many accomplishments during this short ten years.

E4

A Report from the Center's Director

ALAN M. GOLDBERG

Johns Hopkins Center for Alternatives to Animal Testing
615 North Wolfe Street
Baltimore, MD 21205

ABSTRACT

IT HAS BEEN A REMARKABLE TEN YEARS.

I will provide my perspective on topics that CAAT has been involved with and how I visualize the progress and some next steps. I will share with you anecdotes and personal events that have made it fun, sometimes painful, but always rewarding. I will start by looking at our name.

The JOHNS HOPKINS CENTER FOR ALTERNATIVES TO ANIMAL TESTING

I would like to focus on 3 aspects of the name.

Johns Hopkins

I am not certain that the Center would have flourished the way it has in many other institutions. We were able to utilizes the resources, the strengths, and the people. We share a common purpose. We combined a very strong focused research program with a professional service activity and by combining the two we were able to develop a home for the CAAT at the Johns Hopkins School of Hygiene and Public Health.   It is noteworthy that next week the Johns Hopkins School of Public Health will celebrate its 75th Anniversary.

Alternatives

Russell and Burch, in their book *The Principles of Humane Experimental Technique,* described the concept of alternatives in the three R's - refinement, reduction, replacement. The Center has focused on rigorous science with the anticipation that *In Vitro* methods will be used for safety assessment and product development. We have consistently identified that *in vitro* methods are a routine part of the methodology used by the scientific community in the quest for basic knowledge. In that search *in vitro* methods must be coupled with clinical and whole animal studies. I anticipate that *in vitro* methods in safety testing and product development will fully meet the concept of alternatives and be used not only as refinement alternatives and reduction alternatives, but also as replacement alternatives.

Animal

There is no question that the material I read in the press and the fact that successful business strategies have developed based on decreased animal use, tells me what we all already know; humans care deeply about animals. There are many symbols that one could use to show this phenomena - Bugs Bunny is 52 years old and has had a museum exhibit dedicated to him. We have anthropomorphized Bugs, as we have many other animals, so that they speak to us, for us, and with us. Milly, the White House Dog, has written a best seller. Royalties in 1991 were almost one million dollars.

As the word alternative is charged and misunderstood, the words animal welfarist and animal rightist have been more carefully defined. They are not misunderstood. Ten years ago it was clear that animal welfare was the driving force and animal rightists, although present, were by no means as significant. In very short order the animal rightist misinformation and activities raised significant revenues and as a result parts of the welfare movement began to sound like parts of the rightist movement. This shift resulted in a loss of dialogue with industrial and academic groups - a dialogue the welfare community sought. Just about a year ago (Jan./Feb. 1991) a full page ad appeared in the New York Times where many of the major animal welfare organizations dissociated themselves from the rightist movement and the Animal Liberation Front.

Early on the press asked " If animal rightists are one extreme - what is the other extreme?"

Ten (10) years ago I would have answered that question by indicating that there is no other extreme. Scientists have thought out their ethical position, recognize that animals are necessary to advance animal and human well being, there is no other side. The scientific community is already a highly moderated and carefully conceived position. Unfortunately, this is no longer fully true. There are voices saying we have an obligation to use animals since all advances in biomedical research have been the result of animal studies. I do not accept this. Advances in biomedicine and health related studies are the result, not of animal studies alone or *in vitro* studies alone, but the consequence of the proper use of both of these approaches. Clearly, it is the combined approach that led to success in the most widely cited examples - the development of insulin and the polio vaccines.

ETHICAL POSITION OF THE CAAT

- To improve humankind

- A responsibility to nature and our environment, clearly, a responsibility to animals
- A surrogate responsibility to companion and research animals among others. Dick Bartlett and Fred Cheney first presented the concept of animal surrogacy. That is, as humans, we have a surrogate responsibility for companion animals and for those animals that will be used in research. This responsibility is no different than that which we have for our children or for incompetent adults such as severe Alzheimer's Disease patients. Surrogacy provides for informed consent, the basis of human institutional review boards. Federal and State Legislation are the empowering acts.

WE HAVE MADE PROGRESS

One question that I am sure all of us are asked is, "What progress have we made? Have we reduced animal use?"

I generally start by answering that one example is pregnancy testing. Today there are many chemically derived kits that are much less expensive, much more convenient, much quicker and fully replace animal use.

They respond, "That's only one example, are there others?"

I tell them of pyrogen testing and how rabbit use has been replaced with an *in vitro* assay accepted by the regulatory community.

Their response, "That was easy - what have you _really_ done?"

I point out that most hormone assays today and probably all within the very near future will have had the current bioassay that measures them replaced by high pressure liquid comotography (HPLC), a chemical assay.

They say, "But that's just a chemical assay - what have you _really_ done?" and on and on.

There are many different individuals who have now counted the number of *in vitro* papers being presented at meetings such as the Federation meetings (FASEB) or the Society of Toxicology (SOT) meetings. During the last few years, more than 50% of the presentations at these meetings were *in vitro* studies. These are not supplemental or adjunctive test, as some would like us to believe, these are the methods that are being used as independent methodology along with whole animal and human clinical studies.

Last year Procter & Gamble published that in the last 5 years they have decreased their animal use in the household and consumer goods area by 89%. They did this by developing an *in vitro* strategy for product development and safety evaluation. They are not alone.

The LD_{50} is no longer acceptable in pharmaceutical submissions. Further, the U.S. Federal Government, through the IRAG (Interagency Regulatory Animal Group), have stimulated rather significantly the use of refinement and reduction alternatives and by the end of '93, they will have made major efforts at replacement alternatives for Draize eye testing.

We have made progress - incredible progress!

ALTERNATIVES/*IN VITRO* STUDIES - the Jury is in

There appears to be a greater and greater acceptance of the economic impact of the "greening" movement. We are concerned about our environment, rivers, lakes, industrial waste and how many animals are necessary to develop and guarantee safe products.

The Center was by no means the first activity in the alternatives area. Prior to CAAT, there were FRAME (The Fund for Replacement of Animals in Medical Experimentation) in England, the Humane Society of the US (HSUS), and many others. There were several books written on alternatives. In fact, a book on *in vitro* sciences and toxicology was published in 1975. However, a series of events occurred in the late 70's, early 80's that propelled the field. One of these, but only one, was the development of CAAT.

During the last ten years there have been several scientific journals established that deal exclusively with the field of *in vitro* sciences and other major journals in toxicology have sections devoted to the topic. There are easily more than a dozen books devoted to Alternatives and *In Vitro Sciences.*

There are centers dealing specifically with alternatives throughout the world. One can identify four programs in the U.S. and a most significant event is the formation of the European Center for Validation at Ispra, Italy under the direction of the European Communities. There are prizes and gifts awarded to scientists throughout the world for encouraging the development of alternative methods. Last year, I was the very proud recipient of the HSUS Russell and Burch Award. It was significant to me personally, but more importantly, it was significant in that common ground was found to advance science and animal welfare. A dialogue was forged. Lastly, the numbers of for-profit commercial entities that have developed in this field over the last few years is quite astonishing. In fact, alternatives and *in vitro* sciences have clearly become part of our scientific fabric.

VALIDATION

This is one of the least well understood areas but one that will receive intensive activity over the next few years. My concern is that the process of validation and the limitation imposed by formal procedures does not destroy what we are trying to achieve.

The Harvard economist John Kenneth Gailbraith recently wrote a novel titled *A Tenured Professor* . He demonstrates how tenure and the awarding of it, may prevent that which it was meant to preserve. Validation may suffer from the same problems and conflicts. Validation was adequately defined, for the first time, by John Frazier when he stated that validation is the process where a test gets defined <u>for a specific purpose</u>. We must keep this in mind as many of the validation programs continue to develop and try to be things for all substances.

I am hopeful that the validation efforts on going within CAAT and world wide will very shortly produce approaches to combining peer review, publications and scientific acceptance in ways that encourage a continuing development of the discipline.

MECHANISMS VS. CORRELATION

There is no doubt that correlative tests can provide some useful information. I doubt, however, that regulatory acceptance can be developed from correlative tests exclusively. It is recognized that correlative tests can lead to trivial conclusions. Mechanistic based tests, however, are necessary for regulatory acceptance. By mechanism, I mean fundamental scientific underpinning of a chemical biological interaction that allows one to make a true predictive conclusion. It is possible that mechanistically based tests may necessitate a larger number of tests. To some this is difficult and incomprehensible, to others, it is a unique opportunity.

CAAT - ITS FUTURE

We carefully developed a small grant program with the concept that these grants would provide enough impetus, stimulation, and data for investigators to apply to major funding sources which would allow them to complete their work. We follow grantee funding and believe that we are rather successful in actually having this happen. At the SOT meetings just a month or two ago, I saw J. Gandolfi who shared that he had just come back from a study section where he had reviewed several grants. He pointed out to me, and indicated that he had pointed out to those at the study section, that he had seen many of the grants before when they were submitted to CAAT at Johns Hopkins. That is clearly one measure of our impact and success.

One could ask what do Avon and EPA have in common. To us, they are sponsors of program project grants. One in hypersensitivity and the other in neurotoxicity. These are programs aimed at combining the research talents of three, four or even more investigators at different institutions, using different approaches in an attempt to solve the same problem. We anticipate a significant future with the program project approach.

At the School of Public Health we have now established an *In Vitro* Toxicology Program under the direction of Jim Yager, director of the Division of Toxicology. The program will help support the research activities of faculty in the *in vitro* fields. We have a monthly seminar program featuring Hopkins faculty and students and guests to further the scientific dialogue. We also established an education program under the direction of Joanne Zurlo. Both of these programs were established and implemented during the last year.

In eighteen months (Nov. 1993) most of us will participate in a World Congress on Alternatives and Animal Use in the Life Sciences, Education, Research and Testing. This program, which has been brought together by more than 40 people in 25 different countries, will be a major step in increasing the dialogue between the animal welfare community and the scientific community. Many of us in this room will be devoting considerable energies to making that program a next step in sharing our progress and in continuing scientific and ethical discussions.

PEOPLE

My wife has a shirt that reads "life is uncertain, so eat desserts first". However, I've saved the best for last. Clearly and unquestionably for me the most satisfying part of all of these activities have been the people - you.

It is important to remember those who have died. Over the course of the ten years of CAAT, two advisory board members have died. They are Leon Golberg and Larry Ewing. Both of them taught me much and they are missed. Let us remember them.

I would like to start by recognizing my staff. They have been loyal, wonderful, challenging and a pleasure to work with. Please join me in thanking them.

During the last ten years I have interacted with an incredible number of people and many who are not here today sent notes, letters, called and clearly each of those events brought up memories of personal interactions. I will share one of those events with you. Shortly after CAAT was funded by CTFA, I received a telephone call from John Corbert of Britsol-Myers Squibb (then Bristol-Myers). Unfortunately I was not in the office but was traveling. The message was to call him back that evening at home. When I reached him, he was remodeling his basement and told me that Bristol-Myers wanted to fund the Center under the same rules that the CTFA had and that a check for $200,000 would be sent. Would I be able to accept that? Clearly, I said yes and thought this is only a few months into the formation of the Center, we're not going to have any problem getting funded. It is amazing how wrongly I interpreted the data. It wasn't until several years down the road when we began to receive funding from other companies based on our progress and their review of our activities. Our sponsors have continued to grow. They are interactive partners in our activities, I am grateful to them and I thank them all.

Lastly, there is one group of individuals that have been so central to CAAT that I can honestly say "without them there would not be a center". This is the advisory board. They have given of themselves continuously, they have been challenging, thoughtful, and always with enthusiasm. I thank them, I thank you all, it has been fun and I look forward to our future together.

SYMPOSIUM PRESENTATIONS

The Johns Hopkins Center for Alternatives to Animal Testing

Corporate and Federal Sponsors

3M
ARCO
Avon Products, Inc.
BP America, Inc.
Bernice Barbour Foundation, Inc.
Bristol-Myers Squibb Company
Charles River Laboratories, Inc.
CIBA-GEIGY Corporation
The Cosmetic, Toiletry & Fragrance Association

The Geraldine R. Dodge Foundation
The Estee Lauder Companies
Exxon Corporation
Hoffmann-La Roche Inc.
IBM Corporation
Johnson & Johnson
L'Arome (U.S.A.) Inc.
L'Oreal
Mary Kay Cosmetics, Inc.

Environmental Protection Agency
   Health Effects Research Laboratory
National Institutes of Health

Advisory Board

Franklin D. Aldrich, M.D., Ph.D.
IBM Corporation

Donald O. Allen, Ph.D.
University of South Carolina

BP America, Inc.

Melvin W. Balk, D.V.M., M.S.
Charles River Laboratories, Inc.

Myra O. Barker, Ph.D.
Mary Kay Cosmetics, Inc.

Michael S. Dickens, Ph.D.
Avon Products, Inc.

William Dressler, Ph.D.
Clairol, Inc.
(a subsidiary of Bristol-Myers Squibb Company)

Bruce H. Ewald, D.V.M.
CIBA-GEIGY Corporation

Robert Fitzgerald, Ph.D.
Johns Hopkins School of Public Health

John M. Frazier, Ph.D.
Johns Hopkins School of Public Health

Stephen D. Gettings, Ph.D., DABT
The Cosmetic, Toiletry
  and Fragrance Association, Inc.

Gordon A. Glover
The Geraldine R. Dodge Foundation

Alan M. Goldberg, Ph.D.
Johns Hopkins School of Public Health

Gerald B. Guest, D.V.M.
United States Food and Drug Administration

Richard N. Hill, M.D., Ph.D.
United States Environmental Protection Agency

Francis Koschier, Ph.D.
ARCO

Daniel Maes, Ph.D.
Estee Lauder Companies

James P. McCulley, M.D.
University of Texas

A. John Penicnak, Ph.D.
Cosmair (a subsidiary of L'Oreal)

Richard D. Phillips, Ph.D.
Exxon Company

Emil A. Pfitzer, Sc.D.
Hoffmann-La Roche, Inc.

Albert Ritardi
Allied-Signal, Inc.

Bernard Robaire, Ph.D.
McGill University

Noel R. Rose, Ph.D., M.D.
Johns Hopkins School of Public Health

Robert A. Roth, Jr., Ph.D.
Michigan State University

Andrew N. Rowan, D.Phil.
Tufts Center for Animals and Public Policy

Daniel N. Sauder, M.D., FRCP
University of Toronto

Robert A. Scala, Ph.D.
Diplomate, American Board of Toxicology

Solomon H. Snyder, M.D.
Johns Hopkins School of Medicine

Sabine Swierenga, Ph.D.
The Joseph F. Morgan Research Foundation

Eve Lloyd Thompson
Bernice Barbour Foundation, Inc.

Bellina Veronesi, Ph.D.
Environmental Protection Agency
Health Effects Research Laboratory

DeWayne H. Walker, D.V.M., M.S.
3M

Peter A. Ward, M.D.
University of Michigan Medical School

John E. Willson, D.V.M.
Johnson & Johnson

Robert M. Woodard
L'Arome (USA) Inc.

James D. Yager, Ph.D.
Johns Hopkins School of Public Health

Joanne Zurlo, Ph.D.
Johns Hopkins School of Public Health

F. New Technologies

F1

Flow Cytometry—High Speed Approaches to Detecting Cellular Structure, Mechanism, and Function

LARRY A. SKLAR

National Flow Cytometry Resource
Los Alamos National Laboratory
Los Alamos, NM 87544

and

Cytometry, Cancer Center, and Department of Pathology
University of New Mexico
School of Medicine
Albuquerque, NM 87131

ABSTRACT

Flow cytometric technology provides the ability to find, analyze, and isolate cells and chromosomes. This report discusses the development of technology at the Los Alamos National Flow Cytometry and Sorting Resource and its application to a number of biological problems. The problems all involve the characterization of the particles at high rates. The characterization depends typically upon the association of fluorescent molecules with the particles and the applications range from simple ligand binding to cell-cell aggregate detection. A particularly relevant application with respect to alternatives to animal testing is the detection of leukocytes in blood. This technology makes it possible to evaluate the actions of pharmacologic agents on blood cells ex vivo.

INTRODUCTION

Flow cytometric technology provides the capability to analyze thousands of particles - cells or chromosomes - per second by aligning them in a stream and passing them through a laser beam. Particles are characterized on the basis of size, shape, and fluorescent staining (Table I). Recent advances in instrumentation at the Los Alamos National Flow Cytometry Resource (NFCR) now make it possible to define the spectroscopic characteristics of cell associated fluorescent probes including fluorescence spectra and lifetime. These spectroscopic approaches can be used to define the local environment of the fluorophore in the cell. The technology also provides the ability to identify macromolecular assemblies in real-time. It is used to study the kinetics of ligand binding, ligand processing, and cell-cell adheson. Flow cytometry can also be used to define minor subpopulations in complex cell mixtures and is making it possible to examine leukocyte physiology in blood samples where the leukocytes are outnumbered by the red cells and platelets by more than one thousand to one. Together, these applications are providing information about molecular structure, kinetics and mechanism, and novel pharmacological approaches to cellular systems.

Table I. Measurements in Flow Cytometry

Measurement	Utility
Conductivity	Electronic Volume
Forward Light Scatter	Particle Size
90° Light Scatter	Granularity/Surface Morphology
DNA Stains	Cell Cycle/Viability
Fluorescent MoAbs	Cell Markers (Expressed Proteins)
Fluorescent Ligands	Binding Sites
Ion Sensitive Dyes	Cell Activation (Ca^{++}) /Ligand Processing (pH)
Metabolic Indicators	Redox Reactions/Cytoskeleton/Enzyme activities

TECHNOLOGY

NFCR investigators have been at the forefront in several areas of flow cytometric technology. These include a multilaser cytometer used in analysis and sorting cells, two instruments with spectroscopic capabilities, and several instruments for chromosome analysis and sorting. The spectroscopic instruments consist of a Fourier transform cytometer and a phase-sensitive flow cytometer

FLOW CYTOMETRIC ANALYSIS AND SORTING. The development of flow cytometric instruments for automated analysis and separation of cells makes it possible to analyze and isolate cells and organelles (e.g., chromosomes) on the basis of physical, biochemical, and immunological properties. Multiparameter instruments combine electrical and optical sensing techniques for making multiple measurements on cells. Measurements are made on individual cells at high-speeds. The statistical precision is high. Subpopulations are detected and can be separated from heterogeneous mixtures for morphological identification and for functional and biochemical studies.

John Steinkamp and Robb Habbersett developed a three laser/multiparameter flow cytometer for quantitative cell analysis and separation on the basis of eight parameters or characteristics (1). Cells stained with fluorescent dyes are suspended in normal saline and introduced into the flow chamber at rates of up to 3000 cells/sec. As cells pass through the chamber, electronic cell-volume, axial light loss, light scatter, and fluorescence are measured by electrical and optical sensors. Axial light loss (extinction) is the reduction in illumination intensity incident upon a detector caused by a cell passing through an excitation beam. Light scatter is related to the diffractive, reflective, and refractive properties of both the internal and external cellular features. Multicolor fluorescence represents stains bound to cell constituents or from endogenous intracellular components. The axial light loss and forward light scatter detectors are located on the axis of each excitation beam and multicolor fluorescence is measured using a five-channel detector orthogonal to the laser beam-cell stream intersection.

The instrument uses two argon-ion lasers, a krypton-ion laser, and a dye laser as illumination sources. Each laser beam is focused sequentially onto the cell stream. Measurements are processed to provide pulse height, area, and width signals that are made time coincident by analog delay modules. Analog electronics are also used to compute ratios, sums, and differences of signals. Up to eight signals are processed on a cell-by-cell basis and data are stored by a computer in list mode format for display as frequency distribution histograms and two parameter bivariate contour, dot, and isometric plots.

Processed signals also trigger cell-sorting. After measurement, cells emerge in a liquid jet that is broken into uniform droplets, thus isolating them for separation. Sorting is activated by electronically comparing the signal amplitude with preselected boundaries. If the signal amplitude, or combination of amplitudes, fall within the preset ranges, an electronic time delay is activated that triggers a droplet-charging pulse as the cell arrives at the droplet breakoff point. This causes a group of droplets, one of which contains the cell, to be charged and deflected by a static electrical field into a collection vessel. Cells not meeting the preset criteria do not trigger sorting and they pass undeflected into a waste fluid container.

The multiparameter flow cytometer has been used in a wide variety of applications including: 1) the analysis and sorting of cells based of volume measurement; 2) simultaneous analysis of DNA, RNA, and protein using three fluorescent dyes, each excited at a different wavelength; 3) the correlation of cell-volume and fluorescence with time; and 4) the multiparameter analysis and sorting of lung cells, tumor cells, and leukocyte subpopulations. A recent spectroscopic application involving pH sensitive probes is discussed below.

SPECTROSCOPIC CAPABILITIES FOR FLOW CYTOMETERS. Conventional flow cytometry permits analysis of fluorescence intensity at several wavelengths simultaneously. Spectroscopic analysis extends fluorescence flow cytometry in several ways. First, it enhances resolution or separation of multiple chromophores by adding spectral or lifetime analysis. Moreover, since the spectroscopic properties of fluorophores are often sensitive to the local molecular environment, the spectral properties of probes bound to the cell provides insight on local enivronment (ionic composition) and structure (for example, in the case of chromatin and receptor binding pockets). In most fluorescence analysis, the total fluorescence emitted by a particle in flow is resolved into contributions from several emission spectra. These can be the contributions of several fluorochromes or the component spectra of a metachromatic fluorochrome. Conventional systems used in biological applications perform a coarse spectral analysis by dividing the spectrum into a few spectral channels.

Tudor Buican developed a proof-of-principle instrument which demonstrates that Fourier transform spectrometry offers the light throughput, spectral resolution, speed of analysis, and flexibility, required for fluorescence analysis in flow cytometers (2). An FT spectrometer consists of an interferometer that encodes the spectral information into an intensity distribution that varies as a function of time or position, and a computer that extracts the spectral information from this distribution. Although the use of FT spectrometers in flow is desirable because of their high light throughput, the speed at which they usually acquire and analyze spectral data makes them unsuitable for such applications. In order to bring the speed of acquisition of spectral parameters to levels compatible with flow cytometric analysis (100 μsec or less), he developed a novel interferometer that has no moving parts and a data acquisition array processor that can process in real time the high-frequency interferograms produced by the interferometer.

Single cells carried by a stream of fluid intersect an excitation laser beam in the Fourier transform flow cytometer,. The fluorescence emitted while the cells cross the laser beam is collected by a lens and passes through an interferometer driven at a frequency of 85 kHz. The modulated fluorescence waveform (interferogram) is converted into an analog electric signal by a photomultiplier, and then into a digital data stream (typically 8 bits every 120 ns). The data stream is processed in real time by a dedicated array processor in which programmable digital filters extract from the interferogram the contributions of fluorochromes with known fluorescence spectra. The current instrument allows up to eight spectral parameters to be extracted and the computation of the parameters is complete within 170 ns of the cell leaving the laser beam.

The real-time FT spectrometer performs spectral analysis and fluorochrome separation numerically. This leads to an unprecedented degree of flexibility in the use of the instrument. For example, the instrument can operate in several modes which have no equivalent for conventional cytometers. In the spectral analysis mode each computed spectral parameter corresponds to one of several adjacent samples of the fluorescence spectrum. In the fluorochrome separation mode, the instrument computes the individual contributions of several fluorochromes to the total fluorescence emitted by each cell. In the adaptive mode, spectral parameters for a given sample are defined by the instrument through a statistical analysis of the full spectral information obtained from a small fraction of the sample. The adaptive mode is particularly useful when analyzing new types of samples or new fluorochromes. Adaptive analysis can reveal the spectral parameters that are best suited for a given sample/fluorochrome combination and thus eliminate the trial-and-error fliter selection common in flow cytometry.

Some recent biological applications of Fourier transform flow cytometry include: 1) steroid enzyme activity using a new fluorogenic substrate for cytochrome P-450scc enzyme (3); 2) hormone-induced differentiation using the metachromatic lipid probe nile red (4); 3) chromatin structural changes related to cell cycle stage as analyzed by spectral changes in the fluorochromes acridine orange and Hoechst upon binding to DNA; 4) protonation of peptide ligands upon binding to receptor pockets (5).

When fluorochromes have similar excitation and separated emission spectra, they can be resolved using single-laser excitation and multicolor fluorescence detection or Fourier transform cytometry. When fluorochromes have separated excitation spectra, they can be resolved by multilaser excitation coupled with multicolor detection. If fluorochromes have similar spectral excitation and overlapping emission properties, they cannot be resolved by conventional flow cytometry. However, if they have different fluorescence lifetimes, they may be separable using phase-sensitive detection (PSD) methods. John Steinkamp has begun to apply the PSD technology to discriminate signals from fluorochromes having differences in fluorescence lifetimes. This technology is applicable: 1) to measuring and separating signals derived from fluorescent dyes or intrinsic fluorophores that have a common excitation and overlapping emission spectra, but different fluorescence decay lifetimes; 2) to improving the measurement of fluorophores in the presence of background interference caused by cellular autofluorescence, Raman scattering, unbound (free) dye; and 3) to quantifying fluorescence lifetime as a parameter.

A prototype instrument using homodyning technology like that used for cuvette based spectrofluorometry has been developed. Stained cells are analyzed as they flow through a chamber and intersect a high-frequency, intensity-modulated laser beam. The high-frequency, pulse-modulated fluorescence emission signals are shifted in phase from the excitation frequency and demodulated. These signals are processed by PSD electronics consisting of a multiplier, reference phase shifter, and a low-pass filter. Lifetimes have been measured and individual stains present at the same time have been discriminated on the basis of their lifetime characteristics.

INSTRUMENTATION FOR CHROMOSOMES. Dyes that stain DNA make it possible to detect cell nuclei and to analyze cell cycle by flow cytometry. Since the fluorescence of these dyes is intense, it is also possible to detect and sort individual chromosomes. In a technique called bivariate analysis, chromosomes are stained with two DNA specific fluorescent dyes Hoechst-33342 and chromomycin-A3. The 24 human chromosome types can be resolved into 20 groups with chromosomes 9-12 overlapping and several over types partially overlapping. The cytometric analysis of these groupings is called flow karyotyping and is useful clinically in the identification of human diseases which involve chromosome breakpoints and translocations. Chromosome sorting is playing a major role in the Human Genome Program whose goal is to sequence all of the human chromosomes (6).

The Human Genome Program requires chromosome specific DNA libraries which are constructed from purified chromosomes sorted by instruments located in the NFCR. Construction of these libraries require ug quantities of sorted chromosomes. Ten micrograms of DNA corresponds to about 20 million small human chromosomes. Using conventional flow sorters the maximum sample throughput rate is between 1,500 and 2,000 chromosomes per second. At a sort rate of 50 chromosomes per second it takes more than 50 hours to sort ten million chromosomes.

Instruments have been designed to increase the chromosome sample and sorting throughput rates by about an order of magnitude. Increased throughput rate is obtained by increasing the frequency at which droplets are generated, thereby increasing the maximum rate for sorting chromosomes. Generating droplets at higher frequencies requires higher exit jet velocities and correspondingly higher operating pressures. The flow of the chromosome sample in the cytometer is hydrodynamically focused by a sheath flow with an operating pressure about 100 psi and the droplet generating frequency of 142 kHz. Single droplet sorting minimizes the sorted fluid volume and maximizes the concentration of sorted chromosomes.

Stained chromosomes in the sample stream are excited using two large frame argon-ion lasers. The two laser beams are brought in from opposite sides of the flow chamber. Each laser beam is focused onto the chromosome sample stream using a pair of crossed cylindrical lenses. A third argon-ion laser beam is used to monitor the arrival of particles at the sort droplet break off position. Human chromosomes are sorted from chromosome samples with analysis rates in excess of 20,000 chromosomes/sec. The rates, however, depend upon the chromosome concentration. With high concentration samples, sort rates as high as 300 to 400 sorts/sec have been achieved. The purity of sorted human chromosomes ranges from mid eighty to mid ninety percent.

Because of the overlap of individual chromosome types, a chromosome imaging flow system was developed to improve resolution of the chromosome types from one another (7). This system uses a slit scan approach in which the elongated chromosomes flow lengthwise through a thin ribbon of laser illumination. A pulse shape is acquired by digitization of the fluorescence waveform of each chromosome and sort decisions are made of the basis of the waveform. The pulse shape provides additional information resolving chromosome types as it reflect the distribution of dye molecules along the chromosome length.

Scientists associated with the NFCR and Chemistry and Laser Sciences at LANL have developed a "flow cytometer" with ultrasensitive detection capabilities. Single molecules of the fluorochrome rhodamine 6G in solution are detected as they flow through a highly focused laser beam. The instrument uses a pulsed laser and time-gated detection to help discriminate photon bursts emitted by single molecules of R6G from the background. The principles behind ultrasensitive flow cytometry are being exploited as part of a multidisciplinary project to sequence DNA (8) with application to the 3 billion nucleotides which comprise the human genome. The goal is to accelerate the DNA sequencing rate from a typical one, using gel electrophoresis-based techniques, of 100 bases per day to 100-1000 bases per second. The technique involves labeling the nucleotides in a large (40 kb) fragment of DNA with base-specific tags suitable for fluorescence detection, isolating a single strand of the fluorescently labeled DNA, adhering it at one end to a solid support, suspending the supported DNA strand in a flowing sample stream, and sequentially cleaving the labeled bases from the free end of the DNA fragment using an exonuclease. The plan is to detect the cleaved, labeled bases as they flow through the laser beam of the single molecule detector.

KINETICS OF LIGAND-RECEPTOR INTERACTION BY FLOW CYTOMETRY. Flow cytometry is now widely used in kinetic studies of cell activation, ligand binding, enzyme activitiy, and drug transport. Among the most powerful and least exploited capability of flow cytometry is the ability to discriminate free and bound ligand in cells without a wash step. This occurs because cytometers intrinsically monitor the fluorescence associated with a cell and the small volume around it while rejecting the fluorescence signal associated with the large volumes between the cells in the flow stream. Simple ligand binding and other more complex macromolecular assembly events such as antibody recognition of cell surface markers can be monitored with a sensitivity improved by 3 to 6 orders of magnitude over static cuvette methods. A thousand or fewer receptors per cell can be detected by flow cytometry,

Kinetic methods using manual mixing and sample delivery have already been useful in examining binding interactions with time constants in the range of seconds. If the technology were extended into the subsecond time frame, the power of flow analysis could be applied to more ligands, with affinities as low as 1 uM including hormones, peptides and peptidomimetics (Table II). Since macromolecular assembly events occur on cells in subsecond time domains and precede cell activation, such assembly and activation events would be accessible to real-time analysis. Many other biological questions (cell activation, enzyme activities, etc.) demand subsecond kinetic analysis. Therefore, the development of a cytometer with subsecond resolution is now in process with the goal of integrating a rapid (stopped-flow) mixing device with a flow cytometer. Verification of the performance of the instrumentation will use the model receptor system discussed below for which parallel real-time spectrofluorometric and cytometric assays have already been developed.

Table II. SUBSECOND FLOW CYTOMETRY

Assume: $K_d < 10^{-6}$ M for peptides or drugs

$k_{on} \sim 10^7$ M^{-1}sec^{-1} (diffusion limit)

Then: $k_{off} = K_d \times k_{on} < 10$/sec

Equilibration time > 100 msec

APPLICATIONS

This section describes investigations involving the UNM Cytometry group, the NFCR, and several external collaborators. These studies are focused on leukocyte physiology and reflect some important capabilities of flow cytometry. These include: 1)

homogeneous, kinetic analysis of ligand binding; 2) analysis of binding pocket structure using spectroscopy; 3) detection of cell-cell interaction and its molecular basis; and 4) detection of leukocytes in whole blood and its relevance in cell and animal physiology, and alternatives to animal testing.

LIGAND-RECEPTOR INTERACTIONS. We have developed a combination of spectrofluorometric and flow cytometric methods to examine the interactions of a family of fluorescent peptide ligands with their receptors on neutrophils (9,10). The receptors allow neutrophils to participate in host defense by recognizing peptides derived from bacteria. These N-formylated peptides induce the cells to chemotax, adhere, generate free radicals of oxygen and other inflammatory mediators. By taking advantage of the intrinsic ability of flow cytometry to discriminate between fluorescent ligand associated with the cells from the ligand in the surrounding medium we have been able to analyze in real-time the static and kinetic aspects of the ligand-receptor interactions. These include the signal transduction steps mediated by G proteins, and receptor processing events such as desensitization and internalization. The internalization events take advantage of the pH sensitivity of fluorescein (10). Ligands on the outside of a cell are quenched when the pH of the medium is lowered. Ligands on the inside of the cell are protected from the extracellular pH change.

We made use of calibration techniques involving commercial fluorescent bead standards, and the computational power of the Cray supercomputer, to analyze and model individual steps in the signal transduction pathway (9). In brief, our experiments suggest that neutrophil activation proceeds through the following steps: 1) the ligand binds to its receptor at a rate approaching the diffusion limit; 2) a large fraction of the receptors appears to be precoupled to their transduction partners, the intracellular heterotrimeric guanine nucleotide binding proteins; 3) in the presence of physiological concentrations of guanine nucleotide, activation of the G proteins occurs within 100 msecs; 4) the receptor is desensitized within 10 secs of ligand binding which precludes extensive amplification of the transduction signal, i.e., sequential activation of additional G proteins by the activated receptor; 5) the desensitized receptor is internalized with a half-time of ~ 3 minutes. The binding data is consistent with the idea that physically precoupled receptors are responsible for rapid cell reponses and that temporally heterogeneous responses may arise from that fraction of receptors which couple to G proteins slowly over periods of minutes. In addition, we believe that the coupling of receptors and G protein can be regulated in the absence of the ligand by GTP(S) accounting for the well-known ability of GTP(S) to activate response in broken cell preparations.

BINDING POCKET STRUCTURE. Signal transducing receptors which couple to G proteins consist of 7 transmembrane alpha-helical domains with short loops connecting the domains. The binding pocket for ligands for this class of receptors extends an estimated 10-15 A into the receptor. In order to study the topography of the binding pocket of the human neutrophil formyl peptide receptor we have used environmentally sensitive probes conjugated to a family of peptides (N-CHO-Met-Leu-(Phe)$_n$-Lys-PROBE) where n = 1, 2, or 3. When the probe is fluorescein isothiocyanate we find that the probe is quenched upon binding to the receptor for the tetrapeptide (n=1) and pentapeptide (n=2). The hexapeptide (n=3) is not quenched upon binding to the receptor. In contrast, using antibodies which recognize fluorescein, we find that the probe for the hexapeptide is accessible to the antibody; for the shorter ligands, the probe is protected within the binding pocket and inaccessible to the antibody. We interpret these results to indicate that the binding pocket for the ligand is large enough to accomodate at least five but no more than six amino acids (11). Moreover, the probe on the hexapeptide is in the aqueous region just outside the pocket, while on the hexapeptide it is just within. Molecular models suggest that the pentapepide ligand and probe is ~15 A in length.

We have used spectroscopy to characterize the environment in the vicinity of the peptides. The interaction of the pentapeptide is strongly pH dependent. As the pH is decreased, the interaction with the receptor increases, as indicated by more efficient quenching upon binding and decreasing dissociation rate of the ligand. We believe these effects are mediated by a protonation involving an amino acid with a pKa ~ 7, close to the binding pocket, and near the aqueous interface of the receptor. A potential candidate for the interaction is His 90 which is located at the extracellular end of the 2nd transmembrane domain or in the loop connecting the second and third domains. In contrast, the interaction of the tetrapeptide is relatively pH insensitive and may involve contact with a nearby aromatic amino acid residue. We are attempting to verify these assigments by site-directed mutagenesis to the receptor.

Additional experiments to define the interaction between the receptor and the ligand have been performed with a pH sensitive SNAFL labelled pentapeptide. SNAFL, an analog of fluorescein, exhibits distinct excitation and emission spectra for its protonated and unprotonated forms. These distinct species have been identified by both multiparameter and Fourier transform flow cytometric methods (5). In the multiparameter experiments, three laser lines were used: one laser at 488 nm to excite the protonated ligand; one laser at 568 nm for the unprotonated probe; and the laser at 528 nm was used at the isobestic wavelength to measure the total bound ligand. In Fourier transform experiments, the entire spectrum was observed as a function of pH. The SNAFL conjugate was bound to receptors on differentiated HL60 cells which overexpress the receptor. We found that the probe was protonated upon binding over the pH range of about 6.5 to 8.5 compared to free ligand in solution, supporting the idea of a specific site of protonation in the binding pocket.

CELL-CELL INTERACTION. Flow cytometry shows remarkable potential for evaluating cell-cell interactions (12). Cell aggregates (multiplets) are distinguished from singlets on the basis of light scatter, expression of surface antigens, and nuclear staining. In general, the mean channel value of the individual parameters increase linearly as the number of cells in the aggregate increases. We have used flow cytometry to examine aggregate formation in isolated neutrophils and blood and used the data to construct a model of aggregate formation. The experiments show that aggregates form through mass action and that the distribution of sizes of aggregates can be calculated on the basis of rates of aggregation and disaggregation.

Following stimulation, neutrophils begin to aggregate reversibly with one another at a rate which depends upon the cell concentration. After about a minute of aggregate formation, the aggregates are stable in a plateau phase which lasts approximately two minutes. During this plateau phase, few new appregates are formed. Disaggregation begins after about 3 minutes. During the plateau, the administration of antibodies to the adhesive proteins enhances the rate of disaggregation. We interpret this result to indicate that adhesive bonds are breaking and forming within individual aggregates. Antibodies can preclude the reforming of adhesive bonds within the cell-cell contact regions.

By using antibodies to several adhesive proteins, we have obtained evidence that there are two types of adhesive molecules involved in the adhesion events. These are beta 2 integrins and leukocyte selectins (13). We are presently extending this approach by staining distinct cell populations individually. For example, we have examined the ability of cells which lack the adhesive integrins (Leukocyte Adhesion Deficiency disease) to bind to normal neutrophils. The adhesion deficient cells retain leukocyte selectins which permit the deficient cells to stick to control cells even though they don't stick to one another. We can also treat the populations with reagents that interfere specifically with one adhesive protein or the other with goal of determining whether the adhesive molecules are specific receptors for one another. The results of these studies suggests that integrin and selectin are counter-receptors responsible for neutrophil-neutrophil interaction.

CELL PHYSIOLOGY IN BLOOD. The most appropriate milieu for studying leukocyte physiology is blood both because leukocytes change during isolation procedures and because the natural plasma components are retained. We have been motivated over the last few years to examine leukocyte behavior in blood with respect to the following issues: 1) understanding the physiological modulators of leukocyte behavior in blood, particularly the role of bacterial lipopolysaccharides (LPS); 2) defining protocols for the isolation of neutrophils so that they retain the characteristics they exhibited in the blood; 3) understanding the adhesive properties of neutrophils in blood; 4) examining the effect of pharmacologic agents on leukocytes in their native state; 5) assaying leukocyte physiology in clinical samples as prognostic indicators.

Since leukocytes represent less than 0.1% of all the cells in blood, it has been a challenge to detect them in the presence of the overwhelming numbers of platelets and red cells. However, it is possible to detect leukocytes in blood following appropriate staining protocols (13). We have found it useful to stain leukocytes with antibodies to the adhesive integrins or with the vital nuclear stain LDS-751. When the cells are analyzed in the flow cytometer, an electronic threshold is set on the parameter which detects the stained cells. When the data is collected, the red cells and platelets are ignored.

We have found that the expression of receptors on the neutrophil is a very good indicator of the status of the cell. When exposed to minute quantitites of LPS (<100 pg/ml), the cells rapidly upregulate preformed receptors from intracellular compartments. The most impressive upregulation occurs for the adhesive integrins whose level increases more than 10 fold. Remarkably, we find that adhesion occurs even at low levels of integrin and that adhesive properties diminish as the cells are purified. These observations led for a search for a counter-receptor, a molecule which was lost as the cells were isolated. We have tentatively identified the selectins as adhesive molecules which are lost during cell isolation (13).

Why do cells change during isolation? It has been recognized for some time that LPS is a potent modulator of cell function during isolation. By rigorously excluding LPS from the media used for white cell preparation, it has been possible to isolate neutrophils in their native state. These cells express basal levels of cell surface receptors. The detection technology can be adapted to clinical studies to examine leukocyte status as patients progress through sepsis and acute respiratory distress syndrome (ARDS). It has also been possible to evaluate the pathway that LPS uses in upregulating the adhesive receptors (14). These studies show that it involves a serum binding protein for LPS and a cell surface receptor CD14.

Blood has proven to be an important medium for studying the action of anti-inflammatory drugs used in treating sepsis (14). Sepsis is an illness which results from bacterial invasion following surgery or traumatic injury such as burn. We found a unique mode of action of the anti-inflammatory drug methylprednisolone. In native cells methylprednisolone blocks the pathway of receptor upregulation, presumably by blocking its trafficking in native leukocytes. Thus at the same time, the drug reduces inflammation and interferes with the host defense capabilities of the white cells.

CONCLUSIONS

We have described how flow cytometry can be used to detect rare events ranging from individual chromosomes to white cells in blood. We have described how cytometry can be applied to problems of molecular structure using environmentally sensitive probes and spectroscopic techniques. We have described how mechanistic information can be obtained about macromolecular assemblies ranging from ligand binding interactions to the formation of cell-cell aggregates. Flow cytometry will also find application in alternatives to animal testing. In the case of white cell physiology, we can explore the actions of inflammatory mediators and modulators in blood. This makes it possible to examine cells in a relatively native situation. The applications will include an examination of the diagnostic value of leukocyte physiology in patient samples, the evaluation of the biovailability of pharmacological agents, and the use of blood samples as a substitute to whole animal testing.

ACKNOWLEDGMENTS

The work reported here was supported by AI19032, HL43026, GM37696 and RR01315. I would like to acknowledge the contributions of John Steinkamp to the sections on the multiparameter and phase sensitive flow cytometers, Tudor Buican to the section on Fourier transform cytometry, and John Martin, Babetta Marrone, and Dick Keller to the sections on chromosome cytometry.

REFERENCES

1. Steinkamp, J.A., Habbersett, R.C., and Hiebert, R.D. (1991), Improved Multilaser/Multiparameter Flow Cytometer for Analysis and Sorting of Cells and Particles. Rev. Sci. Inst. 62:2751

2. T.N. Buican (1990), Real-Time Fourier Transform Spectrometry for Fluorescence Imaging and Flow Cytometry. SPIE 1205:126

3. Marrone, B.L., D.J. Simpson, T.M. Yoshida, C.J. Unkefer, T.W. Whaley, and T.N. Buican (1991), Single cell endocrinology: Analysis of P-450$_{scc}$ activity by fluorescence detection methods. Endocrinology 128:2654

4. Dive, C., D.J. Simpsonm, T.M. Yoshida, and B.L. Marone (1992), Flow cytometric analysis of steroidogenic organelles in differentiating granulosa cells. Biology of Reproduction, In Press

5. Fay, S.P., Yoshida, T.M., Posner, R.G., Habbersett, R., Domalewski, M.D., Freer, R.J., Pierson, E., Whitaker, J., Haugland, R.P., Magde, D., and Sklar, L.A. (1992), Human Neutrophil Formyl Peptide Receptor-Ligand Interaction Involves A Binding Pocket Protonation. FASEB JOURNAL 6, A1010

6. VanDilla, M.A., Deaven, L.L., Albright, K.L., Allen, N.A., Aubuchon, M.R., Bartholdi, M.F., Brown, N.C., Campbell, E.W., Carrano, A.V., Clark, L.M., Cram, L.S., Fuscoe,

J.C., Gray, J.W., Hildebrand, C.E., Jackson, P.J., Jett, J.H., Longmire, J.L., Lozes, R., Luedemann, M.L., Martin, J.C., Meyne, J., McNinch, J.S., Meincke, L.J., Mendelsohn, M.L., Moyzis, R.K., Munk, A.C., Perlman, J., Peters, D.C., Silva, A.J., and Trask, B.J. (1986), Human Chromosome-Specific DNA Libraries: Construction and Availability. Bio/Technology 4:537

7. M. F. Bartholdi, J. D. Parson, K. D. Albright, L. S. Cram (1990), System for Flow Sorting Chromosomes on the Basis of Pulse Shape. Cytometry 11:165

8. Davis, L.M., Fairfield, F.R., Harger, C.A., Jett, J.H., Keller, R.A., Hahn, J.H., Krakowski, L.A., Marrone, B.L., Martin, J.C., Nutter, H.L., Ratliff, R.L., Shera, E.B., Simpson, D.J., and Soper, S.A. (1991), Rapid DNA sequencing based upon single molecule detection. Genetic Anal., Techniques and Applications 8:1

9. Fay, S.P., Posner, R., Swann, W. and Sklar, L.A. (1990), Real-time analysis of the assembly of ligand, receptor and G-protein by quantitative fluorescence flow cytometry. Biochemistry 30: 5066

10. Sklar, L.A. (1990), Real-Time Analysis of Ligand-Receptor Dynamics and Binding Pocket Structure of the Formyl Peptide Receptor, <u>Molecular and Cellular Mechanisms of Inflammation</u> Vol 3., C.G. Cochrane and M.A. Gimbrone (ed.) Academic Press, 1-23

11. Sklar, L.A., Fay, S.P., Seligmann, B.E., Freer, R.J., Muthukumaraswamy, N., and Mueller, H. (1990), Fluorescence Analysis of the Size of a Binding Pocket of a Peptide Receptor at Natural Abundance. Biochemistry 29:313

12. Simon, S.I., Chambers, J. David, and Sklar, L.A, (1990), Flow Cytometric Analysis and Modeling of Cell-Cell Adhesive Interactions: The Neutrophil As a Model. J. Cell Biol., 111:2747-2756.

13. Simon, S.I., Rochon, Y.R., Anderson, D.C., Smith, C.W., and Sklar, L.A. (1992), Are beta-2 integrin and L-selectin counter-receptors in neutrophil aggregation? FASEB Journal 6, A1689

14. Sklar, L.A., Simon, S., Brandt, M.M., Lynam, E., Weingarten, J., Mathison, J.C., Ulevitch, R.J., Tobias, P.S. Analysis of LPS-PMN Interaction in Blood (1992), J. Cell. Biochemistry, Supp. 16C, 154

F2

Calcium Measurements in the Assessment of *In Vitro* Toxicity

B.F. TRUMP, P.T. JAIN, P.C. PHELPS,
S.H. CHANG, and I.K. BEREZESKY

Department of Pathology
University of Maryland School of Medicine
and
Maryland Institute for Emergency Medical Services Systems
Baltimore, MD 21201

Abstract. Alterations of intracellular ion homeostasis, particularly $[Ca^{2+}]_i$, represent virtually immediate manifestations of acute or chronic cellular toxicity. Increased $[Ca^{2+}]_i$, if uncorrected, leads to altered states of growth and differentiation and, if extreme, to cell death including necrosis or apoptosis. Changes in $[Ca^{2+}]_i$ can be measured using fluorescent probes such as Fura-2 or Fluo-3 combined with transmission or confocal light microscopy, coupled with video intensification microscopy, and image analysis. We have examined $[Ca^{2+}]_i$ changes in a mouse keratinocyte cell line, JB6, which has two strains: clone 30, a non-promotable clone; and clone 41, a promotable clone. As model injuries relevant to cutaneous toxicity, we have studied a series of compounds including benzoyl peroxide, formaldehyde, sodium lauryl sulfate, mercuric chloride, and a calcium ionophore, ionomycin. These results are being compared with similar studies on other cells including hepatocytes, renal proximal tubular epithelium, and cerebellar neurons. In JB6 cells, the magnitude and time of $[Ca^{2+}]_i$ increases can be correlated with dose response curves measuring cell killing, i.e., early, large, and sustained increases of $[Ca^{2+}]_i$ correlate with rapid onset of cell death. Cell death may be mediated by $[Ca^{2+}]_i$-dependent activation of phospholipases, proteases, and endonucleases. Furthermore, based on studies in our laboratory, we propose that sublethal increases of $[Ca^{2+}]_i$ may be important in the regenerative and proliferative responses of epithelial cells, including neoplasia, by the $[Ca^{2+}]_i$-dependent activation of immediate early and stress genes including **c-fos**, **c-jun**, **c-myc**, and **hsp**70. Clearly, assessment of intracellular ions, particularly $[Ca^{2+}]_i$, can serve as a very rapid assay for the prediction of cell toxicity.

I. Introduction

The purpose of this paper is to summarize the utilization of calcium measurements in the assessment of early reactions of the cell to acute and chronic injury. Some years ago, when we began characterizing the events that occur in acute, sublethal, and lethal reactions to injury, it became evident that abnormal regulation of intracellular ions played a very important role in the early events (13,15). Such ions included Na^+, K^+, Cl^-, H^+, and Ca^{2+}. Early on, we were intrigued with the finding that elevations of total calcium (as measured by atomic absorption spectroscopy) correlated with events related to cell death. Prior to this, precipitation of calcium phosphate in dead cells had been termed "dystrophic" calcification by pathologists. At that time, we began to ask whether elevation of calcium might actually occur before cell death, and, if so, whether it might even contribute to the process. Later, it also became evident that ion deregulation was related to cell division and proliferation, and might serve as a link between acute and chronic cell injury, including tumor promotion and carcinogenesis (15).

In all of these studies of cellular and molecular pathobiology, it became increasingly evident that there was a need to correlate morphology, chemical composition, and cell function. Fortuitously, light microscopy was in the process of being revolutionized and many new discoveries such as the development of image intensification microscopy, improvements in light optics, and the development of a variety of fluorescent technologies for detection of chemical activities were available which permitted a variety of physiological and biochemical phenomena to be visualized in 3-dimensional space and time. In the present paper, we will illustrate how this technology can be applied to the study of the toxicological response of cells to injury and more specifically, the response of cells to alterations in the concentration of ionized cytosolic calcium ($[Ca^{2+}]_i$), as shown in Fig. 1.

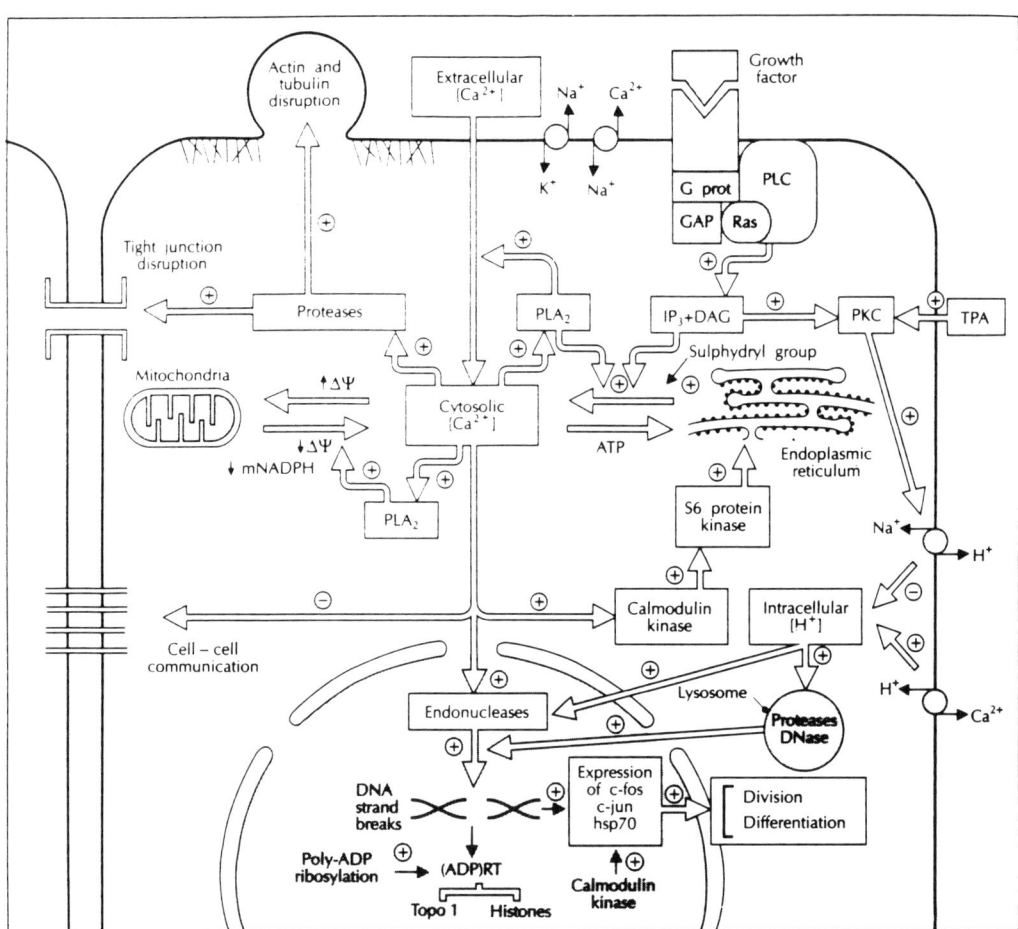

Figure 1. A working hypothesis illustrating the role played by cytosolic $[Ca^{2+}]_i$ concentrations in cell injury, cell death and cell proliferation. (ADP)RT, ADP ribosyltransferase; DAG, diacylglycerol; GAP, GTPase activating protein; G prot, GTP-binding protein; IP_3, inositol trisphosphate; PKC phosphokinase C; PLA_2, phospholipase A2; PLC, phospholipase C; Topo 1, topoisomerase 1; TPA, 12-O-tetradecanoylphorbol-13 acetate; $\Delta\Psi$, mitochondrial membrane potential. Reproduced with permission from Trump & Berezesky, (17).

II. $[Ca^{2+}]_i$ Regulation in the Normal and Abnormal Cell

In most normal mammalian cells, $[Ca^{2+}]_i$ is regulated to levels of approximately 100 nM. As indicated in the hypothesis diagram (Fig. 1), cells exist in an extracellular concentration of ionized calcium ($[Ca^{2+}]_e$) of approximately 1 mM; and thus the cytosol faces a ~10,000-fold outside-inside gradient. This regulation is maintained by membrane transport systems including Ca^{2+}-ATPases in the plasma membrane, the mitochondria, and the endoplasmic reticulum (ER), and also possibly by newly recognized subsets of these membrane systems. Furthermore, $[Ca^{2+}]_i$ is in equilibrium with calcium that is bound to a variety of Ca-binding proteins, such as calmodulin (Cam). Each of these regulatory sites bears important relationships to a variety of cellular phenomena. For example, regulation of the cell membrane is intimately related to transmembrane signalling, (including the effects of a number of hormones and growth factors); mitochondrial regulation involves the generation of ATP through oxidative phosphorylation; and ER phenomena function involves muscle contraction and secondary effects mediated through transmembrane signalling.

$[Ca^{2+}]_i$ is thus poised in a delicately balanced fashion to act as an important primary, secondary, or tertiary messenger for a variety of cell functions, including endocytosis, phagocytosis, secretion, motility, fertilization, cell division, mitotic spindle function, cellular differentiation, and many other activities such as regulation of hormones and growth factors.

It should also be evident from Figure 1, that there are many ways in which toxic and environmental events can adversely affect $[Ca^{2+}]_i$ regulation. These include: (1) interference with the supply of ATP in all the regulatory processes; (2) selective or targeted changes of function of the plasmalemma (8), the mitochondria, or the ER; (3) modification of growth hormone receptors and/or mediating mechanisms, such as the IP_3 pathway; (4) introduction of agents that modify transport proteins which are directly or indirectly involved, such as the Na^+, K^+- or Ca^{2+}-ATPases; and (5) agents that modify the action of mediator molecules, such as calmodulin, phospholipases, Ca^{2+}-activated proteases, and Ca^{2+}-activated endonucleases. Therefore, sustained deregulation of $[Ca^{2+}]_i$ can induce a variety of structural and functional effects through activation of: (1) phospholipases which can modify and/or destroy membrane selective permeability; (2) Ca^{2+}-activated proteases which can modify the effects of a number of functional proteins including those of the cytoskeleton; (3) protein kinases which are involved in a variety of phenomena including gene transcriptional activators; and (4) Ca^{2+}-activated endonucleases which are capable of producing strand breaks in nuclear DNA.

III. Cell Injury and Cell Death

A. Reversible and Irreversible Cell Injury

Injuries to the cell can be classified as lethal or sublethal depending on whether they lead to the death of the cell prior to its expected lifetime (14). Examples of irreversible or lethal cell injury include total ischemia which leads to death of most mammalian cells within a time period of hours. Examples of sublethal injury include fatty metamorphosis in the hepatocytes following a variety of toxins, stimulated autophagocytosis, and carcinogenesis. In the case of irreversible cell injury, the cell passes through three phases: (1) the reversible phase in which the structural and functional changes can be reversed if the injurious stimulus is removed; (2) the phase of cell death; and (3) the changes subsequent to cell death, often termed "necrosis" (14).

B. Classification of Cell Death

1. Types of cell death

There are two general types of cell death, accidental and programmed. Accidental cell death includes the commonly observed types of death that occur following application of chemical toxins, anoxia, ischemia, or xenobiotics;

programmed cell death implies death resulting from genetic or physiological stimuli involved in tissue remodeling or turnover such as those that occur during embryologic development. Types of programmed cell death include _apoptosis_, commonly observed in the immune system, and _terminal differentiation_, such as seen in the maturation of the epidermal cells in the skin. The distinction between accidental and programmed cell death, however, disappears when the stimuli or chemical species that induce the pattern characteristic of programmed cell death are identified and can be administered to cells in either _in vivo_ or _in vitro_ models to induce the same pattern of cell change. An excellent example is corticosteroids, which induce apoptosis in lymphocytes (7,4). Currently, considerable progress has been made in elucidating genetic factors that can regulate programmed cell death such as the bcl-2 gene in mammalian cells (9,11).

C. Role of Ion Deregulation in Cell Injury

Deregulation of cellular ion concentrations including $[K^+]_i$, $[Na^+]_i$, $[Mg^{2+}]_i$, $[Cl^-]_i$, and $[Ca^{2+}]_i$ have been observed to occur very early following injury during the reversible phase (14). Changes in these ions appear to be among the earliest events following injury, often occurring within a few seconds. Early on we noted these changes and subsequently focused particularly on the role of $[Ca^{2+}]_i$ deregulation (15,10), which we found can lead to irreversible cell injury in most cells. More recently, we observed that transient or reversible deregulation of $[Ca^{2+}]_i$ may represent an important factor in the stimulation of regeneration or terminal differentiation. This paper, therefore, focuses on the measurement and significance of change in $[Ca^{2+}]_i$ as a mediator in cell injury and cell death. We also explore the role of sublethal changes in $[Ca^{2+}]_i$, which appear to effect immediate early and stress gene expression in their role in regeneration and tumor promotion.

IV. Regeneration, Tumor Promotion, and Carcinogenesis

At the time of sperm-egg fusion at fertilization, transient or sustained increases of $[Ca^{2+}]_i$ have been found to play a role in cell division and cell differentiation (15). Neoplastic cells have been shown to have higher $[Na^+]_i$ and $[Ca^{2+}]_i$ levels and the use of calcium ionophores has been observed to induce cell division in culture (15). Our recent studies have shown that oxidant stress, which appears to play an important role in tumor promotion and also probably in regeneration, induces increases in $[Ca^{2+}]_i$ prior to induction of immediate early genes such as c-**fos**, c-**jun**, and c-**myc** (1), and also that modifying intracellular $[Ca^{2+}]_i$ by buffering or by eliminating Ca^{2+} from the incubation medium greatly diminishes the induction of these genes (6).

V. Methods for the Measurement of Cellular Calcium

A. Methods for Total Calcium

Total calcium can be analyzed in cells, tissues, and body fluids using atomic absorption spectroscopy on extracts of cells, tissues, or organelles or on dilutions of body fluids. These methods can be coupled with the use of ^{14}C labelled inulin to measure and estimate the size of the extracellular compartment. Measurements of total calcium at the cellular and subcellular level can be performed by energy dispersive x-ray microanalysis of whole cells using the electron microscope to view thin or semi-thin sections of cells, or tissues (16). This method permits assay of calcium in cells and organelles and identification of inclusions or deposits suspected to contain calcium. This method can also be used to measure calcium in precipitates, such as the hydroxyapatite deposits, often found in the mitochondria of injured cells. To prevent extraction of diffusible calcium, the analysis is usually applied to cryosections of rapidly frozen cells or tissues.

B. Ionized Calcium

More recently, methods have become available to measure ionized calcium in cells or organelles. These methods employ fluorescent probes which are calcium chelators and which, when irradiated at the appropriate wavelength, emit photons in the visible range which are proportional in number to the amount of bound calcium. Such probes are typically organic esters of fluorophores that specifically chelate a particular ion (such as Ca^{2+}) and in so doing become fluorescent at a particular wavelength. In the case of Fura-2, irradiation at 340 nm results in the emission of visible light with a peak wavelength of 510 nm (3). In order to normalize for specimen thickness, fluorescence is compared by excitation at a neutral wavelength, such as 380 nm, and then calculating the 340/380 ratioed fluorescence. These probes are loaded into cells in suspension or monolayers by incubation prior to the onset of an experiment (10). During this preincubation period, hydrolysis of the ester occurs in the cytosol through the action of cytosolic esterases, releasing the free acid chelate. Experiments can then be carried out either on cells in suspension using a spectrofluorometer or on monolayer cells using digital imaging fluorescence microscopy (DIFM) coupled with image analysis. In either case, the concentration of intracellular ionized cytosolic calcium is calculated according to the formula, $[Ca^{2+}]_i = \beta \times K_d \times (R - R_{min})/(R_{max} - R)$ where R_{max} is in the range of 1.7-2.2. If more rapid detection of changes is required, photon counting may be employed rather than imaging to produce a continuous curve of the 340/380 ratio. Similarly, more rapid imaging results can be obtained by employing a confocal microscope with which rapid changes in $[Ca^{2+}]_i$ may be followed with concomitant imaging.

VI. $[Ca^{2+}]_i$ Measurement and Assessment of Toxicity

We are currently assessing changes of $[Ca^{2+}]_i$ as possible early indicators of cutaneous toxicity utilizing both mouse and human keratinocytes *in vitro*. The mouse keratinocytes being utilized are from JB6 cell lines, originally isolated by Colburn et al. (2). These murine keratinocytes have the advantage that subclones have been established so that both promotable (clone 41) and nonpromotable (clone 30) clones are available for testing. We are exploring a series of model chemical toxins including mitochondrial inhibitors, modifiers of plasmalemmal integrity, sulfhydryl reagents, and calcium ionophores.

A. Methods

1. Cell culture

Mouse keratinocyte JB6 cells were a gift from Dr. Nancy H. Colburn (National Cancer Institute, Frederick, MD 21701). The toxicity of all compounds (Ionomycin, mercuric chloride, formaldehyde, sodium lauryl sulfate, dimethyl sulfoxide, benzoyl peroxide) was studied in a concentration range of 10^{-15} to 10^{-2} M, using the promotable clone 41 of JB6 cells as described previously (5). The non-promotable clone 30 of JB6 cells, which is presumably more sensitive to toxic effects of oxidant stress, was used to study the possible differential effects of benzoyl peroxide and xanthine/xanthine oxidase. Both clones of JB6 cells were grown in Dulbecco's minimal essential medium (DMEM)/F12, plus 10% fetal calf serum, as described previously (2).

2. Transmission Electron Microscopy

JB6 mouse keratinocytes were fixed with 2% formaldehyde-1% glutaraldehyde in 0.1 M sodium cacodylate buffer (pH 7.3) at room temperature for 2-3 hr. Free-floating cells in the supernatant and scraped cells from the dishes were pooled and centrifuged at 8000 x G for 10 min. After discarding the supernatant, the pellet was resuspended in small aliquots of sucrose-cacodylate buffer, transferred to microfuge tubes, and spun for 5 min. The pellets were then postfixed in 1% buffered osmium tetroxide, stained en bloc with uranyl acetate, dehydrated and embedded in polybed 812 (Polysciences, Warrington, PA). Ultrathin sections were cut, stained with uranyl acetate and lead citrate, and then examined and photographed using a JEOL EX1200 TEM. In some experiments, putative calcium deposits were characterized by x-ray microanalysis.

B. Results

By phase contrast microscopy, control JB6 cells were squamous and polyhedral or elongated with abundant cytoplasm and 1-3 nuclei (Fig. 2a). Well-defined mitochondria, perinuclear lysosomes, and nuclei were observed (5).

Morphological characteristics related to cytotoxic effects included bleb formation, nuclear chromatin condensation, swollen mitochondria, and increased granularity of the cytoplasm. The degree of these morphological changes correlated with the toxicity

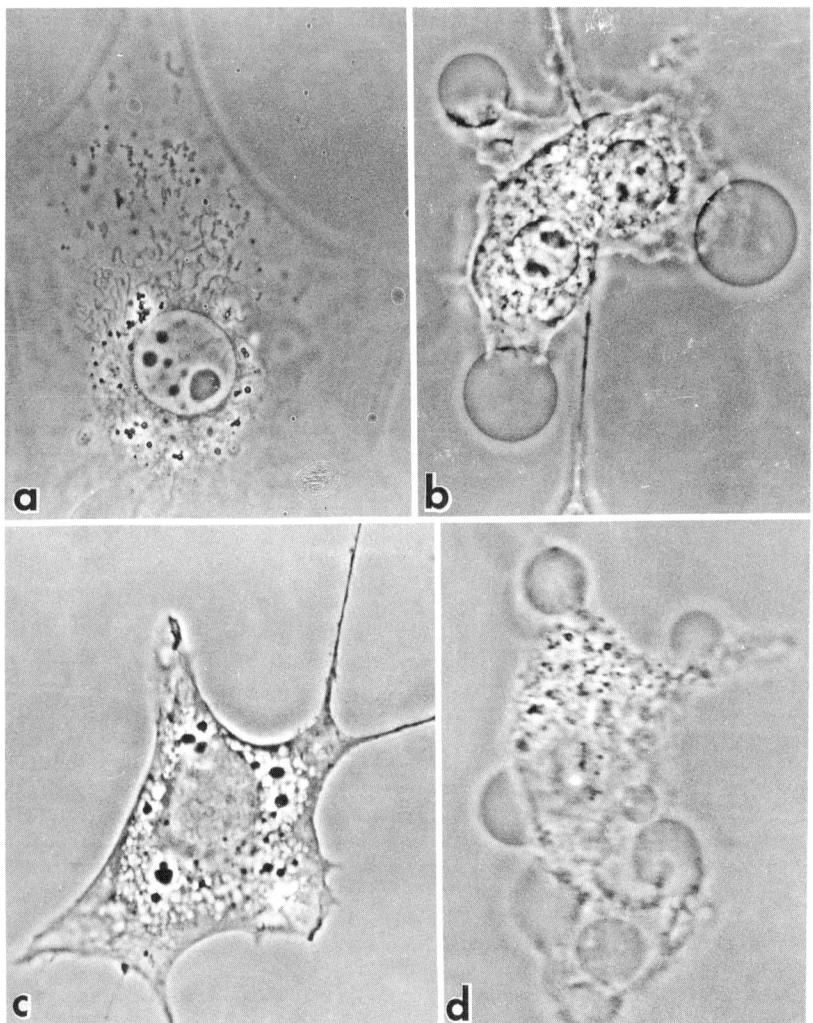

Figure 2. Phase contrast photomicrographs. (a) Control JB6 (clone 41) cell exhibiting a large nucleus containing euchromatin, perinuclear lysosomes and mitochondria. (b) A JB6 (clone 41) cell treated with $HgCl_2$ for 40 min. The cell appears altered with granular cytoplasm and also numerous blebs. (c) and (d) Promotable JB6 (clone 41) cells treated with X/XOD (5 mM). (c) Characteristic long retracting processes are seen prior to the appearance of cytoplasmic vacuoles. (d) Blebs form and cells begin to detach. Vacuolization, granulation, and possibly autophagic vacuoles increase with time. Morphological changes were more intense in non-promotable cells than in promotable cells.

estimated by trypan blue data (5). Bleb formation and the overall necrosis of JB6 (clone 41) cells following treatment with mercuric chloride is shown in Fig. 2b. When JB6 cells (clone 41) are treated by X/XOD (5 mM), they undergo retraction, long, thin remnants of cell processes are characteristically seen (Fig. 2c), and the number of vacuole-like structures increases. Following this, blebs appear on the cell surface and cells begin to detach and appear necrotic (Fig. 2d)

By TEM, JB6 cells exhibited epithelial-like morphology with numerous microvilli at the cell surfaces and junctional complexes between cells; the cytoplasm contained numerous mitochondria, prominent rough ER, well-developed Golgi, and perinuclear secondary lysosomes (Fig. 3). Nuclear chromatin was moderately dispersed.

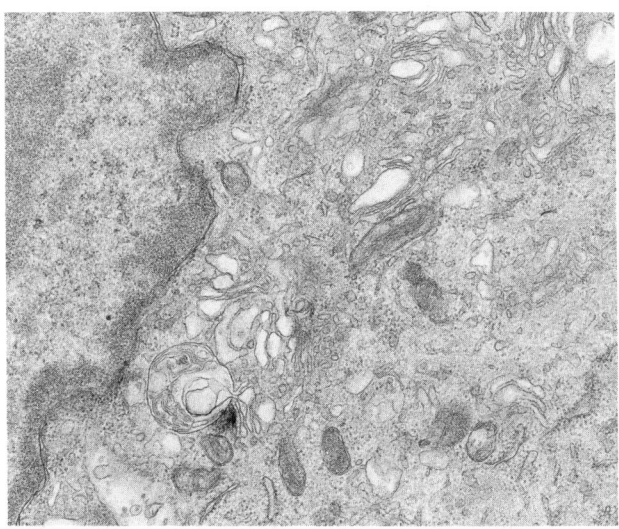

Figure 3. TEM of non-promotable JB6 (clone 30) cell showing perinuclear lysosomes, ER, normal mitochondria, and prominent Golgi regions (25,000X). (Reproduced with permission from Jain et al., (5)).

Following treatment with benzoyl peroxide for up to 4 hrs, non-promotable clone 30 cells showed swollen mitochondria, ER, and nuclear envelopes. In some sections, mitochondria contained dense crystalline aggregates (Fig. 4), which by x-ray microanalysis, were found to contain calcium.

C.   Changes in $[Ca^{2+}]_i$

Ratioed images of untreated Fura-2 loaded JB6 cells are typically found to contain ~100 nM of $[Ca^{2+}]_i$ (Fig. 5a). Maximum increases in $[Ca^{2+}]_i$ were observed when JB6 cells were treated with ionomycin (Fig. 5b). Similar changes were observed when JB6 cells were treated with $HgCl_2$. However, the maximal elevation of $[Ca^{2+}]_i$ was slower and not observed until after 16 min, whereas after ionomycin, the peak was observed by 3 min. Treatment with benzoyl peroxide, an oxidant promotor and weak toxic compound (5) resulted in elevations of $[Ca^{2+}]_i$ that were lower than the levels observed after ionomycin or $HgCl_2$ exposure (Fig. 5c). It was also noted that the extent of $[Ca^{2+}]_i$ elevation by benzoyl peroxide was higher in the non-promotable clone 30 than in the promotable clone 41. However, the amount of $[Ca^{2+}]_i$ increase following treatment with benzoyl peroxide in JB6 (clone 41) cells was still lower than that following treatment with $HgCl_2$ even at a 100-fold higher concentration. These data are in agreement with our hypothesis that $[Ca^{2+}]_i$ elevation, which precedes bleb formation, can serve as an early marker for determining cytotoxicity (12,16).

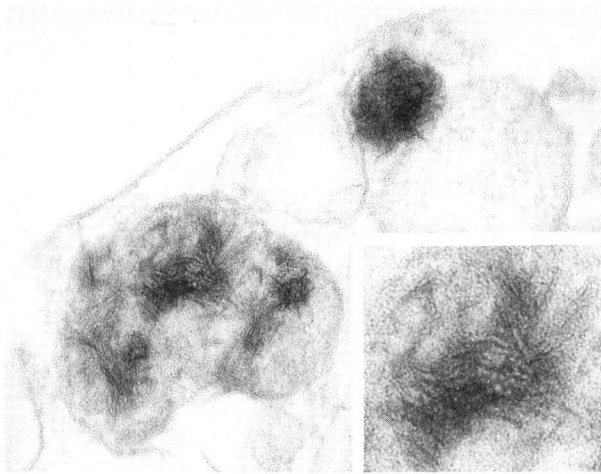

Figure 4. TEM of JB6 (clone 30) cell after 4 hr treatment with benzoyl peroxide (500 µM). The ER, nuclear envelope, and mitochondria become markedly swollen. A mitochondrion is shown which exhibits precipitate formation (99,000X). Inset: Higher magnification of the middle crystal (180,000X), which contains calcium, as verified by x-ray microanalysis. (Reproduced with permission from Jain et al., (5)).

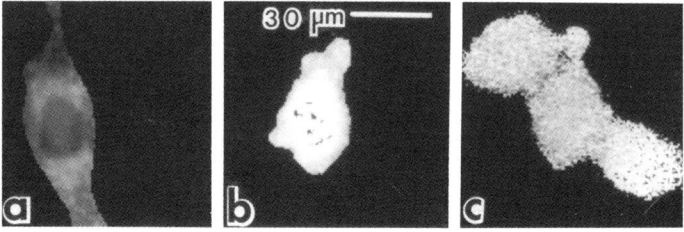

Figure 5. Ratioed images of Fura-2/AM loaded JB6 cells demonstrating $[Ca^{2+}]_i$. These images were generated from fluorescent image pairs collected at 340 and 380 nm excitation using DIFM coupled with image analysis. Ratio value increases are indicated by changes in grey-level intensities ranging from low (dark) to high (white) and indicate increases in $[Ca^{2+}]_i$. (a) Control cells show the presence of about 100 nM $[Ca^{2+}]_i$. (b) After treatment with ionomycin, there is a high elevation of $[Ca^{2+}]_i$. (c) Benzoyl peroxide caused a far lower $[Ca^{2+}]_i$ elevation in JB6 (clone 30) cells. This was also the case in clone 41 cells (not shown).

VII. Discussion

$[Ca^{2+}]_i$ appears to be a major factor in the mechanism of early, prelethal, and lethal toxicity and probably, in the case of sublethal injury, contributes to the entry of cells into the mitotic cycle. Studies in our laboratory on mouse JB6 keratinocytes have shown that a series of model toxins which exert acute lethal injury result in early elevations of $[Ca^{2+}]_i$ which seem to predict later lethal injury. Since lethal injury in JB6 cells *in vitro* appears to correlate with *in vivo* toxicity on animal models, this early indicator may represent a useful *in vitro* screening test with mechanistic implications (5).

Figure 1 illustrates the central role of $[Ca^{2+}]_i$ in a variety of toxic reactions of cells, including injuries that modify the plasmalemma, the mitochondria, or the ER. Thus, deregulation of $[Ca^{2+}]_i$ appears to be a central mechanism through which a variety of degradative and related processes can occur through activation of enzymes including phospholipases, Ca^{2+}-activated proteases, and endonucleases. The relationship of $[Ca^{2+}]_i$ to membrane blebbing, including modification of the cytoskeleton, cell membrane integrity, and changes in DNA and chromatin are illustrated. Furthermore, the suggested ER translocation systems which are modified in cell injury also have a common reaction point with ligands activating transmembrane signalling through the phospho-inositol pathway, which relates to activation of protein kinase C, a target of the phorbol ester class of tumor promotors.

In future studies, we will relate the deregulation of $[Ca^{2+}]_i$ to the activation of immediate early and stress genes, including c-fos, c-jun, c-myc, and hsp70. It is our hypothesis that activation of these genes could also represent important early indicators of toxicity and putative tumor promotors.

VIII. Conclusions

Cell and tissue calcium can be measured by several methods, depending on the desirability of assessing total or ionized calcium. In both cases, methods are available for measurement at the tissue or organ level, as well as the intracellular level. Recent introduction of DIFM, coupled with image analysis and fluorescent probes to measure $[Ca^{2+}]_i$, has meant that observations of $[Ca^{2+}]_i$ can be made on living cells before and after application of a toxic stimulus.

We have summarized the applicability of such methods to the study of cell toxicity and reported on studies on cutaneous toxicities using JB6 mouse keratinocyte cell lines. We have observed that early changes of $[Ca^{2+}]_i$ can, indeed, predict toxicity and that toxicity *in vitro* in JB6 cells shows good correlation with toxicity *in vivo* using data from the literature.

(Supported by JHU/CAAT.) This is contribution No. 3284 from the Cellular Pathobiology Laboratory.

IX. References

1. CERUTTI, P.A. and TRUMP, B.F., (1991), Inflammation and oxidative stress in carcinogenesis. Cancer Cells 3:1-7.

2. COLBURN, N.H., VORDER-BRUEGGE, W.F., BATES, J.R., GRAY, R.H., ROSSEN, J.D., KELSEY, W.H., and SHIMADA, T., (1978), Correlation of anchorage-independent growth with tumorigenicity of chemically transformed mouse epidermal cells. Cancer Res. 38:624-634.

3. GRYNKIEWICZ, G., POENIE, M., and TSIEN, R.Y., (1985), A new generation of Ca^{2+} indicators with greatly improved fluorescence properties. J. Biol. Chem. 260:3440-3450.

4. ISEKI, R., MUKAI, M., and IWATA, M., (1991), Regulation of T lymphocyte apoptosis. Signals for the antagonism between activation- and glucocorticoid-induced death. J. Immunol. 147:4286-4292.

5. JAIN, P.T., FITZPATRICK, M.J., PHELPS, P.C., BEREZESKY, I.K., and TRUMP, B.F., (1992), Studies of skin toxicity *in vitro*: Dose-response studies on JB6 cells. Toxicol. Pathol. 20:000-000, in press.

6. MAKI, A., BEREZESKY, I.K., FARGNOLI, J., HOLBROOK, N.J., and TRUMP, B.F., (1992), Role of $[Ca^{2+}]_i$ in induction of c-fos, c-jun, and c-myc mRNA in rat PTE after oxidative stress. FASEB J. 6:919-924.

7. McCONKEY, D.J., NICOTERA, P., HARTZELL, P., BELLOMO, G., WYLLIE, A.H., and ORRENIUS S., (1989), Glucocorticoids activate a suicide process in thymocytes through an elevation of cytosolic Ca^{2+} concentration. Arch. Biochem. Biophys. 269(1):365-370.

8. PAPADIMITRIOU, J.C., RAMM, L.E., DRACHENBERG, C.B., TRUMP, B.F., and SHIN, M.L., (1991), Quantitative analysis of adenine nucleotides during the prelytic phase of cell death mediated by C5b-9. J. Immunol. 147:212-217.

9. SENTMAN, C.L., SHUTTER, J.R., HOCKENBERY, D., KANAGAWA, O., and KORSMEYER, S.J., (1991), bcl-2 inhibits multiple forms of apoptosis but not negative selection in thymocytes. Cell 67:879-888.

10. SMITH, M.W., PHELPS, P.C., and TRUMP, B.F., (1991), Cytosolic Ca^{2+} deregulation and blebbing after $HgCl_2$ injury to cultured rabbit proximal tubule cells as determined by digital imaging microscopy. Proc. Natl. Acad. Sci. 88:4926-4930.

11. STRASSER, A., HARRIS, A.W., and CORY, S., (1991), bcl-2 transgene inhibits T cell death and perturbs thymic self-censorship. Cell 67:889-899.

12. SWANN, J.D., SMITH, M.W., PHELPS, P.C., MAKI, A., BEREZESKY, I.K., and TRUMP, B.F., (1991), Oxidative injury induces influx-dependent changes in intracellular calcium homeostasis. Toxicol. Pathol. 19:128-137.

13. TRUMP, B.F. and BEREZESKY, I.K., (1984), The role of sodium and calcium regulation in toxic cell injury, Drug Metabolism and Drug Toxicity, J.R. Mitchell and M.G. Horning (Eds.) Raven Press, New York, 261-300.

14. TRUMP, B.F. and BEREZESKY, I.K., (1985), Cellular ion regulation and disease. An hypothesis, Regulation of Calcium Transport in Muscle, A.E. Shamoo (Ed.) Academic Press, Inc., New York, 279-319.

15. TRUMP, B.F. and BEREZESKY, I.K., (1987), Ion regulation, cell injury and carcinogenesis. Carcinogenesis 8:1027-1031.

16. TRUMP, B.F., BEREZESKY, I.K., SMITH, M.W., PHELPS, P.C., and ELLIGET, K.A., (1989), The relationship between cellular ion deregulation and acute and chronic toxicity. Toxicol. Appl. Pharmacol. 97:6-22.

17. TRUMP, B.F. and BEREZESKY, I.K., (1992), The role of cytosolic Ca^{2+} in cell injury, necrosis, and apoptosis. Current Opinion in Cell Biology 4:227-232.

G. *In Vitro* Toxicology and Risk Assessment

In Vitro Toxicology and Risk Assessment

KANNAN KRISHNAN,[1] MICHAEL L. GARGAS,[2] and MELVIN E. ANDERSEN[3]

[1]Département de Médecine du Travail et d'Hygiéne du Milieu
Faculté de Médecine, Université de Montréal
Case Postale 6128, Succursale A
Montréal, PQ, Canada H3C 3J7

[2]ChemRisk, A Division of McLaren/Hart
29225 Chagrin Blvd., Cleveland, OH 44122

[3]Duke University Medical Center
P.O. Box 3210, Durham, NC 27710

Toxicology studies provide both qualitative (hazard identification) and quantitative (dose-response assessment) information on particular toxic effects for the assessment of the risks associated with human exposure to chemicals. Qualitative in vitro studies are used for hazard identification in weight-of-evidence approaches. The potential use of in vitro results for quantitative exposure-dose-response assessments remains to be fully developed. In this aspect, in vitro studies are used to investigate (i) metabolic rates, (ii) mechanisms of action, and (iii) tissue responses, using tissues from various species including humans. However, several questions need to be answered before the results from in vitro studies are acceptable for direct use in risk assessment. For instance, which exposure conditions in the intact animal are likely to cause effects similar to those noted in vitro, and can the shape of the dose-response curve in animals and people be predicted from the in vitro studies? Physiologically-based dosimetry and response models permit extrapolation from in vitro results to predict behavior in the living animal, thus answering these questions. In vitro studies, together with physiological modeling approaches, promise to greatly improve the scientific basis of risk assessment and optimize the value of information obtained in studies in the intact animal.

INTRODUCTION

Risk assessment is the process of estimating the probability and magnitude of potential harmful effects associated with human exposure to chemical, physical or biological agents. Risk assessment is performed in four steps: (i) hazard identification, (ii) exposure assessment, (iii) dose-response assessment, and (iv) risk characterization (1). Once the toxic effects of a chemical are identified ("hazard identification"), the health risks associated with human exposure are characterized ("risk characterization") by combining quantitative information on its exposure levels ("exposure assessment") and on the dose-response relationships for various toxic effects ("dose-response assessment"). In vivo and in vitro toxicology studies provide the qualitative and quantitative information necessary for conducting hazard identification and dose-response assessment. Quantitative risk assessment (QRA) so far has relied primarily upon in vivo animal data, which provide some quantitative basis for estimating health risks associated with human exposure to low levels of chemicals. The estimation of human health risks is conducted following a series of extrapolations, which are based on assumptions and not on any mechanistic considerations. In vitro systems offer an opportunity to investigate the mechanism of action of toxicants and to compare the susceptibility of target cells from several species to toxicants. Before in vitro data on toxicokinetics and toxicodynamics can be used directly in QRA, we need to understand the quantitative relationships between the in vitro systems and the intact organism. This "in vitro-in vivo" link of chemical disposition and toxicity can be achieved when in vitro studies are conducted in conjunction with a physiologically-based modeling approach. This article discusses the role of in vitro studies in hazard identification and dose-response assessment, and the use of physiological models as tools for enhancing the potential of in vitro data to predict in vivo behavior and for use in human health risk assessment.

IN VITRO STUDIES AND HAZARD IDENTIFICATION

Hazard identification involves the determination of whether or not a particular chemical is causally linked to the incidence of adverse health effects. It involves characterizing the nature and strength of the evidence for causation. Essentially this process serves to identify chemicals that can cause an increase in the incidence of adverse health conditions. The hazard potential of a substance is determined by its properties such as acute toxicity, irritation/corrosivity, subacute/subchronic toxicity and chronic toxicity.

Acute toxicity testing of chemicals in vivo is decreasing. Alternative methods, particularly in vitro studies and structure-activity relationships, are contributing to reduced and refined animal use in such studies (2). These alternative approaches help to reduce the unnecessary distress caused to the animal and the large number of animals used in such studies. The potential for continued and increasing use of these alternative methods at the present time emphasize the use of in vitro systems as tools for screening structually-related chemicals, and those that cause acute toxicity by a similar mechanism of action.

Irritation/corrosivity testing of chemicals is also showing a decreasing animal use. A number of battery of tests have been developed which cover various aspects of the complex behavior of in vivo irritant response (3-7). These alternative methods have contributed to important reduction and refinements of animal use, and are headed for replacement of animal use in such studies.

Subacute/subchronic toxicity testing with the primary aim of identifying the target organ(s) continues to rely primarily on in vivo systems. Considerable progress has been made to develop in vitro systems that are predictive of in vivo organ toxicity (e.g., hepatotoxicity (8-11), nephrotoxicity (12, 13), neurotoxicity (14, 15) hematotoxicity (16), thyrotoxicity (17), immunotoxicity (18, 19)). These animal alternative systems most commonly utilize perfused organs, tissue slices, and cell cultures. None of these systems predicts all possible toxic effects associated with any single organ. For example, the commonly used in vitro tests cannot be used to detect a nephrotoxicant acting by certain postrenal and prerenal mechanisms, or a neurotoxicant whose transport is controlled significantly by the blood:brain barrier, or a reproductive toxicant that acts by disrupting hormonal balances, etc. In fact, there is no single battery of tests that allows adequate characterization of the type and magnitude of systemic toxic effects elicited by untested chemicals. Further, there are certain effects that can only be monitored effectively in the intact animal (e.g., effect on physiological parameters, behavioral effects). Despite these shortcomings, in vitro tests can assist in prioritizing and ranking the relative toxicity of structurally-related chemicals, thus contributing to a reduction and refinement of animal use in subacute/subchronic toxicity studies.

Chronic toxicity studies relate to the following endpoints: cancer, genetic effects and teratogenic effects. The use of in vitro tests in screening chemicals based on short-term end points helps prioritize research needs, thus contributing to reduction of animal use in these areas (20-24). However, negative results obtained in these predictive assays is not accepted as adequate demonstration of the lack of potential of the chemical to induce such effects. Ideally, one would not want to take a chance of overlooking a chemical that may in fact be carcinogenic or teratogenic in vivo, especially in humans. Therefore, until high-fidelity in vitro models are developed and validated, in vivo testing for chronic effects is inevitable.

Any acceptable alternative in vitro test should (i) produce reasonably consistent and reproducible results wherever and whenever it is carried out, (ii) provide information on all the endpoints covered by the animal study (or part thereof) that it is intended to replace, and (iii) exhibit general applicability over a wide range of compounds of different structure and physicochemical properties (25). Such properly-validated non-animal tests, which are also quantitative and mechanistically-based, should not have to be used just as a prescreen before carrying out a definitive test using an empirical and descriptive animal procedure, the relevance and reliability of which have not been scientifically established (26).

The quantitative in vitro approaches can have a significant impact on the dose-response assessment portion of the risk assessment process. This impact mainly arises from the utility of in vitro studies to (i) elucidate the mechanisms of action and (ii) determine interspecies variability in metabolism and tissue responses, thus reducing the uncertainty associated with such extrapolations. However, the potential use of in vitro results in conducting quantitative exposure-dose-response assessments remains to be fully developed.

IN VITRO STUDIES AND DOSE-RESPONSE ASSESSMENT

Dose-response assessment refers to the process of estimating the incidence of response for various exposure levels in animals and people. The original NAS report which used the expression "dose-response assessment" does not explicitly address the issue of tissue dose. Considering the very high doses used in qualitative toxicology studies (e.g., cancer bioassay), it is conceivable that tissue dose may not be proportional to the administered dose throughout the range of exposure levels but is more complex due to nonlinearities in pharmacokinetics (i.e., absorption, distribution, metabolism and excretion). In these cases, tissue disposition of chemical may change from one exposure level to another, and the basis of this exposure level-dependent behavior must be ascertained to accurately predict response incidence across exposure levels. Because of the need to clearly distinguish the concepts of exposure level and dose to critical tissues, we emphasize the use of the more comprehensive expression, namely, "exposure-dose-response assessment" (27). Thus, the conventional dose-response really refers to exposure-response involving the characterization of the relationship between exposure levels and tissue responses. On the other hand, exposure-dose-response refers to the determination of the quantitative relationship between exposure levels and tissue dose, and further the relationship between the tissue dose and observed/expected responses in animals and people.

Such a comprehensive approach allows to examine systematically the steps involved in chemical toxicity. The steps of the exposure-dose-response paradigm shown in Figure 1 can be grouped to represent three processes, namely, chemical disposition (toxicokinetics), toxicant-target interaction (mechanism of action) and tissue response (toxicodynamics). Information on toxicokinetics and toxicodynamics of chemicals obtained from conventional animal studies are used in QRA only after conducting extrapolations. The high dose to low dose extrapolation of toxicokinetic behavior of chemicals is conducted by linear extrapolation, and the tissue dosimetry is considered to be similar for all routes of exposure in all species. The interspecies extrapolation of toxicokinetics is performed on the basis of body weight or body surface. Regarding the toxicodynamics of chemicals, a threshold model to derive RfD (reference dose) or RfC (reference concentration) in case of systemic toxicants, and a non-threshold model (linearized multistage model) in case of

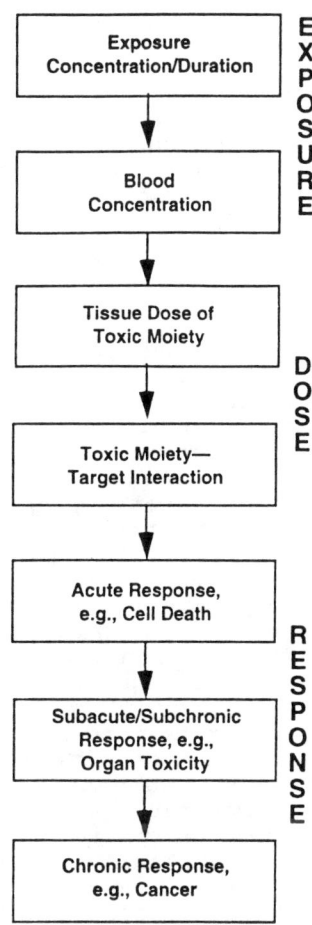

Figure 1. The "Exposure-Dose-Response" paradigm for chemical carcinogens and systemic toxicants.

carcinogens are used for low dose extrapolation. This mandated extrapolation approach results from the use of assumptions and empirical relationships in place of understanding of the mechanisms of toxicokinetics and toxicodynamics of particular chemicals (28).

In vitro studies have the potential of contributing to the understanding of the mechanistic basis of these processes, thus reducing the uncertainty associated with the conventional extrapolation procedures. However, several questions need to be addressed before the results of in vitro studies are acceptable for direct use in QRA. For instance, what exposure conditions in the intact animal are likely to cause effects similar to those noted in vitro, and can the shape of the exposure-dose-response curve in animals and people be predicted from the in vitro studies? Physiologically-based modeling approaches permit extrapolation of in vitro results to predict chemical disposition and toxicity in the intact animal, thus answering these questions.

Physiological modeling is the process of developing mathematical descriptions of the interrelationships among the mechanistic determinants of the events of interest (29, 30). This approach involves (i) identification of the mechanistic determinants (i.e., physicochemical, physiological, biochemical and molecular factors) of the exposure-tissue dose-response continuum, and (ii) encoding the interrelationships among the mechanistic determinants in mathematical equations. The solution to these equations by analytical or numeric methods predicts the behavior of the biological system under a specified set of experimental conditions. The predictions may be related to dosimetry, toxicant-target interactions, or tissue response. The extent to which the predictions coincide with subsequent experiments is a test of "correctness" of the proposed mechanisms. In this sense, these mathematical models are actually quantitative statements of our proposed hypothesis of toxic action. These models then become central factors in maintaining the risk assessment focus of ongoing research. Experiments, designed based on these working hypotheses, confirm, refute or alter the model description. These physiological models provide a basis with which to use in vitro data to predict chemical disposition and toxicity in intact animals.

In vitro-In vivo Extrapolation of Toxicokinetics

In vitro studies providing qualitative and quantitative information on the toxicokinetics of a chemical primarily include studies on absorption, distribution, and metabolism. Most common of these are the metabolism studies conducted to determine the intrinsic clearance for organ(s) of interest. A variety of in vitro systems find use in such experiments including, perfused organs, tissue slices, tissue homogenates, cultured cells, isolated cells and subcellular fractions (31). These various in vitro systems represent diverse levels of biological complexity, thus differing in their ability to metabolize chemicals by particular pathways. These in vitro systems have in general not been used to predict quantitatively the kinetics in vivo, but rather to provide qualitative information about relative proportion of a chemical metabolized by particular metabolic pathways in several species including humans. Often the in vitro assays have been conducted using substrate concentrations that have no relevance to the in vivo exposure situations. Further, the in vitro system represents a closed system which does not account for organ blood flows, extrahepatic metabolism, intratissue transport, etc. that are encountered in vivo. These problems can be addressed when in vitro data are analyzed within a physiological modeling framework, and when the model is used as a tool to plan such experiments. The physiological model can be run to determine the concentration of the parent chemical in the venous blood leaving liver, and this concentration range can be used for incubation studies. Further, metabolic data collected in the "closed" in vitro system can be incorporated into a physiologically-based computer model which provides the framework of an "open" animal system comprising of organs, blood flows, tissue specific localization of enzymatic activity, intratissue transport, etc.

The potential utility of physiological models in enhancing the value of in vitro constants to predict in vivo behavior has been investigated only to a limited extent. These predictions were mostly conducted in concentration ranges where the first order kinetics prevailed, and therefore the ratios of V_{max} and K_m were used. Some of the chemicals for which in vitro-derived rate constants incorporated within a physiological model described adequately the disposition kinetics in one or more species include: 1-b-D-arabinofuranosyl cytosine, ethanol, ethoxybenzamide, diisopropyl fluorophosphate and parathion (32-36).

The success in in vitro-in vivo extrapolation of clearance has principally been attained for nonvolatile chemicals that are metabolized by membrane-bound oxidases or soluble cytosolic enzymes. In vitro-derived metabolic rate constants reported for certain lower molecular weight volatile chemicals that are metabolized primarily by the membrane-bound mixed function oxidases system do not correlate well with constants obtained in vivo (37). For example, the clearance of methylene chloride (MC) by oxidative metabolism estimated in vitro using rat liver microsomes is lower than the actual clearance estimated by in vivo methods. The examination of the in vitro- and in vivo-derived metabolic rate constants reveal that the Vmax correlates well but there are differences of upto four orders of magnitude in the Km between the two approaches (Table 1). Use of these in vitro Km values in a PBPK model would severely underestimate the amount of MC metabolized via the oxidative pathway at low concentrations. Such a description would have the MFO pathway competing less efficiently with the GSH pathway, thus overpredicting the metabolite production via the GSH pathway. Products from the GSH pathway have been correlated with tumor outcome (38), and this parameter mis-specification would lead to substantial errors in assessing risk posed by low level exposure to methylene chloride.

Table 1. Comparison of in vitro and in vivo-derived metabolic rate constants for methylene chloride (37).

System	Method	Vmax (μMol/hr/335g rat)	Km (μM)
In vitro	Microsomal[a]	9.14	50100
In vitro	Microsomal[b]	9.12	1420
In vivo	Gas uptake[c]	21.9	4.76

[a] Kubic and Anders (39)
[b] Reitz et al (40)
[c] Gargas et al (41)

The maximal metabolic rates observed with several chemicals in an in vitro vial equilibration technique utilizing enriched homogenate fractions from both fed and fasted male Wistar rats and those determined with an in vivo gas uptake approach using fed male F-344 rats have recently been compared (Table 2). The scale-up of the in vitro Vmax to the whole organism was conducted based on the mass recovery of the particular fraction. The difference in magnitude of the Vmax values between the in vitro values obtained using homogenates from fasted rats and the in vivo values obtained using fed rats was attributed to induction of specific isoenzymes of P-450. The magnitude of these fed-fasted increases is yet to be demonstrated in vivo. In vitro Kms using enriched homogenates have been reported for only three compounds. Unlike the MC example using microsomes, in this case,

Table 2. Comparison of in vitro and in vivo-derived Vmax for several chemicals (37).

Compound	In Vivo[a]	In Vitro (Fed Rats)[b]	In Vitro (Fasted Rats)[b]
Benzene	19.62	8	16.56
Toluene	37.85	10.57	18.34
m-Xylene	35.06	12.26	18.66
Styrene	37.48	16.64	20.98
Chloroform	26.46	11.5	25.07
Carbon tetrachloride	1.21	1.11	2.68
1,1-Dichloroethane	35.25	11.15	25.48
1,1,1-Trichloroethane	1.46	0.292	0.546
1,1,2-Trichloroethane	26.83	12.26	25.48
1,1,1,2-Tetrachloroethane	18	4.73	14.92
1,1,2,2-Tetrachloroethane	33.25	7.77	18.2
1,1-Dichloroethylene	35.99	18.16	30.62
Trichloroethylene	38.92	11.04	25.94
Tetrachloroethylene	0.5	0.292	0.865

[a] Gargas et al (41)
[b] Nakajima and Sato (42)

there was a good agreement between in vitro- and in vivo- derived Km values (Table 3).

Table 3. Comparison of the Michaelis Constant, Km derived from in vivo[a] and in vitro[b] studies (37).

Compound	In Vivo Km (μM)	In Vitro Km (μM)
Benzene	3.8	4.2
Toluene	3.8	3.3
Trichloroethylene	1.9	3.8

[a] Gargas et al (41)
[b] Nakajima and Sato (42); Sato and Nakajima (43)

The identification of in vitro approaches for determining metabolic rate constants that give values consistent with those operative in vivo is critical for eventually predicting human dosimetry. Recent studies are indicative of hepatocytes being the better in vitro system, providing rate constants that compare well with the in vivo situation (44-46). Such approaches need be applied for greater number of prototype chemicals, representing specific pathways of metabolism, and validated with appropriate in vivo pharmacokinetic data. For validation of the in vitro system, the in vitro-derived intrinsic clearance should be incorporated along with separately determined values of reversible plasma/blood binding and blood flow rate into a physiological model of organ elimination to get an estimate of the drug's clearance by the organ of interest (47, 48). In using a similar approach for chemicals showing relatively lower membrane permeabilities, the diffusional clearance in addition to the intrinsic metabolic clearance should be assessed (49). By making the organ clearance a part of the "open" animal system with a PBPK description, it becomes feasible to predict chemical kinetics for various exposure scenarios in the intact animal.

In vivo approaches exist for determining metabolic rate constants in animals (41, 50), but are not always feasible for application in humans. The default position is to use scaling of the in vivo kinetic constants in rodents when extrapolating to humans. Scaling of these constants has been performed allometrically (51). The reliability of this procedure is not known. It is therefore preferable to determine the metabolic

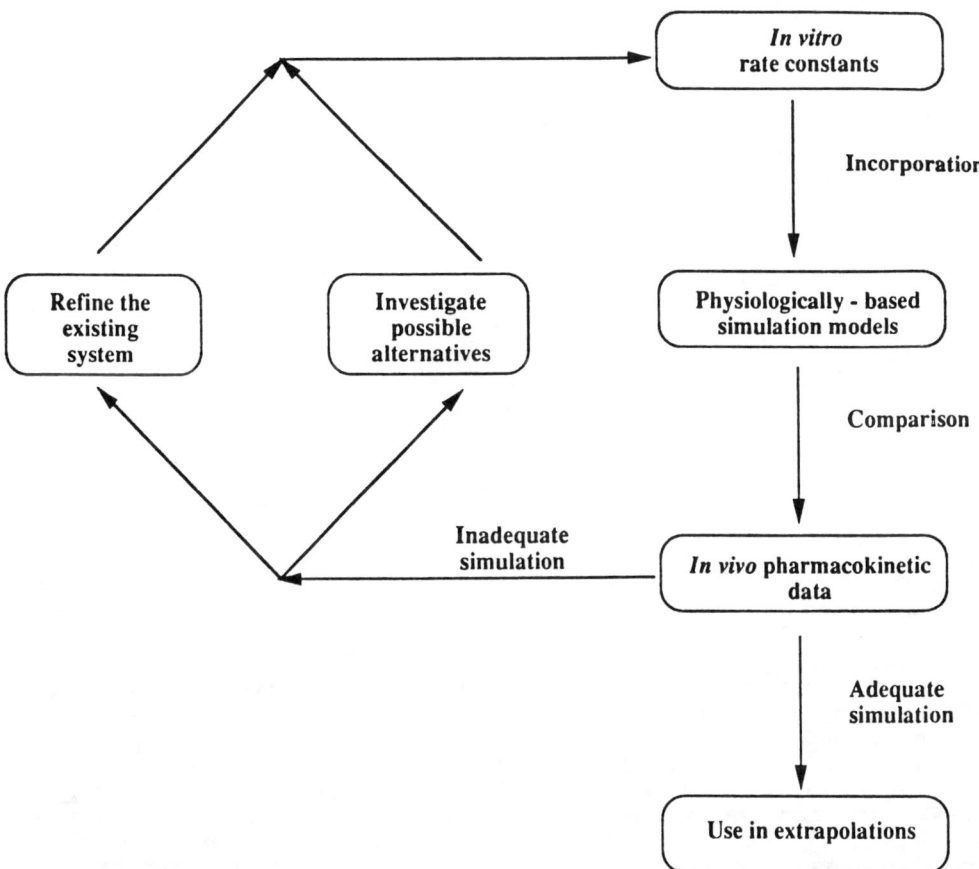

Figure 2. Schematic of the steps involved in using the physiological modeling approach to identify in vitro systems that are predictive of in vivo behavior.

rates in vitro using an appropriate system to predict human dosimetry. However, more focussed research is necessary to quantitatively understand the basis of in vitro-in vivo extrapolation of metabolism in various model systems in animals (Figure 2). Until the ideal in vitro system(s) is(are) identified and understood, we will have to rely on indirect estimations of in vivo metabolic rates from human in vitro data based on the relationship between the in vitro and in vivo rate constants observed in the rodents (40) (Figure 3).

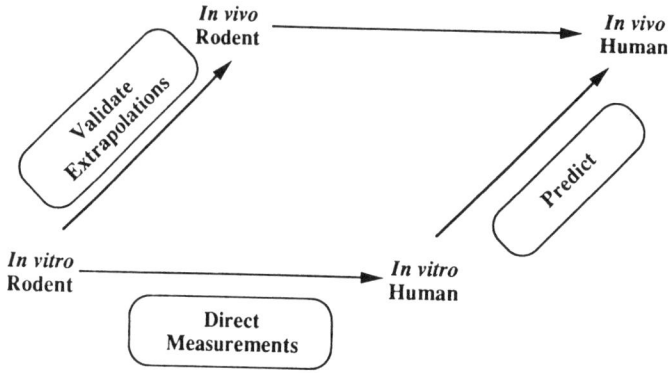

Figure 3. The parallelogram approach of in vitro-in vivo extrapolation using animal and human data.

In vitro-In vivo Extrapolation of Mechanism of Action

The elucidation of mechanism of toxic action of chemicals is critical to the process of QRA. The understanding ("qualitative") of the mechanistic basis of toxicant-target interaction indicates whether or not such a mechanism is operative in a particular species, and if so the relative importance in the species of interest (i.e., humans) in comparison to another (e.g., rat). An example of in vitro studies resolving mechanistic issues as related to interspecies extrapolation is that of trichloroethylene. It was found that trichloroethylene did not induce peroxisome proliferation in cultured human hepatocytes (52), thus providing a mechanistic basis to suggest that this chemical does not represent a hepatocarcinogenic hazard to humans.

For in vitro toxicology efforts to have a direct and significant impact on the QRA process, the mechanistic toxicology studies should be conducted within the framework of a physiological model of the mechanism of toxic action for each chemical. Such an approach would lead to the direct use of in vitro data to predict the extent of toxicant-target interaction in the intact animal and humans at various doses administered by different routes. The underlying hypothesis of such a quantitative modeling approach is that the interrelationships between certain physicochemical, biochemical, physiological, molecular and cellular processes determine the magnitude of a specific type of toxicant-target interaction.

The physiologically-based descriptions of mechanisms of action thus integrate the critical biological determinants of dosimetry and toxicant-target interaction, leading to the initiation of tissue response. For carcinogens exhibiting DNA-reactivity, the relevant initial target tissue interaction is the formation of DNA adducts. With ethylene oxide, for example, the rate of change in the amount of DNA adducts in the various tissues (dA_{eo-dna}/dt) of rats and mice is believed to be related to the concentration of the chemical in the tissue (C_{t-eo}), tissue DNA concentration (C_{dna}), tissue volume (V_t), the concentration of the adduct at any given time (C_{eo-dna}), and the rate constants for the formation (K_f) and removal (K_r) of the particular adduct in each tissue (27):

$$dA_{eo-dna}/dt = K_f C_{t-eo} C_{dna} V_t - K_r C_{eo-dna} V_t$$

The concentration of tissue DNA adducts is determined by dividing the amount of the adduct by tissue volume. Whereas K_f and K_r can be estimated from both in vitro and in vivo studies, the tissue concentration of the chemical can be predicted with a physiologically-based pharmacokinetic model (53).

Another example of a biologically-based mathematical description of the mechanism is the one developed for carbon tetrachloride (54). Reactive metabolites of this chemical bind to cellular macromolecules, and the accumulation of alkylated macromolecular adducts (with attendant decrease in the concentration of functional macromolecules) is believed to initiate events leading to cell death. In this case, the level of chemically-stable adducts is related to both the rate of carbon tetrachloride metabolism and the degradation rates of the altered macromolecules. Differential equations used in this case to describe the change in adduct levels with time are of the following form:

$$d[Adduct]/dt = P_1 \, dA_{met}/dt - K_1[Adduct]$$

where

P_1 is the proportion of metabolite binding covalently
k_1 is the rate constant or adduct degradation or repair

To predict cell death that ensues the accumulation of these adducts in this case, the sensitivity to cell death is described as a normal or lognormal distribution based on adduct level in the cell.

In each example above, toxicant-target interaction is described mathematically by equations that include the critical determinants of dosimetry and initial tissue interactions. For interspecies extrapolation of the mechanism of action of a chemical, quantitative information on the critical biological determinants (e.g., rates of formation and degradation of macromolecular adducts, and the relative sensitivity of cells from different species) needs to be obtained for the animal species of interest. Such information can frequently be obtained by using cells or tissues in vitro. Once the in vitro techniques are determined to faithfully predict in vivo interactions in animals, similar in vitro studies using human tissues can be performed to provide the required parameters for the models to conduct interspecies extrapolations.

In vitro-In vivo Extrapolation of Toxicodynamics

There may not be a high fidelity in vitro model for predicting effects such as cancer and other chronic diseases in vivo. However, if the mechanism of toxicity is described quantitatively based on physiological modeling of in vitro data, this alone can contribute to important reductions in uncertainties in the QRA process. Some of the toxic effects induced early-on by chemicals (e.g., cytotoxicity) can be quantitated and integrated with other determinants to make predictions of the chronic diseases (e.g., cancer) (55).

For example, chloroform-induced cell death is described with the rate of metabolism via a statistical distribution of cell sensitivities (56). Specifically, a normal distribution was used to calculate the proportion of cells susceptible to dying at any given rate of chloroform metabolism. In general terms, the linking relationship for the proposed biochemical mechanism by which liver cells are killed by chloroform is:

$$dN_h/dt = -SENS\ N_h\ K_{(death)}$$

where

SENS = normal or log normal distribution of cell sensitivity to cytotoxicity as a function $(dA_{met}/dt)/V_l$. This provides an estimate of the proportion of cells at risk at any time and can be derived from in vitro experiments.
N_h = Total number of viable hepatocytes.
$K_{(death)}$ = Rate at which cells at risk die
V_l = Liver volume

The extrapolation to people then requires quantitative information on the rates of metabolism of chloroform to phosgene and the liver volume. The rate is determined by Vmax and Km, liver chloroform concentration and blood flow. Information on the kinetic constants of chloroform oxidation in people versus mice, together with a PBPK model permits prediction of the exposure conditions under which people will develop liver toxicity from this chemical. Because oxidation rates of these volatile chemicals are greater in mice than in people, people are expected to be at less risk than mice for hepatotoxic effects of chloroform. This conclusion is not necessarily expected to be valid with cytotoxic chemicals with other biochemical mechanisms of hepatotoxic action.

While describing toxic effects, it is necessary to consider the repair and recovery processes. Model parameters representing such processes are crucial for developing adequate descriptions of the overall toxic effect in the intact animal, and can only be ascertained from in vivo studies. When high fidelity in vitro systems are devised to mimic such in vivo effects, careful consideration should be given to evaluate the need for any correction factors for incorporation into the in vitro - in vivo extrapolation algorithm.

SYMPOSIUM PRESENTATIONS

IN VITRO TOXICOLOGY AND RISK ASSESSMENT

The integration of the in vitro toxicology and physiological modeling efforts can result in the direct use of in vitro data in QRA. This approach consists of (i) developing a physiologically-based description and (ii) conducting in vitro studies of toxicokinetics, mechanism of action, and toxicodynamics of the chemical.

The implementation of this integrated approach ideally should begin with the formulation of a physiologically-based description of the toxic processes of interest. This preliminary model can serve to organize the thoughts of the investigator(s) such that clearly defined hypotheses of the mechanism of disposition and action of the chemical are generated and presented in a mathematical form. The latter requires that we specify the critical determinants of the process and the proposed nature of the interrelationships among these determinants with respect to each endpoint of interest. For example, the schematic presented in Figure 4 depicts the working hypotheses of disposition and action of a volatile organic chemical. Such a preliminary model formulated by the integration of the quantitative information already existing in the literature, serves both to identify datagaps, and as a tool to plan in vitro experiments (e.g., determination of incubation concentrations).

This preliminary model formulation is followed by the pursuit of the necessary in vitro and in vivo studies as identified by the investigator(s). This step involves the determination of the metabolic and binding rate constants using in vitro preparations, and the generation of concentration-response relationships of the mechanism of action (e.g., adduct formation) or early effects (e.g., cytotoxicity) in vitro. The metabolic rate constants incorporated into a physiological pharmacokinetic model translate exposure concentration into tissue dose, and the physiological model of the mechanism of action provides the magnitude of the interaction between the toxic moiety at the tissue and the tissue macromolecules. The physiological model can provide answers to such questions as what exposure concentration would provide the tissue/blood concentration of the chemical or adducts comparable to the in vitro incubation conditions?

The in vitro-derived metabolic rates should be validated or refined with specific in vivo pharmacokinetic data. Similarly tissue repair rates etc. that need to be investigated in the intact animals should be obtained to complete parameter estimation. Then, the simulations of the physiological response model constructed with in vitro data can be compared with experimental observations of the toxic effects to validate or refine the model (Figure 5). During this process, if the experimental results differ from the predicted outcome, then the model has to be modified. Just as our ideas change with new experimental data/observations, these models are dynamic constructs that can be continually updated by new information and the revised models used in turn as guides in another iteration for designing new research studies. The finished product of this biologically- and mechanistically- based approach is a computer model that can be used for extrapolations of toxicokinetics and toxicody-

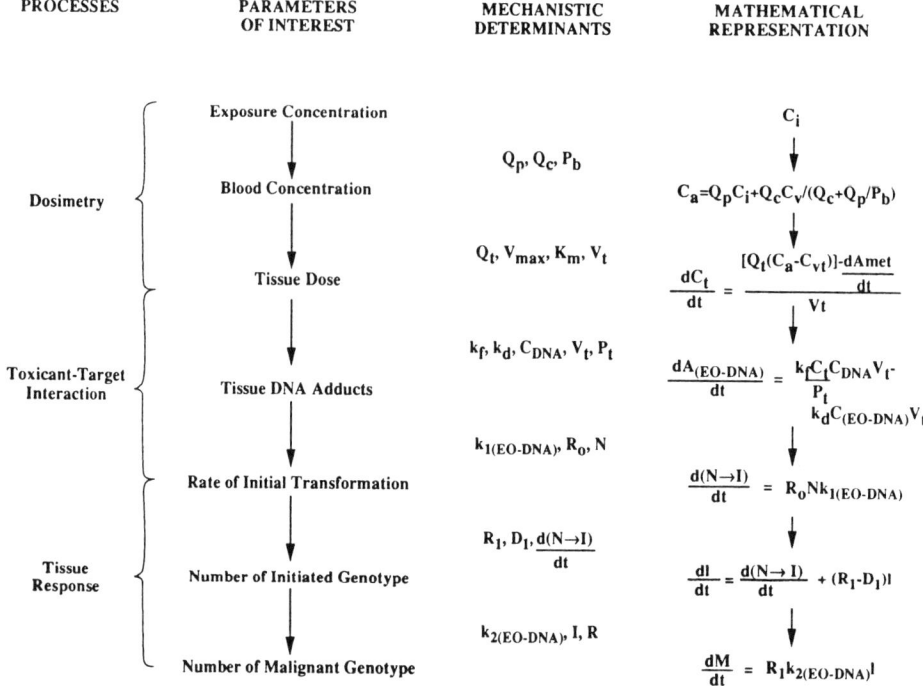

Figure 4. Biologically-based description of the exposure-dose-response continuum to estimate tumor incidence for any exposure concentration of a volatile organic chemical (EO) detoxified by metabolism, based on working hypotheses of its mechanisms of disposition, target interaction (e.g., DNA reactivity) and tissue response. All the mathematical representations of the phenomena of interest are linked to each other sequentially via at least one term. Concentration of the chemical in arterial blood (C_a) is determined from the interrelationship between the breathing rate (Q_p), inhaled concentration (C_i), cardiac output (Q_c), venous blood concentration (C_v) and blood:air partition coefficient (P_b). Rate of change in the tissue concentration of the chemical (dC_t/dt) is calculated from the tissue blood flow rate (Q_t), arteriovenous concentration difference (C_a-C_{vt}), the rate of metabolism ($dA_{met}/dt = V_{max} \cdot C_{vt}/(K_m+C_{vt})$), and the volume of the tissue (V_t). The rate of change in the amount of the DNA adducts formed by the chemical ($dA_{(EO-DNA)}/dt$) is represented by the difference between the rate of formation (a function of constant (k_f), concentration of the chemical in the venous blood leaving the tissue (C_{vt}), volume of the tissue (V_t) and the tissue concentration of DNA (C_{DNA}) and degradation (a function of the adduct removal rate constant (k_d), concentration of adduct at anytime ($C_{(EO-DNA)}$) and the volume of the tissue (V_1)). The cancer response arising from exposure to this chemical is hypothesized to be the end result of two critical events (N -> I; I -> M) that correspond to mutations, one converting the normal cell (N) to an intermediate cell (I), and the second mutation converting the intermediate cell to a malignant genotype (M). Birth rates of normal and intermediate cells are R_0 and R_1 and death rates are D_0 and D_1, and the mutation frequencies between cell types are represented as a function of the DNA adduct levels

Figure 4 (Contd.)

($k_{x(EO-DNA)}$). Predicted cancer incidence is a stochastic function of the numbers of these various cell types over time. Of the parameters required for this quantitative exposure-dose-response model, physiological parameters can be obtained from biomedical literature, all physicochemical and some biochemical parameters can measured in vitro. Certain biochemical determinants for the tissue response model need to be estimated from in vivo experiments.

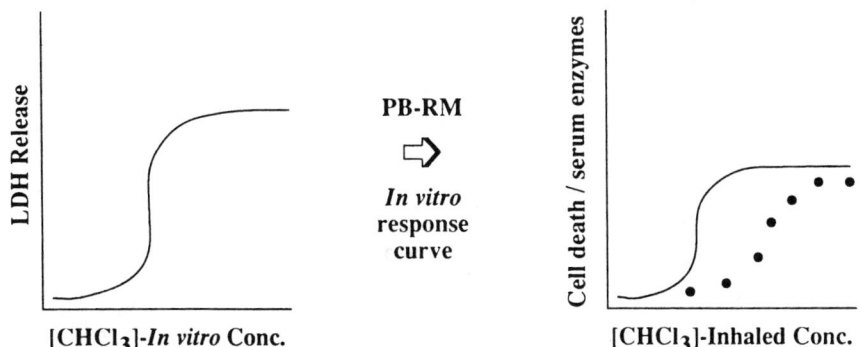

Figure 5. Illustration of the use of physiologically-based response model (PB-RM) in predicting the in vivo response based on the concentration-response curve obtained in vitro.

namics from high dose to low dose, from one exposure route to another and for various exposure scenarios in several species.

This integrated "biological modeling-in vitro experimentation" approach holds promise to enhance the credibility and applicability of in vitro data in the quantitative risk assessment process. The in vitro-in vivo extrapolation has already been conducted successfully with the physiological modeling approach for certain pieces of the exposure-dose-response paradigm. However, there is still a need to develop strategies for integrated "physiological modeling-in vitro toxicity testing" of a variety of prototype chemicals, and validate and extend them to other similar chemicals. Overall, this approach provides a framework to predict the shape of the dose-response curve in the intact animal and humans, based on concentration-response relationships obtained in vitro.

REFERENCES

1. NATIONAL ACADEMY OF SCIENCES (1983), Risk assessment in the federal government: managing the process. National Academy of Sciences, Washington, D.C.

2. PHILLIPS, J.C., GIBSON, W.B., YAM, J., ALDEN, C.L., and HARD, G.C., (1990), Survey of the QSAR and in vitro approaches for developing nonanimal methods to supersede the in vivo LD50 test. Fd. Chem. Toxicol. 28: 375.

3. FLINT, O.P., (1990), In vitro alternatives to ocular toxicity testing: report of a meeting organized by the Industrial In Vitro toxicology group. In Vitro Toxicol. 3: 281.

4. SOTO, R.J., and GORDON, V.C., (1990), An In vitro method for estimating ocular irritation. Toxicol. In Vitro 4: 332.

5. REINHARDT, C.A., (1990), In vitro predictive tests for eye irritants. Toxicol. In Vitro 4: 242.

6. HOTCHKISS, S.A., CHIDGEY, M.A.J., ROSE, S., and CALDWELL, J. (1990), Percutaneous absorption of benzyl acetate through rat skin in vitro: validation of an in vitro model against in vivo data. Fd. Chem. Toxicol. 28: 443.

7. DYKES, P.J., EDWARDS, M.J., O'DONOVAN, M.R., MERRETT, V., MORGAN, H.E., and MARKS, R., (1991), In vitro reconstruction of human skin: the use of skin equivalent as potential indicators of cutaneous toxicity. Toxicol. In Vitro 5: 1.

8. TYSON, C.A. (1987), Correspondance of results from hepatocyte studies with in vivo response. Toxicol. Ind. Health 3: 459.

9. TYSON, C.A., GEE, S.J., HAWK-PRATHER, K., and STORY, D.L., (1989), Correlation between in vitro and in vivo toxicity of some chlorinated aliphatics. Toxicol. In Vitro 3: 145.

10. GOETHALS, F., DEBOYSER, D., GONZALEZ, C., and ROBERFROID, M., (1988), Use of isolated hepatocytes for studying the biochemical mechanism oif steatosis and cholestasis. Alt. Meth. Toxicol. 6: 159.

11. FENTEN, J.H., FOSTER, B., MILLS, C.O., COLEMAN, R., and CHIPMAN, J.K., (1990), Biliary excretion of fluorescent chlorophiles in hepatocyte couplets: an in vitro model for hepatobiliary and hepatotoxicity studies. Toxicol. In Vitro 4: 452.

12. GANDOLFI, A.J., and BRENDEL, K., (1990), In vitro systems for nephrotoxicity studies. Toxicol. in vitro 4: 337.

13. BRADLEY, M.O., NOBLE, C. and SINA, J.F., (1988/89), An in vitro nephrotoxicity assay useful for drug development. In Vitro Toxicol. 2: 171.

14. ATTERWILL, C.K., (1990), Neurotoxicology in vitro: model systems and practical applications: comparative studies with the cholinergic neurotoxins in primary brain cultures and in rabbit retina in vitro. Toxicol. In Vitro 4: 346.

15. DAVENPORT, C.J., and MORGAN, K.T., (1988/89), In vitro neurotoxicology: industrial applications. In Vitro Toxicol. 2: 207.

16. NAUGHTON, B.A., SIBANDA, B., TRIGLIA, D., and NAUGHTON, G.K., (1991), Rat bone marrow cell proliferation and differentiation as an index of the effects of xenobiotics in vitro. Toxicol. In Vitro 5: 389.

17. DUFFY, P.A., and YARNELL, S.A., (1991), Use of primary

canine thyroid monolayer cultures to investigate compounds that are thyrotoxic *in vivo*. Toxicol. In Vitro 5: 373.

18. DEARMAN, R.J., and KIMBER, I., (1991), Immunotoxicity and allergy: opportunities for *in vitro* analysis. Toxicol. In Vitro 5: 519.

19. STEER, S., LASEK, W., CLOTHIER, R.H., and BALLS, M., (1990), An *in vitro* test for immunomodulators? Toxicol. In Vitro 4: 360.

20. ENNEVER, F.K. and ROSENKRANZ, H.S. (1988), Methodologies for interpretation of shortterm test results which may allow reduction of the use of animals in carcinogenicity testing. Toxicol. Ind. Health 4: 137.

21. PETERS, P.W.J., and PIERSMA, A.H., (1990), *In vitro* embryotoxicity and teratogenicity studies. Toxicol. In Vitro 4: 570.

22. BOREK, C., ONG, A., and MASON, H., (1987), *In vitro - in vivo* ststems in multistage carcinogenesis. Toxicol. Ind. Health 3: 347.

23. DOOLITTLE, D.J., MULLER, G., and SCRIBNER, H.E., (1987), The *in vitro-in vivo* hepatocytes assay for assessing DNA repair and DNA replication: studies in the CD-1 mouse. Fd. Chem. Toxicol. 25: 399.

24. TENNANT, R.W., MARGOLIN, B.H., SHELBY, M.D., ZEIGER, E., HASEMAN, J.K., SPALDING, J., CASPERY, W., RESNICK, M., STASIEWICZ, S., ANDERSON, B., and MINOR, R., (1987), Prediction of chemical carcinogenicity in rodents from *in vitro* genetic toxicity assays. Science 236: 933.

25. VAN DEN HEUVEL, M.J., and FIELDER, R.J., (1990), Acceptance of *in vitro* testing by regulatory authorities. Toxicol. In Vitro 4: 675.

26. BALLS, M., and CLOUTIER, R.H., (1991), Comments on the scientific values and regulatory acceptance of in vitro toxicity tests. Toxicol. In Vitro 5: 535.

27. ANDERSEN, M.E., KRISHNAN, K., CONOLLY, R.B., and McCLELLAN, R.O., (1992), Mechanistic toxicology research and biologically-based modeling: partners for improving quantitative risk assessments. CIIT Activities 12 (1): 1.

28. KRISHNAN, K., and ANDERSEN, M.E., (1991), Physiological modeling and cancer risk assessment. In: Rescigno, A. and Thakkur, A.K. (Eds.), New trends in pharmacokinetics, Plenum Press, NY. pp335-354.

29. ANDERSEN, M.E., (1991), Physiological modeling of organic compounds. Ann. Occup. Hyg. 35: 309.

30. KRISHNAN, K., and ANDERSEN, M.E., (1991), The role of physiological modeling in reducing animal use in toxicology research. Alternative Methods in Toxicology 8: 113.

31. WALKER, C.H., (1981), The correlation between *in vitro* and

in vivo metabolism of pesticides in vertebrates. Progr. Pest. Biochem. 1: 247.

32. DEDRICK, R.L., FORRESTER, D.D., and HO, D.H.W., (1972), In vitro - in vivo correlation of drug metabolism - deamination of 1-B-D-arabinofuranosylcytosine. Biochem. Pharmacol. 21: 1.

33. DEDRICK, R.L., and FORRESTER, D.D., (1973), Blood flow limitation in interpreting Michaelis constants for ethanol oxidation in vivo. Biochem Pharmacol. 22: 1133.

34. LIN, J.H., HAYASHI, M., AWAZU, S., and HANANO, M., (1978), Correlation between in vitro and in vivo drug metabolism rate: oxidation of ethoxybenzamide in the rat. J. Pharmacokinet. Biopharm. 6: 327.

35. GEARHART, J.M., JEPSON, G.W., CLEWELL, H.J.III., ANDERSEN, M.E., and CONOLLY, R.B., (1990), Physiologically based pharmacokinetic and pharmacodynamic model for the inhibition of acetylcholinesterase by diisopropyl fluorophosphate. Toxicol. Appl. Pharmacol. 106: 295.

36. SULTATOS, L.G., (1990), A physiologically based pharmacokinetic model of parathion based on chemical specific parameters determined in vitro. J. Amer. Coll. Toxicol. 9: 611.

37. GARGAS, M.L., (1991), Chemical-specific constants for physiologically-based pharmacokinetic models. CIIT Activities 11 (3): 1.

38. ANDERSEN, M.E., CLEWELL, H.J.III., GARGAS, M.L., SMITH, F.A., and REITZ, R.H., (1987), Physiologically based pharmacokinetics and the risk assessment process for methylene chloride. Toxicol. Appl. Pharmacol. 87: 185.

39. KUBIC, V.L., and ANDERS, M.W., (1978), Metabolism of dihalomethane to carbon monoxide III. Studies on the mechanism of the reaction. Biochem. Pharmacol. 27: 2349.

40. REITZ, R.H., MENDRALA, A.L., PARK, C.N., ANDERSEN, M.E., and GUENGERICH, F.P., (1988), Incorporation of in vitro enzyme kinetic data into the physiologically based pharmacokinetic model for methylene chloride: implications for risk assessment. Toxicol. Lett. 43: 97.

41. GARGAS, M.L., ANDERSEN, M.E., and CLEWELL, H.J.III., (1986), A physiologically based simulation approach for determining constants from gas uptake data. Toxicol. Appl. Pharmacol. 86: 341.

42. NAKAJIMA, T., and SATO, A., (1979), Enhanced activity of liver drug-metabolising enzymes for aromatic and chlorinated hydrocarbons following food deprivation. Toxicol. Appl. Pharmacol. 50: 549.

43. SATO, A., and NAKAJIMA, T., (1979) A vial equilibration method to evaluate the drug-metabolizing activity for volatile hydrocarbons. Toxicol. Appl. Pharmacol. 47: 41.

44. BISGAARD, H.C. and LAM, H.R., (1989), In vitro and in vivo

studies on the metabolism of 1,3-diaminobenzene: comparison of metabolites fromed by the perfused rat liver, primary rat hepatocytes, hepatic rat microsomes and the whole rat. Toxicol. In Vitro 3: 167.

45. KEDDERIS, G.L., MURPHY, J.E., BATRA, R., HELD, R., CARFAGNA, M.A., and GARGAS, M.L., (1992), In vivo and in vitro kinetic analysis of furan biotransformation by F-344 rats. Toxicologist 12: 348 (Abstract 1360).

46. SATO, H., SUGIYAMA, S., MIYAUCHI, S., SASWADA, Y., IGA, T., and HANANO, M., (1986), A simulation study of the effect of a uniform diffusional barrier across hepatocytes on drug metabolism by evenly or unevenly distributed uni-enzyme in the liver. J. Pharm. Sci. 75: 3.

47. WILKINSON, G.R., (1987), Clearance approaces in pharmacology. Pharmacol. Rev. 39: 1.

48. ANDERSEN, M.E. (1982), Recent advances in methodology and concepts in characterizing inhalation pharmacokinetics in animals and man. Drug Metab. Rev. 13: 799.

49. MIYUCHI, S., SUGIYAMA, Y., SAWADA, Y., MORITA, K., IGA, T. and HANANO, M., (1987), J. Pharmacokinet. Biopharmaceut. 15: 25.

50. GARGAS, M.L., and ANDERSEN, M.E., (1989), Determining kinetic constants of chlorinated ethane metabolism in the rat from rates of exhalation. Toxicol. Appl. Pharmacol. 99: 344.

51. KRISHNAN, K., and ANDERSEN, M.E., (1991), Interspecies scaling in pharmacokinetics. In: Rescigno, A. and Thakkur, A.K. (Eds.), New advances in pharmacokinetics. Plenum Press, NY. pp334-354.

52. ELCOMBE, C.R., ROSS, M.B., and PRATT, I.S., (1985), Biochemical, histological and ultrastructural changes in rat and mouse liver following the administration of trichloroethylene: possible relevance to species differences in hepatocarcinogenicity. Toxicol. Appl. Pharmacol. 79: 365

53. KRISHNAN, K., GARGAS, M.L., FENNELL, T.R., and ANDERSEN, M.E., (1992), A physiologically-based description of ethylene oxide dosimetry in the rat. Toxicol. Ind. Health 8: 121.

54. PAUSTENBACH, D.J., CLEWELL, H.J.III., GARGAS, M.L., ANDERSEN, M.E., (1988), A physiologically based pharmacokinetic model for inhaled carbon tetrachloride. Toxicol. Appl. Pharmacol. 96: 191.

55. ANDERSEN, M.E., KRISHNAN, K., CONOLLY, R.B., McCLELLAN, R.O. (1992), Biologically based modeling in toxicology research. Arch. Toxicol. Suppl. 15: 217.

56. REITZ, R.H., MENDRALA, A.L., CORLEY, R.A., QUAST, J.F., GARGAS, M.L., ANDERSEN, M.E., STAATS, D.A., and CONOLLY, R.B., (1990), Estimating the risk of liver cancer associated with human exposures to chloroform using physiologically based pharmacokinetic modeling. Toxicol. Appl. Pharmacol. 105: 443.

Part 2
Poster Abstracts

A. Dermal Toxicity

A1

Inflammatory Mediators from Reconstituted Human Skin Models Treated with Formulated Cosmetic Products

William E. Dressler, Ph.D.[*], Thomas J. Stephens, Ph.D.[†],
Hillary Kasbarian, Ph.D.[†] and E. Tiffany Spence, B.S.[†]

[*]Clairol, Inc., Stamford, CT 06922; [†] Thomas J. Stephens & Associates, Inc. Carrollton, TX 75006

An oxidative (permanent) haircolor base alone, a haircolor base plus dye, and a haircolor base plus dye mixed with peroxide were evaluated in two reconstituted human skin models for patterns of inflammatory mediator release. The models were a dermal equivalent containing mast cells (LDMMC™ from Organogenesis, Inc.) and a full thickness equivalent (Skin^2 Model 1300 from Advanced Tissue Sciences, Inc.). The models were exposed topically to the test materials for two to six hours. Results showed that the presence of an intact stratum corneum essentially eliminated cytotoxicity as detected by MTT conversion. The combination of haircolor base plus dye and peroxide appeared to increase the amount of PGE_2, IL-6 and GM-CSF detected in spent media from treated tissues. These patterns were not observed upon analysis for IL-1 α, IL-8, histamine and serotonin. TNF α was not detected in the spent media of any test material treated tissues or vehicle control tissues. Patterns of mediator release may prove useful in evaluating the potential for skin irritation and allergic contact dermatitis.

A2

EXPRESSION OF THE ANTIGEN PRESENTING CELL MOLECULE, B7 IN NORMAL HUMAN SKIN. Anthony A. Gaspari, Department of Dermatology, University of Rochester School of Medicine and Dentistry, Rochester, NY, USA.

Functional antigen presenting cells (APC) express class II MHC as well as a recently described molecule, the B7/BB-1 antigen, which is an important molecule for productive signalling between APC and CD28+ T-cells. The B7/BB-1 antigen is likely to be a source of co-stimulatory activity for T-cell activation. Since Langerhans cells are resident functional APC of the epidermis, the purpose of this investigation was to determine the distribution of the B7/BB-1 antigen in normal human skin (NHS). Immunoperoxidase staining of formalin fixed, paraffin embedded NHS derived from 5 different individuals revealed the presence of infrequent strong positive supra-basal dendritic epidermal cells (EC) that reacted with the monoclonal antibody BB-1. There was weak reactivity of small populations of keratinocytes (KC) with this monoclonal antibody. Flow cytometric analysis of trypsinized, freshly isolated epidermal cell suspensions derived from NHS revealed that approximately 10% of EC reacted with BB-1, whereas the frequency of CD1+ or HLA-DR+ or HLe1+ cells (i.e., LC) was only 1-2%. Since the number of BB-1+ EC exceeds the number of epidermal LC, this suggested that other populations of EC such as KC may express the BB-1 antigen. Indeed, cultured normal human KC that had been passaged 2-3 times (devoid of LC) reacted with BB-1. The significance of BB-1 expression by KC and possibly LC remains to be determined.

A3

Use of Multiple Endpoints for Assessing Chemical Insult in an Organotypic Skin Culture. R. Gay, M. Swiderek, A. Ernesti, D. Nelson and A. M. Kligman (1) Organogenesis Inc., Cambridge, MA and (1) Department of Dermatology, University of Pennsylvania.

Living skin equivalents (LSE) are co-cultures of human dermal fibroblasts in a collagen lattice with overlying layers of stratified human epidermal keratinocytes. LSE were used to evaluate the relative dermal irritation potential of selected chemicals using a variety of endpoints. Time and dose-dependent changes in cellular viability, the release of the proinflammatory mediators, prostaglandin E2 and interleukin-1-alpha, and tritiated water penetration through the LSE were evaluated. Irritants from different chemical classes were rank ordered using several criteria including the effective concentration which inhibited 50% (EC50) of thiazolyl blue conversion (MTT) at a constant exposure time and the time required to inhibit 50% MTT conversion (ET50) at a set concentration. The extent to which the barrier function of the LSE was damaged, as assessed by water penetration through the LSE, was also used to grade the irritation potential of different test chemicals. The correlation between in vitro rankings an in vivo dermal irritation scores was dependent on chemical class and the in vitro assay method. In the case of anionic surfactants, good agreement was seen between ET50 scores, rates water penetration through the LSE and the ability of these irritants to induce erythema and dryness in human skin.

A4

An *In Vitro* Cytotoxicity Test on JB6 (clone 41) Mouse Epidermal Cells: A Potential Model for Prediction of *In Vivo* Toxicity. Jain, P.T., Berezesky, I.K. and Trump, B.F. Univ of Maryland Sch of Med., Dept of Pathology, and MIEMSS, Baltimore, MD 21201.

The objective of the present experimentation was to study the development of *in vitro* alternatives using available new technology and, thus, to develop better models to predict *in vivo* toxicity in animals and/or man. A broad range of model toxic compounds included mercuric chloride ($HgCl_2$), sodium lauryl sulfate (SLS), formaldehyde, dimethyl sulfoxide (DMSO), benzoyl peroxide (BOP), and ionomycin, which have proven to be positive in the Draize test or in cutaneous toxicity, were evaluated for their toxicity on mouse epidermal JB6 cells in culture. Cell death was evaluated after 15, 30, 45, 60 min or 24 hours of treatment using the trypan blue exclusion method, while morphological changes were evaluated using phase contrast microscopy. Dose and time-dependent cell death and morphological changes, at the light and electron microscopic levels, were observed in concentration ranges of 10^{-14} to 10^{-2} M. Arbitrary rankings was assigned to the tested compounds based on: (1) IC50 values estimated from the present data; (2) *in vivo* toxicity reported by the Registry of Toxic Effects of Chemical Substances. Good correlation between *in vitro* and *in vivo* toxicity arbitrary rankings were observed. Thus, these findings demonstrate that JB6 cell cultures may be used for predicting *in vivo* toxicity, particularly that of rodent skin; furthermore, it was observed that increases of cytosolic ionized calcium and expression of immediate early genes may be early predictors of cell toxicity. In conclusion, the *in vitro* mouse JB6 cells may serve as a potential model for screening a variety of toxic compounds which will, thus, lower the number of animals used for this purpose. (Supported by JHU/CAAT.)

A5

Prediction of Eye Irritancy by a combined method of In Vivo Primary Rabbit Skin Irritation Test and In Vitro Cytotoxicity Test

Hajime Kojima, Atsushi Sato, Satoru Miyamoto, Yoshifumi Kawai, Izumi Ishii and Hiroaki Konishi

Biochemical Research Institute, Nippon Menard Cosmetic Co., LTD. 4-66, Asakusa, Ogaki, Gifu-ken, Japan

We compared in vivo Draize rabbit eye irritation scores (Draize scoes) with primary rabbit skin irritation scores(skin scores), and also compared Draize scores with in vitro cytotoxicities of cultured cells to the 16 surfactants. Cytotoxicities of the surfactants were measured by newtral red assay 48 hr after treatments.

There is a good correlation between Draize scores and skin scores, and also cytotoxicities, but correlation coefficient is low.

Therefore, we combined both data to compair it with Draize scores.

These results suggested that the combined method of primary skin irritation tests and cytotoxicity test are useful to predict precisely of eye irritancy.

A6

Evaluation of the Skin Irritation Potential of Petroleum Based Compounds in a Reconstituted Human Skin Model

Francis J. Koschier, Ph.D.*, Randy N. Roth, Ph.D.*, Thomas J. Stephens, Ph.D.†, E. Tiffany Spence, B.S.†, Hillary Kasbarian, Ph.D.† and Mary Ann Duke, B.A.†

*ARCO, Los Angeles, CA 90017;
†Thomas J. Stephens & Associates, Inc., Carrollton, TX 75006

Seven petroleum based test materials were evaluated for their skin irritation potential using full thickness reconstituted human skin models (Skin^2 Model 1300 from Advanced Tissue Sciences, Inc. and Living Skin Equivalent from Organogenesis, Inc.). Test materials were dosed undiluted in triplicate onto the epidermal side of the tissues and incubated in polyethylene bags designed to minimize cross-contamination and the loss of volatile constituents. The endpoints measured were MTT reduction, and the presence of LDH, PGE_2 and IL-1 α in spent media from treated and untreated tissues. Data from these tests were correlated with Draize PDII scores using Cooper's criteria. Results showed that all endpoints measured (with the exception of IL-1 α in ATS' Skin^2 Model 1300) approximated the skin irritation potential of the test materials. Significant levels of IL-1 α could not be detected in the spent media of tissues after a four hour exposure. This incubation period may be too short for significant IL-1 α release. The orientation of the tissues in the dosing chamber may be a critical factor as measured by MTT and LDH release. Further refinement of the dosing chamber may provide scientists with a novel method for evaluating volatile test materials in tissue culture.

A7

APPLICATION OF THE SKINTEX™ SYSTEM TO THE EVALUATION OF COSMETIC PRODUCTS. Kruszewski, F.H.[1], Dickens, M.S.[1], Gordon, V.C.[2], and Renskers, K.J.[1]. [1]Avon Products, Inc., Suffern, NY, and [2]Ropak Laboratories, Irvine, CA.

A total of 133 cosmetic and personal care product formulations and raw ingredients were evaluated with the SKINTEX™ System to determine the potential of this *in vitro* alternative test to predict the *in vivo* responses from rabbit skin irritation studies and human patch tests. The SKINTEX™ System is a non-animal, biochemical test developed by Ropak Laboratories, Irvine, CA. It's designed to approximate the Draize rabbit skin irritation assay as a tool for the evaluation of dermal toxicity. Agreement between assays, or concordance, exists when the SKINTEX irritation judgement matches that assigned by the *in vivo* test. Avon Products, Inc. provided all test samples, which included raw ingredients and products from 14 different classes, and represented a range of *in vivo* dermal irritancy from non-irritant to moderate irritant. The SKINTEX protocols utilized were the Upright Membrane Assay (UMA) and, when appropriate, the Alkaline Membrane Assay (AMA).

SKINTEX results were compared with rabbit dermal irritation data (single occlusive patch), which was obtained from the historical records of Avon Products, Inc. A strong positive correlation between SKINTEX results and the *in vivo* assay was demonstrated by an overall concordance rate of 83.5%. The assay error was 16.5%, of which 7.5% was due to an overestimation of sample irritancy (false positives) and 9.0% was attributed to underestimation (false negatives).

SKINTEX data for a subset of 68 products and raw ingredients, were additionally compared with human dermal irritation data (single insult patch). Human data were also obtained from the historical records of Avon Products, Inc. A strong positive correlation between SKINTEX results and the human assay was demonstrated by an overall concordance rate of 88.2%. The assay error was 11.8% which was totally attributed to an overestimation of sample irritancy (false positives). Overestimation could be supported in part by the inability of the protocols to accurately classify test samples with very low irritation potential. Underestimation of sample irritancy may be generally associated with interference by ethoxylated materials and high concentrations of specific types of surfactants or other ingredients.

A8
Potential Irritation by Dermatological Vehicles Assessed with In Vivo and In Vitro Tests.

S. Matsumoto, J. Cheng, R. Oda, S. Sabatine, C. Anger
Dept. of Microbiology and Cytotoxicity,
O. Angelov, J. Andersen, D. Sullivan, B. Brar
Dept. of Safety Evaluation, Allergan, Inc., Irvine, CA 92713-9534
G. Ewing, J. Trogden, P. Laskar
Herbert Laboratories, Inc., Irvine, CA 92713-9534

Cream and gel vehicles for dermatological products are designed to cause minimal irritation and they present special challenges for toxicological evaluation. Twelve vehicles were chosen to represent a range of chemical compositions. The vehicles were administered to New Zealand albino rabbits in a single dermal application under occlusive bandage for 24 hours with two days of observation for skin reaction (erythema and edema). The vehicles were tested in parallel using in vitro cytotoxicity assays which included two differentiated human skin models, Testskin (Organogenesis, Inc.) and Skin^2 (Advanced Tissue Sciences, Inc.). The results for the in vivo and in vitro tests were compared and analyzed in terms of the composition of the vehicles.

A9
INTERACTION OF BENZOPSORALEN WITH NCTC 2544, HELA AND HL60 CELLS.
P.P. Parnigotto, M.T. Conconi, M. Moras, V. Bassani, A. Chilin
Department of Pharmaceutical Sciences - University of Padua - Italy

4-hydroxy-methyl-4',5'-benzopsoralen (compound 1) and 4-hydroxy-methyl-4',5'-tetrahydro-benzopsoralen (compound 2) has been studied on NCTC 2544, HeLa and HL60 cells with the aim to evaluate their citotoxic activity. In inhibition growth assay after an exposure period of twenty-four hours ID50 values (µM) for compound 2 are 12.77±0.46 in HeLa cells, 6.45±0.21 in HL60 cells and higher than 59.2 in NCTC 2544 cells respectively. In confluent cultures of NCTC 2544 cells the minimal concentration (µM),causing irreversible cell damage, for compound 2 is higher than 59.2 after an exposure period of seventy-two hours. From our data the compounds examined are more active on malignant cells in respect to non-malignant ones. These results are consistent with the lack of erythemas on guinea-pig skin in vivo,as reported in a previous work. We think that the use of various cell lines subjected to simple and quick assays as proposed in this work may help to obtain information about the degree of toxicity of some biologically active agents on skin cells,agents which can been screened, and in the same way may offer a valuable tool for the prediction of skin irritancy.

A10
EVALUATION OF AN IN VITRO PHOTOIRRITATION ASSAY
R.J. Soto, J.S. Griesemer, and V.C. Gordon, J. Acevedo
S.C. Johnson & Son, Inc., Racine, WI and In Vitro International, Irvine, CA

An in vitro assay was evaluated by comparing results to human phototoxicity irritation scores for ten personal care formulations. The SOLATEX™ in vitro assay (SIA) was selected for evaluation based on previous literature. Formulas tested consisted of deodorants, skin lotions, hair conditioners, hair conditioners, and shampoo formulations. A positive phototoxic response in humans was an immediate wheal and flare response following UV-A light exposure or intense erythema and edema within 24 to 48 hours. A positive response in SIA was a net irritation increase of 50 optical density units above background after exposure to UV light. Results predicted 100% (10/10) of the non-photoreactive formulas at the concentrations tested in humans. Dose-response curves generated in multiple vehicles demonstrated non-reactivity at doses as high as twice the concentration tested on humans. A major advantage of SIA is the ability to screen unknown materials prior to human use.

A11
An in vitro Skin Model for the Study of Keratinocyte Responses to Irritants
Sandra R. Slivka, Frank Zeigler and Ronnda L. Bartel
Advanced Tissue Sciences, Inc. (formerly Marrow-Tech); La Jolla, CA 92037.

We have developed an in vitro skin model to study the responses of keratinocytes exposed to substances which are irritants of skin in vivo. This model consists of keratinocytes and fibroblasts derived from foreskin. The fibroblasts are seeded onto nylon mesh and grown for 14 or 26 days until a dermal model is formed. The matrix of this dermal model contains collagen (types I and III), fibronectin, and glycosaminoglycans. Keratinocytes are seeded onto this dermal model and grown 12-14 days in calcium containing medium until 3-5 layers of differentiated keratinocytes are formed or for 28 days until a fully differentiated epidermis is formed. This skin model is laser cut into squares and placed in multiwell culture dishes. Irritants in DMEM with 2% fetal calf serum were incubated with the model for 24-48 hours. The resultant conditoned culture medium was assayed for interleukin 1 alpha (IL-1α) and tissue-type plasminogen activator (t-PA) by ELISA. To test for cytotoxicty, the model squares were incubated with the vital dye MTT. Exposure to the tumor promoting phorbol ester (PMA) (1μM), a known irritant, results in the release of both IL-1α and t-PA. This increase can be detected at 24 hours without any observed decrease in cell viability as measured by reduction of the mitochondrial dye MTT. Tumor necrosis factor alpha (40 U/ml) potentiates the PMA-induced release of IL-1α without stimulating IL-1α release itself. Since IL-1α is an important regulator of immune and inflammatory responses and t-PA is elevated in many skin disorders, we believe that these assays using this in vitro skin model are useful for predicting irritant responses of keratinocytes in skin in vivo.

A12
Cytotoxicity Testing Using A Three-Dimensional in vitro Model of the Human Dermis and Six Different Assay Systems
Dennis Triglia, Sonia Sherard Braa, Inger Kidd and Tracy Donnelly
Advanced Tissue Sciences, Inc. (formerly Marrow-Tech); La Jolla, CA 92037.

A three-dimensional in vitro model of the human dermis, developed at Advanced Tissue Sciences, has been used as a substrate in a number of cytotoxicity and irritancy tests. The Dermal Model consists of metabolically and mitotically active, neonatal foreskin-derived fibroblasts (grown on nylon mesh) and naturally-secreted collagen and extracellular matrix proteins. This model has been used effectively to study the toxic effects of a variety of compounds and formulations. Utilizing six in vitro alternative assays (Neutral Red vital dye uptake [lysosomal function], MTT reduction [mitochondrial function], lactate dehydrogenase release [membrane integrity], glucose utilization [metabolic activity], Prostaglandin E_2, and IL-6 release [inflammatory mediators]), we have obtained dose-dependent toxicity data for surfactants, shampoos, industrial solvents, alcohols, metals, pesticides, metal-cutting fluids and industrial microbicides. Correlation of the in vitro data to existing eye and skin irritation data is very good, demonstrating the utility of this model in conjunction with six different assays as potential in vitro alternatives to animal testing. Multiple endpoint toxicity testing of test agents from diverse classes may be used to further elucidate the actual mechanisms of induced toxicity.

A13
A Three-Dimensional in vitro Human Skin Model for Toxicity Testing of Topically Applied Test Materials
Dennis Triglia, Tracy Donnelly, Inger Kidd and Sonia Sherard Braa
Advanced Tissue Sciences, Inc. (formerly Marrow-Tech); La Jolla, CA 92037.

A three-dimensional, in vitro human skin model, developed at Advanced Tissue Sciences, has been used as a substrate for the toxicity assessment of topically-applied, undiluted or high concentrations of raw materials and finished products similar to those used in human or animal skin patch tests. The Barrier Function Model consists of several layers of actively dividing, metabolically active, neonatal foreskin-derived, human fibroblasts grown on nylon mesh in the presence of ascorbate, and a basal layer of epidermal keratinocytes, several layers of differentiated keratinocytes and a stratum corneum. The substrate is placed atop a MilliCell polycarbonate culture insert (3 µm pore size) and serum-free, DMEM-based medium is placed below. Test articles are applied undiluted (or diluted in medium or solvent) onto the stratum corneum; the culture is assayed for cytotoxicity using the MTT viability assay and the medium beneath the insert is assayed for release of PGE_2 (inflammatory mediator) and lactate dehydrogenase (membrane integrity). We have tested petrochemicals, cosmetics, personal care and household products and have obtained excellent correlation of the multiassay in vitro data with in vivo skin and eye irritation data. The ability of this human skin model to accomodate topically-applied, undiluted test materials could result in the establishment of a multiassay in vitro toxicological database by several different industries.

A14

__Development of a Three-Dimensional in vitro Oral Mucosa Model__
Michael P. Zimber, *Linda Odioso, Frank Zeigler, *Matthew Doyle, Dennis Triglia and Ronnda Bartel
Advanced Tissue Sciences, Inc. (formerly Marrow-Tech); La Jolla, CA 92037
*Procter and Gamble; Cincinnati, OH 45239.

An in vitro oral mucosa model has recently been developed using a three-dimensional co-culture technique previously described for the growth of skin cells. In brief, this process utilizes fibroblasts and epithelial cells enzymatically isolated from normal human gingiva and expanded in monolayer culture. The fibroblasts are seeded onto nylon mesh where they proliferate and deposit extracellular matrix, forming a stromal support tissue. The epithelial cells are then innoculated onto the stromal tissue and allowed to grow in culture for up to one month. The growth progression of these cultures was followed histologically. The stromal component of the cultures contained fibroblasts suspended within a network of extracellular matrix. About 14 days after the epithelial cells were seeded, the tissue morphology was similar to that of junctional oral epithelium in vivo (i.e., 2-5 layers of non-keratinized epithelial cells). When the cultures were allowed to grow for an additional 10-14 days, the epithelium underwent keratinization and resembled the parent gingival tissue. The oral mucosa model was used as a substrate for assessing the in vitro toxicity of a number of oral hygiene products. Cultures were exposed overnight to various concentrations of over a dozen products; viability was assessed using the MTT assay, and release of lactate dehydrogenase gave an indication of cell membrane integrity. In addition, this in vitro oral mucosa model may be used for efficacy studies for oral hygiene and health care products.

B. Genotoxicity

B1

DEVELOPMENT AND APPLICATION OF HUMAN CELL LINES EXPRESSING INDIVIDUAL OR MULTIPLE HUMAN CYTOCHROME P450s. Cl. Crespi[a], BW Penman[a], R Langenbach[b], HV Gelboin[c], DT Steimel[a], FJ Gonzalez[c], [a]GENTEST Corporation, Woburn, MA 01801; [b]NIH/NIEHS, RTP, NC 27709; [c]NIH/NCI, Betheseda, MD 20892.

Cytochrome P450-mediated metabolism is often responsible for the toxic and genotoxic effects of xenobiotics. These enzymes are found at highest levels in liver but are also present in extrahepatic tissues. Expression of cytochromes P450 is usually present in primary cell cultures but lost during the establishment of cell lines. We have taken a cDNA transfection/expression approach to engineer human B-lymphoblastoid cell lines to stably express cytochromes P450. These approaches provide an alternative to the use of animal-derived tissues in toxicity and genotoxicity assays or metabolite analyses. Recently, two novel cell lines have been developed. The first cell line, designated MCL-5, was engineered to stably express five cDNAs encoding human CYP1A2, CYP2A6, CYP2E1, CYP3A4 and microsomal epoxide hydrolase. The level of P450 expression was 1.5-3 pmole/mg microsomal protein. This cell line was utilized as a target cell for mutagenicity assay and mutagenic activity was observed at ng/ml concentrations of five procarcinogens. A second cell line, designated h2D6v2, was engineered to express high levels of human CYP2D6, an important drug metabolizing enzyme. CYP2D6 expression levels were found to be 150-200 pmole P450/mg mirosomal protein. This expression level is near the total P450 level present in human hepatocytes and indicates that high levels of stable cytochrome P450 can be achieved in human lymphoblasts. The eventual integration of these two advances to attain high level expression of multiple cDNAS should result in the development of a verstatile xenobiotic metabolizing system which can be utilized in a variety of <u>in vitro</u> assays either as a target cell or present in co-cultures with other target cell types.

B2
THE ASSESSMENT OF A MICRONUCLEI-INDUCTION ASSAY TO EVALUATE THE IN VITRO GENOTOXICITY OF RESPIRABLE DUSTS.

Denis Nadeau and Denis Lane, Laboratoire de Biochimie et de Toxicologie Pulmonaires, Département de Biologie, Faculté des Sciences, Université de Sherbrooke, Sherbrooke, Québec, Canada.

In this study, Chinese hamster ovary cells (CHO-K1) were selected as targets to serpentine and amphibole asbestos fibres, UICC chrysotile (CHR) and crocidolite (CRO) respectively. The well known carcinogens benzol [α] pyrene (BP) and methylcholanthrene (MC) were used to validate the assay. The CHO-K1 cells were initially seeded at a density of 1×10^4 cells/assay. After the exposure, $2 - 3 \times 10^3$ cells/assay were scored for the presence of micronuclei. These were revealed by the DNA-dependant fluorochrome Hoechst 33258. At a dosage of 0.1 to 1.0 μg/ml, these two genotoxic chemicals induced dose-dependant increases in the percentage of CHO-K1 cells containing micronuclei (≈ 2 and ≈ 3 times over control levels for BP and MC respectively). When the cells were exposed to 1 and 3 μg of CHR/ml, significant increases in the incidence of the micronuclei were also observed (≈ 3.5 times over controls). At 10 μg/ml, the serpentine fibres were too cytotoxic. While there was no significant effect of the CRO fibres at the 1 μg/ml level, doses up to 10 μg of the amphibole fibres/ml however increased the percentage of micronucleated cells by ≈ 2 times over control values. An increase in multinucleated and multilobed nuclei was also observed in the fiber-exposed cells. These results suggest that the in vitro induction of micronuclei in CHO-K1 cells could be useful in a battery of tests to evaluate the genotoxic potential of respirable dusts. One of the main advantage of the assay is that it requires only a 20 hrs-exposure of the cells to the toxicants and, after 3.5 days total incubation time, the cells are ready to be analysed. Moreover, its simplicity is such that, for respirable dusts, the assay could easily be adapted to more relevant targets such as pulmonary mesothelial cells. (Supported by l'Institut de l'Amiante, Montréal, Québec, Canada).

C. Hepatotoxicity

C1

NEW METABOLITE PROFILE OF TOLBUTAMIDE IN MALE AND FEMALE RATS. A STUDY WITH PRECISION-CUT LIVER SLICES AND ISOLATED HEPATOCYTES.

P. Dogterom and G. Zbinden, Institute of Toxicology, Swiss Federal Institute of Technology and University of Zürich, CH-8603 Schwerzenbach, Switzerland.

During the last few years, the use of liver slices for metabolism and toxicity studies has got renewed attention, since it is possible now to make precision-cut liver slices. Several advantages of these slices over isolated hepatocytes are: the liver architecture is intact, there is no need for enzymatic treatment, and there is a better access to tissue from larger species, including man.
We have compared the metabolism of tolbutamide in isolated hepatocytes and precision-cut liver slices derived from male and female Wistar and Sprague Dawley rats. Tolbutamide is an hypoglycemic agent and it is well known that there are marked species differences in metabolism and hepatotoxicity. According to literature data tolbutamide is metabolized by oxidation of the methyl group (hydroxy- and carboxytolbutamide) in rat and man; in dogs the molecule splits to generate tolylsulfonamide, a substance that is hepatotoxic in the dog.
Freshly isolated hepatocytes (about 2 mg protein / ml) and precision-cut liver slices (weighing about 25 mg / slice) were incubated for 5 hours in Williams E medium, supplemented with various concentrations of tolbutamide. Cells were incubated at 37°C in a rotary shaker; slices were placed individually on baskets in 24-well plastic culture plates on a gyratory shaker and maintained at 37°C.
In hepatocytes and liver slices, the metabolite profile of tolbutamide differed from literature data. In cells and slices from male and female rats the major metabolites were hydroxytolbutamide and tolyl sulfonamide with small amounts of carboxytolbutamide. In addition, in cells and slices from male rats, tolylsulfonylurea was also found. In all experiments, linear increases of metabolites over time were observed. No differences in metabolite profiles were found between the two rat strains. Quantitative, but no qualitative differences in metabolite formation existed between hepatocytes and precision-cut liver slices. The *in vitro* technique of precision cut liver slices may be a useful addition, besides other *in vitro* techniques, in predicting whole animal metabolism for compounds subject to hepatic biotransformation and thus can support the selection of proper animal species for drug safety studies.

C2

IN VITRO CULTURE OF FISH HEPATOCYTES AND THEIR USE TO ASSESS MARINE POLLUTION.
M. Faisal and B.J. Rutan
Virginia Institute of Marine Science, School of Marine Science, The College of William and Mary. Gloucester Point, VA 23062.

Pollution of the marine environment with polycyclic aromatic hydrocarbons (PAH) is widespread. Fish caught from waters whose sediments are highly contaminated with PAH exhibited high prevalence of liver cancers. To investigate this phenomenon, several unsuccessful trials to culture parenchymal liver cells of several fish species were attempted. Therefore, the present study was designed to investigate the optimal culture conditions of liver cells derived from fish indigenous to the Chesapeake Bay. To obtain the optimal growth of hepatocytes, modification of the enzyme digestion procedure and several physicochemical culture characteristics such as growth medium, osmolality, temperature, and gas requirements was necessary. Hepatocytes of spot and Atlantic menhaden remained viable, exhibited differentiated hepatic functions, and continued active mitosis making subculture possible. Cells of some of these cultures have been cloned and subcultured and evidence indicates that these cells have a high potential for becoming immortal. Furthermore, we examined the effects of organic extracts of ten sediments collected from the Elizabeth River, Virginia, containing varying levels of PAH, on the viability and macromolecular synthesis of hepatocytes *in vitro*. Our results indicate that PAH at relatively high concentrations are cytotoxic, while low concentrations induce a sharp increase in the rate of DNA synthesis. There are, however, discrepancies among the methods used to assess cytotoxicity.

C3

Use of histological and biochemical criteria for assessing the hepatocellular alterations in rat liver slices.

Goethals F., Allaeys V., Caillau E., Buc-Calderon P. and Roberfroid M.
Unité de Biochimie Toxicologique et Cancérologique, Université Catholique de Louvain, BCTC 7369, B-1200 Brussels, Belgium.

The most popular methods for in vitro hepatotoxicity evaluation employ suspensions or culture of isolated hepatocytes. However, there are certain disadvantages associated with the use of these systems including the need of proteolytic enzymes for cell isolation and loss of tissue organization.

Rat liver slices provide a complementary in vitro system that preserves the architecture of the tissue, the cellular heterogeneity and intercellular communications. Fresh rat liver slices of reproducible thickness (250µm) were producing using a mechanical slicer (Trends Pharmacol. Sci., 8, 11-15, 1987) and incubated for 8h in the presence or absence of hepatotoxicants. The biochemical integrity of liver slices was assessed by the measurement of a number of cell functional parameters : ATP, GSH and glycogen content, protein synthesis.

Several culture media were tested in order to improve the maintenance of glycogen and cytochrome P_{450} content which are known to be sensitive to culture conditions. Using the optimal conditions, the hepatic glycogen levels remained stable for 4h. The cytochrome P_{450} content and the activities of 7-ethoxy resorufin-O-demethylase and aminopyrine-N-demethylase respectively decreased to 80% and 50% of their initial value after 8h of incubation. In addition, the histopathological changes which occured in the liver slices treated with hepatotoxicants were demonstrated using various staining (hematoxylin/eosin, PAS, Brachet).

C4
CULTURED HUMAN HEPATOCYTES - A MODEL FOR DRUG METABOLISM / TOXICITY STUDIES
G M Hawksworth, L Abernethy, S Barnard, J A Coundouris, M H Grant, C K Lindsay & V Maitland   Depts of Biomedical Sciences and Medicine & Therapeutics, University of Aberdeen, U.K.

Human hepatocytes in primary culture would provide a suitable system to investigate the regulation and induction of drug metabolism and mechanisms of xenobiotic-induced toxicity if the problems of limited availability of material and the progressive loss of oxidative enzyme activities with time in culture could be overcome. Human hepatocytes can be cryopreserved by cooling at 1^0C/min to -80^0C or -126^0C in a 25% vitrification solution (DMSO, acetamide, propylene glycol and polyethylene glycol 800) in Leibovitz medium with maintenance of cytochrome P450 dependent activities and intracellular nucleotides post thawing. Percoll density centrifugation to remove damaged cells improved plating efficiency after cryopreservation. When cultured in a cysteine-free medium cytochrome P450 dependent activities and conjugating enzymes were maintained at 70% fresh cell values over 72h. Rat cytochromes P450 IA1 and IA2 can be induced by 1,2 benzanthracene in culture medium containing 2% DMSO or when plated on an extract of EHS sarcoma to levels seen after induction in vivo (40 fold). Inhibition by cycloheximide and immunoblotting against an antibody raised against P450 IA1 that recognises P450 IA1 and IA2 confirmed that this was due to de novo protein synthesis. Induction of ethoxyresorufin-O-deethylase (selective for induced P450 IA1) in two human hepatocyte cultures was only 1.5 fold. Constitutive enzyme activities are better maintained in human hepatocyte cultures compared with rat cultures, but the inducibility may be less.

C5
Liver crude membrane fractions from rat liver improve the maintenance of liver specific functions in long term, serum free rat hepatocyte cultures.

Bashar Saad, Hanspeter Schawalder and Peter Maier
Institute of Toxicology, Swiss Federal Institute of Technology and University of Zürich
CH-8603 Schwerzenbach, Switzerland

Rat hepatocyte cultures on collagen lose the capacity to express liver specific functions over time in culture. The influence on this degradation process by an alternative substratum, the crude membrane fractions (CMF) prepared from the liver of the same rat strain, was investigated. Freshly isolated rat hepatocytes were cultured on CMF:collagen type I (100:1) coated flasks and in serum-free culture medium. Cells adhered firmly, exhibited minimal spreading, remained grouped in columns or in cell islands. Hepatocytes secreted substantially higher amounts of albumin and stabilized the total P-450 content at 72% and at 40% of freshly isolated cells on day 1 and day 9 in culture, respectively. The 7-ethoxyresorufin O-de-ethylase and the aldrin-epoxidase activities were maintained at more than 50% of freshly isolated hepatocytes on day 6. Exposure to 3mM Phenobarbital from day 3-6 doubled the total P450 content compared to untreated cultures; exposure to $25\mu M$ 3-methylcholanthrene induced the corresponding cytochrome P-450 isoform activity 20-fold compared to untreated cultures and 6-fold compared to freshly isolated cells. The crude membrane fraction preparation provides therefore simple and reproducible culture conditions suitable for pharmacotoxicological studies in long-term cultures of rat hepatocytes.

C6
THE ENHANCED RESPONSIVENESS OF HEPATOCYTES TO GROWTH FACTORS AS A RESULT OF ESTROGEN TREATMENT. **N Ni** and J D Yager. Division of Toxicological Sciences, Johns Hopkins University School of Hygiene & Public Health, Baltimore, MD

Previous work in this laboratory has demonstrated that ethinyl estradiol is a potent promoter of hepatocarcinogenesis and that it stimulates liver DNA synthesis. Additional studies have shown that estrogens act as a co-mitogen in hepatocytes by enhancing the stimulation of DNA synthesis induced by epidermal growth factor. Work by others has suggested an important role for transforming growth factor alpha (TGF-α) in liver growth.

The goal of this study was to examine the effects of estrogen treatment on TGF-α responsiveness in cultured rat hepatocytes. Hepatocytes were isolated from female F344 rats by collagenase perfusion and cultured on collagen-coated dishes for 48 hrs. in the presence of various concentrations of TGF-α $\pm$ estradiol (E2). TGF-α caused a concentration-dependent enhancement of hepatocyte DNA synthesis that reached 38-fold over control at 20 ng/ml. Estradiol alone at 30 μM stimulated DNA synthesis about 2-fold, while TGF-α and E2 together acted synergistically, causing a 61-fold increase.

These result indicate that the estrogens can also act as co-mitogens with an endogenous liver growth factor. The role of this interaction in estrogen-induced liver growth is under further investigation. Supported by NCI grant CA 36701.

C7
EFFECT OF CULTURE CONDITIONS ON THE MAINTENANCE OF XENOBIOTIC METABOLISM IN PRIMARY RAT HEPATOCYTES *IN VITRO*. J Zurlo, L M Arterburn*, E E Stickler, R M Barry*, J M Frazier and J D Yager. Division of Toxicological Sciences, Johns Hopkins School of Hygiene & Public Health, Baltimore, MD and *W.R. Grace & Co.-Conn., Research Division, Columbia, MD.

We have investigated the role of specific culture conditions on the maintenance of several forms of cytochrome P450 and two phase II enzymes in primary rat hepatocytes. Our goal was to determine the conditions for maximal basal and inducible activities of these enzymes. Hepatocytes were isolated from male F344 rats by the two-step collagenase perfusion method and cultured on collagen-coated plates. Hepatocytes were cultured in various media, differentiating agents, and on several types of cell culture plastic. Fluorometric assays were performed to measure ethoxyresorufin-O-deethylase (EROD) (P4501A1/2) and pentoxyresorufin-O-dealkylase (PROD) (P4502B1/2); HPLC analysis was performed to measure the 6-hydroxylation of chlorzoxozone (P4502E1) and the 3-hydroxylation of diazepam (P4503A). Glutathione-S-transferase and UDP-glucuronyl transferase activities were also determined. The highest baseline activities of all of the enzymes were maintained when the cells were cultured in modified Chee's essential medium on Nunc Permanox plates in the presence of 1μM dexamethasone (DEX). Baseline activities of most of the P450 enzymes examined were also enhanced by dimethylsulfoxide (DMSO) at 1% in the medium. EROD activity was maximally induced *in vitro* by exposure to ß-naphthoflavone (ßNF) at 25μM for 48 hr. PROD activity was maximally induced *in vitro* after 96 hr of exposure to 2mM phenobarbital (PB). DEX augmented both types of induction. EROD induction by ßNF was also enhanced by DMSO, while this agent had little effect on PROD induction by PB. Initial northern blot analyses showed a correlation between the mRNA levels and the observed EROD activity. Induction studies on the remaining enzymes are currently under way. Four different cytotoxicity assays were also performed on hepatocyte cultures treated with $CdCl_2$, and all yielded a similar EC_{50}. Taken together, the results suggest that these cells can potentially serve as a reliable in vitro hepatotoxicity test system.

D. Mechanisms

D1
TOPIC: GLUTATHIONE DEPLETION INCREASES THE CYTOTOXIC EFFECT OF FUMONISIN IN VITRO

Azuka Charles, G. D. Osweiler, D. L. Reynolds, M. Howard and Y. Niyo. Veterinary Diagnostic Laboratory, Veterinary Pathology and Veterinary Medical Research Institute, Iowa State University, Ames, Iowa 50011

A colorimetric assay employing tetrazolium salt (MTT) was used to evaluate the effect of glutathione (GSH) depletion on the cytotoxic response of four cultured cell-lines to Fumonisin (FB). The following cell lines were used: normal mouse liver (BNL), normal rat liver (CL2), rat lung (L2) and pig kidney (LL CPK$_1$). Cellular GSH was depleted by exposure of cells to Diethyl malate (DEM) (0.5 uM) for four hours, after which the cells were exposed to a solution containing FB. The cytotoxic response to FB was characterized in the normal and the GSH depleted cells by calculating the Lethal cytotoxic Dose for 50% of the cells (LCD$_{50}$). The LCD$_{50}$ for the normal cells were 1085, >2000, 280 and 1020 ug/ml for BNL, CL2, L2, and LLCPK$_1$, respectively. The values for GSH depleted cells were 95, 96, 78 and 155 ug/ml. Examination of treated cells by light microscopy revealed cytoplasmic vacuolation, cytoplasmic acidophilia, cell shrinkage, nuclear pyknosis and cell lysis. These results show that FB toxicity can be increased by GSH depletion and suggests that GSH is involved in the modulation of FB toxicity in cultured cells.

D2

Inhibition of protein synthesis in hepatocytes during hypoxia: an early cytotoxic event or an adaptative cellular response ?

V. Lefebvre(*), M. Van Steenbrugge, I. Goffin, M. Roberfroid and P. Buc-Calderon (Unité BCTC, UCL 739, Université Catholique de Louvain, 1200 Bruxelles, Belgium).

Many energy-dependent functions, such as biosynthetic activity or ionic homeostasis are modified when cells or tissues become hypoxic, thus leading in some cases to cellular death. However, it remains to be clarified which of the changes induced by hypoxia are or not related to cell death. By using isolated rat hepatocytes as experimental model, the biochemical effects of hypoxia were studied in cells incubated either in normoxia or in hypoxia. Our main findings are: 1) protein synthesis is totally and immediately stopped, while intracellular ATP content decreases progresively when cells are incubated in hypoxia; 2) hypoxic cells are more sensitive to H_2O_2-mediated injury; and 3) addition of fructose protects against hypoxic cell injury. Due to the rapidity of the changes in protein synthesis, it appears that cells respond to oxygen limitation rather than to ATP depletion. The rationale of such a mechanism is to lead cells in a state of "metabolic arrest", thus keeping ATP for more critical cellular functions. Such a hypothesis implies the existence of an "oxygen sensor" indicating cells whether to stop or to reinitiate their biosynthetic activities.

(*) V.Lefebvre is Research Assitant of the National Fund for Scientific Research (Belgium).

D3

Toxicity of formate in dissociated primary neural cultures: Dorman DC, Bolon B, Morgan KT, CIIT, RTP, NC, 27709. Formate is suggested as the toxic metabolite of methanol (MeOH) responsible for both blindness and metabolic acidosis. Tissue acidosis may have an important role in the development of neurotoxicity. For example, astrocytic alterations induced by lactic acid result from decreased extracellular pH rather than direct effects (Norenberg MD, et al., J Neuropath Exper Neurol 46: 154-166, 1987). Using a neural cell culture system, we determined that formate neurotoxicity is not induced by extracellular pH alterations. Primary, dispersed cerebrocortical cultures (1.7 X 10^6 cells/ml) containing both neuronal and glial elements were prepared from gestational day 15 fetal CD-1 mice. Cells were plated in Primaria® multiwells using Eagle's MEM supplemented with 10% heat inactivated horse serum, glutamine (2 mM), glucose (total 21 mM), and $NaHCO_3$ (26 mM), and then incubated at 37C in a humidified atmosphere (5% CO_2). Exposure of mature cultures (15-30 day-old) to formate was conducted for 8 hr at 37C using a 25mM Tris-buffered control salt solution of the following composition (mM): NaCl 120, $MgCl_2$ 0.8, $CaCl_2$ 1.8, KCl 5.4, and glucose 15. The effect of variable formate concentrations (0 - 240 mM) throughout a range of extracellular pH (pH 6.0 - 7.5, adjusted at 37C) on cytotoxicity, as determined by LDH and ^{14}C-adenine leakage, indicated that formate, unlike lactate, results in direct neurotoxicity (2 way ANOVA; $p \leq 0.05$). The approximate cytolethal dose50 of formate (pH = 7.2) was 60 mM. Less than 10% cytotoxicity was observed in control cultures (0 mM formate) between pH 6.3 and 7.5. Similar exposures with MeOH (0-8% v/v) revealed no change in MeOH-induced cytotoxicity after 1.5 h pretreatment with the formaldehyde (HCHO) scavenger, semicarbazide (10 mM), suggesting that HCHO does not play a role in neurotoxicity. This system may be used to examine mechanisms of neurotoxicity *in vitro*. Research supported in part by NRSA ES05558.

D4

MECHANISMS OF BUTYLATED HYDROXYTOLUENE HYDROPEROXIDE-STIMULATED TOXICITY AND CHANGES IN GENE EXPRESSION IN MOUSE EPIDERMAL CELL LINE PA.
K Z Guyton, L J Prestigiacomo, N E Davidson and T W Kensler. Division of Toxicological Sciences, Johns Hopkins School of Hygiene & Public Health, and Johns Hopkins Oncology Center, Baltimore, MD.

The food antioxidant butylated hydroxytoluene (BHT) has several known toxic and carcinogenic properties, including potency as a tumor promoter in a number of tissues initiated with diverse agents. The extensive metabolism of BHT and its secondary products may mediate these activities. The oxidative metabolite BHT hydroperoxide (BHTOOH) is a tumor promoter in mouse skin; a radical-derived quinone methide has been previously shown to mediate this activity *in vivo*. In order to explore its mechanisms of action, several effects of BHTOOH which are associated with promotion have now been characterized in an *in vitro* model system. BHTOOH enhances growth and induces genes critical to proliferation in keratinocyte cell line PA. At higher doses, BHTOOH is also toxic to keratinocytes; this toxicity may provide the basis for the differential effects of BHTOOH on a heterogeneous cell population *in vivo*. Initiated cells have developed phenotypic attributes which favor their survival and growth, such as elevated glutathione levels, which afford greater resistance to the toxic effects of tumor promoters such as BHTOOH. Thus, in addition to directly stimulating the target cells in skin, BHTOOH may also create a selective advantage for the initiated cell population *in vivo* through its toxic effects on normal keratinocytes. Taken together, these studies may lead to the elucidation of pathways for BHTOOH-stimulated alteration of gene expression as well as mechanisms for *in vivo* tumor promotion by BHTOOH.

D5

REGULATION OF CATALASE GENE EXPRESSION BY COPPER. P.J. Lapinskas, and V Culotta. Division of Toxicological Sciences. Department of Environmental Health Sciences, Johns Hopkins University, School of Public Health and Hygiene, Baltimore, MD 21205.

The mechanism of cellular copper toxicity is thought to involve the generation of hydroxyl radical ($\cdot$OH) via a cupric ion-catalyzed Fenton reaction. The production of $\cdot$OH is decreased by the combined action of three oxygen radical scavanging enzymes, namely superoxide dismutase (SOD), catalase (CAT) and glutathione peroxidase (GSHPO). In S. cerevisiae, the activity of all three enzymes is induced when cells are exposed to toxic Cu ions. Induction of SOD was recently found to occur at the level of gene expression and involves ACE1, the same "Cu-fist" transcription factor that regulates yeast metallothionein. By northern analysis, we have investigated whether catalase is regulated by Cu through a similar or novel mechanism. Expression of both the peroxisomal catalase (CAT A) and the cytosolic isoform (CAT T) was measured in wild type and mutant yeast cells defective for the ACE1 factor. Our data indicates that the CAT A gene is not regulated by copper. In contrast, CAT T mRNA levels are induced by copper and surprisingly, this induction is independent of the ACE1 factor, indicating a novel mechanism of Cu regulated gene expression. Recent studies using CAT T promoter/Lac Z fusion constructs demonstrate that Cu induction of CAT T occurs at the level of transcriptional initiation. The trans acting factor(s) and cis acting regulatory sequences involved in Cu regulation of CAT T are currently being investigated.

D6
IN VITRO STUDIES EXAMINING THE ROLE OF COPPER AND GLUTATHIONE IN HYDROQUINONE-INDUCED CYTOTOXICITY TO PRIMARY BONE MARROW STROMAL CELLS

Yunbo Li and Michael A. Trush

Division of Toxicological Sciences, The Johns Hopkins School of Hygiene and Public Health, Baltimore, MD

Hydroquinone (HQ) has been shown to induce cytotoxicity and dysfunction of bone marrow stromal cells both *in vivo* and *in vitro*. The further activation of HQ to electrophilic benzoquinone (BQ) by peroxidases in the bone marrow has been suggested to be critical for the induced cytotoxicity. In this study, we have investigated the roles of copper ions (Cu^{2+}) and glutathione (GSH) in HQ-induced cytotoxicity to primary bone marrow stromal cells from DBA/2 mice. In phosphate buffered saline (PBS), HQ undergoes autoxidation slowly to BQ, while the presence of Cu^{2+} (1, 2.5, 5, 10 µM) strongly accelerates the oxidation of HQ to BQ in a concentration-dependent manner. Reaction of HQ with Cu^{2+} also caused depletion of oxygen and the concomitant generation of H_2O_2. The oxidation of HQ in the presence of Cu^{2+} could be blocked by the Cu^+ specific chelator bathocuproine. Adding 10 µM Cu^{2+} to bone marrow stromal cell cultures significantly enhanced HQ-induced cytotoxicity. The enhanced cytotoxicity of HQ by Cu^{2+} could be prevented by adding GSH and dithiothreitol (DTT), while adding catalase to the cultures did not offer any protection.

Further investigation of the role of cellular GSH showed that treatment of the cells with 100 µM HQ in the absence of exogenous copper caused a significant depletion of cellular GSH, which preceded the loss of cell viability. In addition, pretreatment of the cells with the GSH synthesis inhibitor buthionine sulfoximine dramatically enhanced HQ-induced toxicity. Supplementing the cells with DTT or L-cysteine but not GSH significantly inhibited HQ-induced cytotoxicity. Interestingly, bathocuproine inhibited HQ-induced toxicity to stromal cells in the absence of extracellular Cu^{2+}, suggesting a possible role of intracellular copper in the activation of HQ to BQ. The above results indicate that Cu^{2+} may be a factor involved in the activation and toxicity of HQ and that GSH plays a role in preventing HQ-induced cytotoxicity.(Supported by ES03760, ES05131 and ES03819)

D7
ANALYSIS OF THE REACTIVE OXYGEN SPECIES (ROS) ASSOCIATED TO THE RESPIRATORY BURST OF PULMONARY ALVEOLAR MACROPHAGES (PAM) EXPOSED IN VITRO TO MAN-MADE FIBRES (MMF).

Denis Nadeau and Denis Lane, Laboratoire de Biochimie et de Toxicologie Pulmonaires, Département de Biologie, Faculté des Sciences, Université de Sherbrooke, Sherbrooke, Québec, Canada. J1K 2R1

One of the events implicated in the toxicity of many fibrous materials has been the induction of ROS from target cells. Since there is a growing concern about the relative safety of MMF, the purpose of this study was therefore to investigate the production of ROS by dust-challenged PAM, as measured by lucigenin- and luminol-amplified chemiluminescence. Rat PAM monolayers (2 x 10^5 cells) were exposed to three known cytotoxic dusts: two mineral MMF, namely JM100 glass fibres and the HSA grade of the aluminium silicate Fiberfrax®, and UICC crocidolite asbestos fibres. The luminescence with both amplifiers was recorded every five minutes for a total incubation period of five hours. Both MMF induced a massive lucigenin-amplified chemiluminescence (> 1000 mV·min.) when compared to the luminol-amplified chemiluminescence. Effectively, the ratio of the total chemiluminescences (luminol/lucigenin) was below 0.5 for both MMF tested at 50 and 250 µg of dust/ml. For the crocidolite-exposed cells, we observed a reversal of profile: the luminol-amplified chemiluminescence ($\approx$ 1000 mV·min.) was greater than the one detected in the presence of lucigenin (ratio luminol/lucigenin of $\approx$ 3 and $\approx$ 2 for 25 and 100µg of dust/ml, respectively). This study confirm that MMF can induce the production of ROS from PAM. Moreover, since the lucigenin-amplified chemiluminescence is believed to be quite specific for the detection of superoxide anions while the luminol-amplified chemiluminescence appears to be dependent on the presence of more than one type of ROS (e.g. hydrogen peroxide, hydroxyl radical, etc...), these results also suggest that differences in the nature and level of dust-induced cellular ROS could have some biological relevance (Supported by l'Institut de l'Amiante, Montréal, Québec, Canada).

E. Methods Development

E1

Evaluation of a Group of Petrochemicals Using Clonetics' NeutralRed Bioassay to Predict Irritancy. R. BARSTAD, J. Janus, J. Lauten, N. Accomando, A. Triana. Clonetics Corporation, 9620 Chesapeake Drive, San Diego, California 92123-1324

The normal human keratinocyte based NeutralRed Bioassay (NRB), adapted from the procedure of Borenfruend and Puerner, is one of several in vitro alternative cytotoxicity tests. We have previously demonstrated that this assay can predict the irritancy of several different classes of compounds (personal care products, shampoos, perfumes, insoluble talcs, alcohols, metal salts, burn ointments). The current study examines the irritation potential prediction capability of the NRB with a group of 52 petrochemicals for which Draize data were available (supplied by Mobil Oil Corporation). The water insoluble compounds were eluted overnight into Keratinocyte Growth Medium (KGM) before application to the cultured keratinocytes and testing in the NRB.

* The neutral red uptake (NRU) assay correctly identified (irritating or non-irritating) 48 of the 52 compounds.
* Three of the compounds were classified as irritating by NRU but had Draize scores in the non-irritating range (false positive).
* One compound was classified as non-irritating by NRU but had a Draize score in the irritating range (false negative).

Eight compounds, which were previously tested in the NRU, were tested in the neutral red release assay (NRR). Tested were three false positives, one false negative, three true positives, and one true negative.

* The three false positives were correctly identified as negative.
* The three true positives were correctly identified as positive.
* The true negative tested correctly as negative.
* The false negative tested incorrectly negative.

Further studies indicated the reason for the false negative was failure of the toxic constituent(s) to elute into KGM.

E2

Evaluating teratogen exposure utilizing hsp 27 cDNA. N. Bournias-Vardiabasis, Hopkins, K. California State University, San Bernardino, CA. and Boris Wang. Prenatal Diagnosis Center, Beverly Hills, CA.

A molecular based in vitro teratogen assay has been developed utilizing human chorionic villi cells and a heat shock-hsp 27-DNA probe. It has already been established in Drosophila embryonic cultures and in a number of mammalian systems, that exposure of embryonic cells to teratogens results in specific induction of a subset of heat shock proteins. In this project, we are investigating the induction of hsp 27 mRNA after teratogen exposure by dot blot hybridization analysis. The hsp 27 probe is biotinylated then total RNA isolated from chorionic villi cells is blotted onto nitrocellulose paper and probed with the biotinylated probe. The visualization of the mRNA-DNA hybrid is accomplished with standard SA-AP protocol. In preliminary trials, teratogen treated chorionic cells have been shown to express higher levels of hsp 27 mRNA while chorionic cells cultured in the presence of nonteratogen express low levels (similar to control cultures) of hsp 27 mRNA. It is hoped that successful development of this assay can eventually be applied at the clinical level and allow for the first time, the ability to assess teratogen exposure in the developing embryo. Such in vitro assay would certainly be welcomed as an alternative to animal testing and would be particularly helpful to pregnant women exposed to environmental contaminants at work, women who consume alcohol while pregnant and other at risk groups of women. Finally, this assay relies on a non-radioactive detection protocol which certainly makes it more attractive if it is ultimately used in a clinical setting. Supported in part by a CAAT grant to NBV.

E3

A NON-INVASIVE BIOTEST FOR OCCUPATIONAL EXPOSURE TO WEAK OR NON-MUTAGENIC TOXICANTS. M. J. W. Chang, M. T. Chou, and R. S. Lin. Chang Gung Medical College and National Taiwan University, TAIWAN, ROC

As a parallel to the Ames test used to monitor an exposure to mutagens, two CHO cytotoxicity assays, viability (%V) and colony formation efficiency (CFE), were evaluated as a potential non-invasive biotest to monitor exposure to weak or non- mutagens. Wistar rats were given either dimethylformamide (DMF) or aniline HCl (AH) intraperitoneally. 24-hour urine samples were collected for d0, d1, and d2 and kept at -30°C. Frozen urines were quickly thawed and centrifuged at 10,000 x g for 20 min to eliminate particulates. Urinary creatinine was determined and used for dose calculation. Data were expressed as % of saline control and evaluated against d0 by Student's t-test. It was found that (i) both DMF and AH had minimal toxicity on CHO cells, (ii) both tests could detect an exposure to DMF or AH at various dose levels, (iii) within a dose group, individual variation in metabolism was observed, and (iv) CFE was more sensitive as a biotest for exposure than %V, detecting an exposure to DMF at a dose as low as 1% LD50 (47.2 mg/kg) and AH, 12.5% LD50 (73 mg/kg). Based on these results, it is tentatively concluded that both tests have the potential to be a non-invasive biotest to monitor occupational exposure to weak or non- mutagenic toxicants. (Supported partially by a grant CMRP 279 and a project EPA/ROC 81-J204-09-09.)

E4

AN IN VITRO MODEL FOR STUDYING COCHLEAR TOXICITY. W.J. Clerici and L.D. Fechter. Division of Toxicological Sciences, The Johns Hopkins School of Hygiene and Public Health, Baltimore, MD.

The cochlea provides several cell types for the study of toxic injuy. These include receptor cells (inner hair cells), effector cells (outer hair cells), support cells (Deiter, Hensen, Claudius) as well as primary sensory neurons (spiral ganglion cells). Morphological, electrophysiological and motile properties have been studied in various cochlear cell types in response to parmacological manipulations and may present a model in which different cell types and their functions may be studied following toxic challenge. We have previously shown that trimethyltin (TMT) and triethyltin (TET) administered in vivo impair cochlear function acutely at the inner hair cell/spiral ganglion cell synapse, and subsequently at the outer hair cell. Outer hair cells are motile elements which influence stiffness of the cochlear partition, and, thereby, sensitivity to acoustic stimulation. In this study outer hair cells in primary culture were exposed to TMT or TET and the effect on cell length examined. Results showed that both TMT and TET produced dose dependent shortening of outer hair cells at concentrations between 30μM and 1mM, and appear equipotent in terms of this effect when given in vitro. This model may prove useful for studying the effects of toxic exposures that affect auditory function at the level of the cochlea. (Supported in part by NIH grants ES02852 and ES03819).

E5

AN *IN VITRO* ASSAY TO EVALUATE ALBUMIN BINDING OF TOXICANTS.
J M Frazier and S Dacosta, Division of Toxicological Sciences The Johns Hopkins University, Baltimore, MD. 21205

The *in vitro* toxicity of various toxicants is influenced by the presence of albumin in the culture medium. The observed effect is attributed to the binding of the toxicant to albumin, thus reducing the active concentration of the toxicant in the culture medium. Theoretically, this effect on *in vitro* toxicity can be used to evaluate the binding of a toxicant to albumin. The current study was designed to determine the binding affinity of cadmium to albumin. Hepatocytes were isolated from Fisher 344 rats by the two step procedure of Seglen and plated for 4h in 96 well micro titer plates coated with rat tail collagen. At t=0 hepatocytes are exposed to various concentrations of cadmium (0.1-1000 μM Cd) in the presence of 0-1000 μM bovine serum albumin (BSA) for 1 h. The plates were washed and fresh, cadmium-free media added. Hepatocytes were incubated for an additional 19 h and toxicity evaluated by a standard MTT assay. BSA concentrations greater than 3.1 μM significantly reduced cadmium toxicity. At the highest BSA level, the EC50 was shifted by more than two orders of magnitude. These data can be analyzed by assuming: (1) equal toxicity occurs at equal free cadmium concentrations, (2) there is one cadmium binding site on each BSA molecule, and (3) all reactions are simple mass action effects and reversible. Based on this data, the dissociation constant for the cadmium-BSA complex is 4.1 ± 1.2 μM. This method can be used to estimate the binding of other toxicants to albumin.

E6

Using Real-Time/Kinetic Viability Assays to Measure Acute Toxicity In-Vitro. John F. Hamberger, M.A., Jeanette Schepper Vaughan, M.A., and David A. Porter, Ph.D., Cell Biology Department, Bausch & Lomb, Rochester, NY 14692.

Many procedures used in measuring acute toxicity *in-vitro* are based upon endpoint analysis. These approaches do not readily account for the kinetics by which toxic effects may occur. The importance of a kinetic analysis is evident in an ocular environment in which toxic substances may be naturally and rapidly diluted to lower concentrations with reduced toxicity. Our laboratory determined the toxicity of various serially diluted alcohols *in-vitro* using real-time/kinetic viability assays. These assays utilize L929 mouse fibroblast suspensions or monolayers and test solutions preloaded with propidium iodide. After exposure to test solutions, fluorescence of dead cells was measured over time with a fluorescent spectrophotometer or fluorescent microwell plate reader and percent viability calculated. Preliminary results indicate that alcohols with higher molecular weights exhibited higher toxicity than lower molecular weight alcohols overall.

E7

IN VITRO DIFFERENTIATION USING BLASTOCYST-DERIVED EUPLOID EMBRYONAL STEM (E8) CELLS OF THE MOUSE: A NEW APPROACH TO IN VITRO TERATOGENESIS TESTING
G. Klein, A.Pöting and H. Spielmann
Federal Health Office (Bundesgesundheitsamt), ZEBET, Berlin, Germany

To develop a mammalian *in vitro* system for teratogenicity testing we used a pluripotent stem cell line. The cells can be maintained in an undifferentiated state buy cultivation on a feeder layer of embryonic fibroblasts. When cultured in suspension the cells spontaneously differentiate into complex organized embryoid bodies which resemble mouse early postimplantation embryos. After transfer to a normal tissue culture dish the embryoid bodies attach to the surface via outgrowths of previously formed endoderm cells. Continued culture of these aggregates gives rise to a variety of cell types e.g. muscle, nerve cartilage etc.
Culture conditions were established which allow a reproducible differentiation of ES cells. This was achieved by controlling the initial size of cell aggregates and by varying the composition of the culture medium and the time of cultivation in suspension,. The following steps of differentiation could be standardized: formation of spontaneously beating cardiac muscle, nerve and blood cells and in addition cartilage formation. Morphological and biochemical methods were used to define parameters of differentiation for each of the embryonic cells types. Established embryotoxic chemicals will be tested in ES cultures in order to validate this *in vitro* system for teratogenicity testing.

E8

A NOVEL CYTOTOXICITY SCREENING ASSAY USING A MULTI-WELL FLUORESCENCE SCANNER: CORRELATION WITH LDH RELEASE AND DRAIZE EYE SCORES. Anna-Liisa Nieminen, Pipsisewa Merrick, Robert A. Harper*, Gregory J. Gores, John M. Bond, Roberto Imberti, Brian Herman and John J. Lemasters. Department of Cell Biology & Anatomy, University of North Carolina, Chapel Hill, NC and *Division of Research and Development, Helene Curtis, Inc., Chicago, IL.

Each year, thousands of new chemical compounds are synthetized by the chemical and pharmaceutical industries which require screening for potential toxicity. To reduce the cost and animal usage of toxicity screening, an inexpensive and reliable *in vitro* cytotoxicity screening assay is needed. Here, we describe a new assay using a multi-well fluorescence scanner for screening cytotoxicity to cells cultured in 96-well microtiter plates. The assay is based on binding of propidium iodide (PI) to nuclei of cells whose plasma membranes have become permeable due to cell death. Increases of PI fluorescence measured with a multi-well fluorescence scanner were linearly proportional to the number of permeabilized cells and to release of lactate dehydrogenase into the culture medium. To validate the PI cytotoxicity assay with different cell types, cultured hepatocytes, neonatal cardiac myocytes and kidney cells were exposed to toxic chemicals. Kinetics of cell killing with each cell type were similar to nuclear staining with PI or trypan blue. Irritancy potential of 7 commercial shampoos was also evaluated in cultured human keratinocytes. The concentration of shampoos causing 50% loss of cell viability after 15 minutes (V_{50}) of incubation was determined by probit analysis. Log V_{50} measured in human keratinocytes showed a strong negative correlation (r=-0.95, p<0.001) with Draize eye scores in rabbits. In conclusion, a high capacity cytotoxicity screening assay was developed for cells cultured in 96-well microtiter plates. With this assay, cell viability was monitored continuously in a nondestructive manner in a variety of cell types after exposure to toxic chemicals. Moreover, the assay was highly predictive of Draize eye scores for surfactant-containing shampoos in human keratinocytes. Supported, in part, by a gift from Helene Curtis, J1433 from ONR and AG07218 from NIH.

E9

An *In Vitro* Model for Investigating the Effects of Xenobiotics on the Differentiation of Monocytic Cells

Stephen J. Rembish[1], Ruth W. Craig[2] and Michael A. Trush[1]

[1] Division of Toxicological Sciences, Johns Hopkins School of Hygiene and Public Health; Baltimore, MD
[2] Department of Physiology, Johns Hopkins School of Medicine; Baltimore, MD

The human myeloblastic leukemia cell line, ML-1, can be differentiated along the monocyte/macrophage pathway by treatment with 12-O-tetradecanoyl-phorbol-13-acetate (TPA) and therefore may be useful in examining the effects of xenobiotics on this process. When ML-1 cells are induced to differentiate they exhibit characteristics of monocyte-like cells including morphological changes, expression of the cell surface markers CD14 and CD11b, a decrease in myeloperoxidase content and an increase in NADPH oxidase activity. They also exhibit an increase in mitochondrial activity as shown by increased oxygen consumption, increased lucigenin-derived chemiluminescence (CL), a measure of mitochondrial superoxide anion production, and increased MTT reduction, which is a measure of Complex I (NADH dehydrogenase) activity. Since mitochondria are important to the function of mature macrophages, we studied the effects of a non-toxic dose of the antibiotic chloramphenicol (CAP) on differentiating ML-1 cells. CAP blocks mitochondrial protein synthesis while sparing cytoplasmic protein synthesis, resulting in incomplete formation of the electron transport chain due to the absence of the peptide subunits synthesized in the mitochondria. CAP treatment of TPA-differentiated ML-1 cells results in decreased mitochondrial function as measured by oxygen consumption, CL and MTT reduction, while surface markers and assays of cellular function that do not require mitochondrial protein synthesis are not affected. These results indicate that although the differentiation of ML-1 cells may appear to be normal, their function may be impaired due to incomplete development of the mitochondrial electron transport chain. We propose that this *in vitro* model may be useful in studying the effects of xenobiotics on myelopoietic stem cells which may lead to compromised monocytic cells and in turn an alteration in host defense mechanisms. (Supported by ES03760, ES03819, ES07141 and CA54385.)

E10

"SPECIFIC APPLICATIONS OF *IN VITRO* TECHNOLOGIES FOR PRODUCT DEVELOPMENT"

Paul M. Silber and Charles E. Ruegg
In Vitro Technologies, Inc. 5202 Westland Boulevard, Baltimore, MD 21227

A wide variety of *in vitro* models have been developed to predict the interactions of chemicals with biological systems. However, there is considerable confusion about how these methods should be integrated into industrial product safety and development programs. Thus, the purpose of this presentation is to address specific strategies for using *in vitro* technologies to achieve these goals. Specific applications for *in vitro* methodologies in the product development process include:

a. prescreening a large number of chemically related prototypes to predict safety and/or efficacy prior to conducting animal or human studies;

b. comparing drug metabolite profiles among different species *in vitro* (including humans) to aid in the rational selection of the most appropriate animal model for preclinical studies;

c. providing an efficient tool for evaluating product reformulations following the observation of toxicity during a preclinical or clinical study;

d. studying chemical interactions with human tissues *in vitro* to bridge the gap between preclinical and clinical studies;

e. significantly reducing the time, cost, and number of animals required for the product development process.

Together these strategies provide valuable tools for increasing product development efficiency and solving problems encountered in preclinical and clinical studies.

E11

Human Bronchial Cell Culture System. J. Stengel, J. Janus, J. Cortesi, M. Coleman, J. Reseau. Clonetics Corporation, 9620 Chesapeake Drive, San Diego, CA, 92123-1324

Clonetics Corporation, through an SBIR grant, has established a commercially available serum-free system, BronchialPack, for the culture of normal human bronchial epithelial cells (NHBE). BronchialPack contains viably cryopreserved or actively proliferating cells, optimized serum-free culture medium, and all of the reagents, instructions and support necessary for researchers to prepare subcultures in their laboratories. The lung, in particular the bronchial epithelium, is a major site for tumor formation. It is one of the first points of contact for airborne allergens or carcinogens and is therefore vulnerable to airborne diseases. In addition, the bronchial epithelium is seriously affected by respiratory diseases characterized by derangements in mucociliary clearance such as cystic fibrosis and asthma. In culture, serum has been shown to mask the effects that toxic compounds have on NHBE cells, and in fact inhibit the growth of NHBE cells by inducing terminal squamous differentiation. Considerable research has focused upon these cells as a model for the study of lung cancers. They are used as a model to study differentiation and proliferation and as a model to study *in vitro* transformation or *in vitro* transfection and the pathogenesis of human lung carcinomas.

BronchialPack was specifically designed as a flexible control/model system for the study of diseases of the human respiratory system. The product will also have applications as an *in vitro* model to study inhalants (such as mucolytic compounds) or toxins (such as tobacco products) on NHBE. It gives researchers the ability to easily study cell growth and differentiation at the cellular and molecular level, the efficacy of pharmaceutical agents and the cytotoxic effects of test agents.

F. Neurotoxicity

F1
MULTICENTRE INITIAL VALIDATION OF A TIERED SYSTEM FOR THE IN VITRO DETECTION OF NEUROTOXICITY.
C.K. Atterwill. Hatfield Polytechnic, Celltox Centre, Division of Biosciences, College Lane, Hatfield, Herts. AL10 9AB. United Kingdom

Many cell culture models are available for the in vitro assessment of neurotoxicity. We have been investigating the use of three culture types: neuroblastoma cell lines, primary cultures of rat and chick midbrain, and organotypic whole brain reaggregate cultures. A tiered system (Atterwill, 1989) has been proposed involving hierarchical testing through three layers of different neural complexities. This scheme is currently undergoing validation under the auspices of FRAME/EC using 40 test chemicals (including neurotoxicants plus non-neurotoxicants). Three different centres will be involved, and the trial is scheduled to be completed in mid 1993. To determine the performance and suitability of these culture models studies on selected neurotoxins have been performed:- ECMA, vincristine, aluminium, glutamate, MPTP and T_3-deprivation. Aspects of this work are described, including mechanistic investigations in rat brain reaggregate cultures. In vitro exposure of xenobiotics through a tiered testing system (ranging from simple cell-based assays measuring cytotoxicological parameters to more complex markers in organotypic cultures may permit detection of CNS neurotoxicity in both 'screening' and mechanistic contexts. The degree of simplicity, automaticity and transportability of the tests requires consideration as will the possibility of endpoints for specific classes of chemicals, e.g. cholinesterase for organophosphorus insecticides. Factors such as extrapolation from CNS to the PNS, metabolic activation, the blood-brain-barrier, degree of neural cell activation, repair mechanisms, and developing vs adult nervous systems will be considered.

F2

CYTOTOXIC EFFECTS OF ORGANOPHOSPHORUS ESTERS AND OTHER NEUROTOXIC CHEMICALS ON CULTURED CELLS
Amy C. Nostrandt, Teresa K. Rowles, and Marion Ehrich, Virginia-Maryland Regional College of Veterinary Medicine, Virginia Tech, Blacksburg, Virginia 24061-0442.

The capability of a neuronal cell line to respond to 5 neurotoxic chemicals was assessed by using alterations in viability, morphology, acetylcholinesterase (AChE) activity, and free intracellular calcium ion concentration ($[Ca^{2+}]_i$) as indices of cytotoxicity. Differentiated SY-5Y cells were used as the test system for examination of these effects, as they were particularly useful for the study of early effects of a neuropathy-inducing organophosphate (OP), mipafox. Other compounds studied for their cytotoxic effects in SY-5Y cells were: paraoxon, another organophosphorus ester; aldicarb, a carbamate; ß, ß'-iminodipropionitrile (IDPN), a compound which induces a peripheral neuropathy; and carbachol, a cholinergic agonist. Results indicated that acetylcholinesterase inhibition was the most sensitive indicator of neurotoxicity of the OPs and the carbamate. Inhibition of AChE was observed within 10 minutes of toxicant exposure and at concentrations of these compounds that did not affect viability at 24 hours, and at concentrations which did not affect morphology or $[Ca^{2+}]_i$ until days later. For compounds that did not have as notable an effect on AChE (IDPN and carbachol), continuous exposures over several days were needed before cytotoxic effects were noted. These results indicate that toxic effects of esterase inhibitors may be more easily detected in the differentiated SY-5Y cell culture system than toxic effects of other chemicals.

F3

ACRYLAMIDE TOXICITY STUDIED IN CULTURE NEUROBLASTOMA CELLS
Lena Odland, Lennart Romert*, Cecilia Clemédson and Erik Walum, Dep. of Neurochemistry and Neurotoxicology, * Dep.of Genetic and Cellular Toxicology, Stockholm University, S-106 91 STOCKHOLM, Sweden.

Acrylamide is a well-known neurotoxic compound that produces central and periferal distal axonopathy. Degenerative changes of this type can be induced in the neuroblastoma cell line C 1300, clone NlE 115 and has been extensively studied in our laboratory specially regarding acrylamide interference with the cellular metabolism. In this study we continue to elucidate the mechanism of acrylamide induced neurite degeneration in N1E 115 cells.

Acrylamide concentrations were chosen not to be cytotoxic but merely cause an inceasingly severe neurite degeneration. The rate of protein synthesis was decreased in a concentration dependent manner in response to acrylamide exposure (0,1-2,5 mM). Detoxification of acrylamide in vivo occurs mainly through conjugation with glutathione catalysed by glutathione-S-transferases. Cells grown in presence of acrylamide showed a concentration dependent decrease in glutathione content. In the highest acrylamide concentration tested this was compained with an increased glutathione-S-transferase activity. Despite the reduced level of glutathione and a possible impaired protection of the plasma membrane to oxidativ stress no elevated level of lipidperoxidation could be registered in acrylamide treated cells.

The parameters measured in this study represents basal cell functions. Acrylamide may thus cause axonopathy through interference with such functions of special importance for maintenance of the axonal structure and function.

F4

EARLY MORPHOLOGIC CHANGES IN SH-SY5Y NEUROBLASTOMA CELLS AFTER EXPOSURE TO A NEUROPATHY-INDUCING ORGANOPHOSPHORUS COMPOUND, MIPAFOX
Delana Taylor, Teresa K. Rowles[*], Amy C. Nostrandt, and Marion Ehrich, Virginia-Maryland Regional College of Veterinary Medicine, Virginia Tech, Blacksburg, Virginia 24061, *Department of Animal Science, University of Tennessee, Knoxville, Tennessee 37901.

We are developing an in vitro model for organophosphorus toxicity testing using SH-SY5Y human neuroblastoma cells. Certain organophosphorus compounds are neurotoxic as they have the capacity to inhibit activity of acetylcholinesterase and/or induce a delayed neuropathy. In vivo, organophosphorus induced delayed neuropathy, (OPIDN), is preceded by inhibition of neurotoxic esterase activity. Biochemical studies indicate that neurotoxic esterase activity of SH-SY5Y cells can be inhibited by mipafox. To enhance the validity of an in vitro model for delayed neuropathy, morphologic changes were evaluated after exposure to several organophosphorus compounds, including mipafox.

Cultures of SH-SY5Y cells were exposed to a $5 \times 10^{(-5)}$M concentration of mipafox. Time lapse videomicroscopy was used to record changes from 0-12 hours post-treatment. Immediately after addition of mipafox to the media, cells exhibited unusual blebbing activity in cytoplasmic membranes and the degree of intracellular motion was greater than in controls. Light microscopic changes at 24 hours post-treatment included variations in staining intensity and swollen cell bodies with vacuolated cytoplasm. These changes did not occur in stained controls.

These studies on intact cells indicate early neurotoxic damage to cell membranes previously undetected in experiments describing the action of mipafox.

F5

A MULTIPLE CELL-CULTURE TOXICITY TEST SCHEME FOR THE IDENTIFICATION OF NEUROTOXIC COMPOUNDS
Erik Walum, Department of Neurochemistry and Neurotoxicology, Stockholm University, S-106 91 STOCKHOLM, Sweden

Several in vitro neurotoxicity test procedures have been developed. However, very few test batteries have been proposed. Such test schemes must most likely be hierarchical and multioptional in order to be able to cope with the large number of possible mechanisms of neurotoxicity. Although the regenerative capacity of the nervous system is low, lesions can be compensated for by a number of dynamic functions. Therefore, cellular tests included in primary screens of a multiple system should be based on determinations of cell physiological parameters rather than on measurements of single biochemical reactions. A general purpose neurotoxicity test system has been described by Walum et al (1990, ATLA 18, 153-179). It has now been modified and further developed. First basal cytotoxicity is determined in a human neuroblastoma cell line. In a second step, differential cytotoxicity is assayed in highly developed primary cultures of neuronal and non-neuronal cells. In order to find out if the compound is likely to produce axonopathy a test procedure in mouse neuroblastoma cells is carried out. Toxicokinetic information is obtained from hepatocyte/target cell and endothelial cell/astrocyte co-cultures. To disclose alterations in cell physiology, studies of cell respiration, membrane permeability and calcium homeostasis is suggested. When information from these test-steps is taken into consideration together with available data on in vivo toxicity, toxicokinetics and physical/chemical data one may find it necessary to proceed to more neuronal specific determinations or mechanistically oriented studies.

F6

An *in vitro* model of drug neurotoxicity in the developing nervous system.
Arthur D. Weissman and Benjamin L. Crenshaw, Neuroscience Branch, Addiction Research Center, NIDA, P.O. Box 5180, Baltimore, MD 21224.

Amphetamine-like drugs exert a profound effect on monoamine systems in the brains of mature animals. These changes generally appear as deficits in neurochemical function (e.g. neurotransmitter uptake) that relate in part to the neurotoxicity of these drugs. *In utero*, these drug effects may be quite different rom that observed in the adult animal due to their interaction with an immature central nervous system. *In vivo*, prenatal amphetamines cause alterations in monoamine levels and uptake that persist into adulthood. These effects can be modeled in neuronal cell cultures and perhaps provide a means to study the mechanisms of drug actions on the central nervous system. NG108-15 neuroblastomaglioma cells were exposed *in vitro* for various lengths of time and to drug concentrations of 10^{-9} to 10^{-3} M. Cultures were studied by both light microscopy using trypan blue exclusion and [^{3}H] thymidine uptake for evidence of altered growth patterns. The pharmacology of drug action was also characterized in these cells, using radiolabeled drugs and competition with specific monoamines. Specific dose-related inhibition of cell division was seen with most of the substituted amphetamines and this effect, in general, peaked at eight hours after exposure. This inhibition was still evident at four days with drugs which we observed in our previous studies to be the most toxic, such as imipramine and fenfluramine. Serotonin and some of the amphetamine compounds appeared to paradoxically stimulate growth at lower doses. *In vivo*, the impact from prenatal amphetamine is most profound on the serotonin system and may either stimulate neuronal growth or produce neurotoxicity, depending on the level of exposure. This *in utero* drug treatment effect may be a function of the plasticity and compensatory responses of the developing nervous system. This effect may be reflected in cultures where neuronal cells respond differentially to a low or high dose of amphetamine-like compounds.

G. Ocular Toxicity

G1

Evaluation of Two In Vitro Methods As Predictors of Ocular Irritation of Shampoo Formulations. Lauren Bernhofer, Chandni Juneja and Charles W. Stott. JOHNSON & JOHNSON Consumer Products, Inc., Skillman, New Jersey.

Two cytotoxicity assays were evaluated with respect to their ability to distinguish between the ocular irritation potentials of seventeen mild shampoo prototypes which had been previously evaluated by the rabbit eye test. The two procedures were the agar overlay test using L929 cells and the protein inhibition assay with primary normal human epidermal keratinocytes. In the former, the test formulations were applied full strength in paper discs to the agar surface for 24hr. The radius of the zone of lysis was the parameter used for comparison. In the latter, NHEK cells were incubated with dilutions of the test formulations in culture media for 24hr. Total cell protein was determined, using the Bradford dye reagent and used to calculate the median inhibitory concentration, the EC_{50}. Comparison of the results of each of these two test methods with the in vivo data showed poor correlation for either method. These cytotoxicity methods were not capable of predicting the corneal responses to repeated application of mild shampoo formulations.

G2

SURFACTANTS TOXICITY DETERMINED IN VITRO BY SILICON MICROPHYSIOMETER

Catroux P.*, Eber A.C.*, Panfili P.**, Dossou K.G.*, Rougier A.*, Humphries G.**, Cottin M.*

L'OREAL Basic Research Center*, Aulnay sous Bois, France and MDC**, Menlo Park, USA

Monitoring the physiological state of cultured cells with the Silicon Microphysiometer has been suggested to provide a better endpoint to evaluate the ocular irritancy potential in vitro.

Present study was undertaken to determine the effects of 19 surfactants and 17 water-soluble surfactant based formulations (shampoos, lotions) with well-known in vivo irritancy data.

Fibroblast like cells (L929) were cultured on Transwell membrane in a low-buffered medium. After their basal acidification rate has been determined, cells were subjected to a single dose or successive increasing concentrations of products.

The MRD 50 (concentration of product that decreases the metabolic rate by 50%) was extrapoled and compared with the in vivo maximal average score (MAS).

The chief results of this study show a strong correlation between MAS and MRD 50, more particularly with the raw materials ($r=0.89$, $p < 10^{-6}$). Thus, they provide supports to consider Silicon Microphysiometer as an interesting method for the study of the eye irritancy potential of these products.

G3

EVALUATION OF THE EYTEX SYSTEM FOR USE AS A PREDICTOR OF OCULAR IRRITANCY OF SHAMPOOS

D. Decker and R. Harper
Helene Curtis Inc., Chicago, IL 60639

ABSTRACT: The Eytex in vitro assay was used to evaluate 42 adult and baby shampoos. The assay, which is based on protein denaturation and/or precipitation, was chosen because it provides rapid, quantitative results at a relatively low cost. The protein reagent is a highly ordered macromolecular matrix which contains an active oligomeric protein as well as other small proteins. In response to irritants the conformation of the active protein changes as a result of its molecules binding with the other protein components. The adult shampoos in this study are composed mainly of alkyl sulfate surfactants (ethoxylated and non ethoxylated). The baby shampoo's primary components are branched chain ethoxylated alkyl as well as amphoteric surfactants. All shampoos were diluted 1:10 in deionized water and tested with two different protocols; the rapid membrane assay (RMA) protocol for the adult products and the high sensitivity assay (HSA) for the baby shampoos. All samples were tested in two, and in some cases, three separate experiments and the qualified Eytex scores were averaged. The correlation of the Draize scores to the Eytex scores was statistically significant ($r^2=0.90$). The Eytex scores were used to establish irritation classes similar to the standard Draize classification scheme (minimal, mild, moderate, severe). When the Draize eye irritation class was compared to the Eytex irritation class for a given shampoo, the correlation for the baby shampoo data was 100% and 87% for the adult shampoo data. While the Eytex data does not relate to data obtained with the Draize method concerning wash out and recovery, the Eytex in vitro assay for ocular irritancy is highly predictive of the maximum 24 hr. Draize eye scores for the shampoos examined in this study.

G4

A 10-COMPANY COLLABORATIVE EVALUATION OF ALTERNATIVES TO THE EYE IRRITATION TEST USING CHEMICAL INTERMEDIATES, D.M. GALER (WARNER-LAMBERT CO.), R. CURREN (MICROBIOLOGICAL ASSOCIATES, INC.), S.C. GAD (G.D. SEARLE & CO.), P. GAUTHERON (MERCK SHARP & DOHME CHIBRET RESEARCH CTR.), B. LEONG (THE UPJOHN COMPANY), K. MILLER (MICROBIOLOGICAL ASSOCIATES, INC.), E. SARGENT (MERCK & CO.), P.V. SHAH (HOFFMANN-LAROCHE), J. SINA (MERCK SHARP & DOHME), R.G. SUSSMAN (WARNER-LAMBERT CO.)

Programs for the evaluation of in vitro alternatives to the eye irritation test have most often focused on series of structurally or functionally related compounds. These studies have generally been used to correlate ranking of irritation in the alternative systems to ranking of irritation potential in vivo. It is not yet possible to use the available tests to categorize the irritation potential of individual compounds without regard to chemical class. Ten (10) companies participated in a collaborative study to evaluate currently available alternative models with a set of generally unrelated compounds. The following tests were selected for evaluation: the Bovine Corneal Opacity/Permeability (BCOP), EYTEX™ (Ropak Laboratories), Neutral Red Uptake Bioassay in Normal Human Epidermal Keratinocytes (Clonetics Corporation), MTT Assay using TESTSKIN Living Dermal Equivalent (Organogenesis Inc.), Microtox Bioassay (Microbics Corp.) and the Chorioallantoic Membrane Vascular Assay (CAM-VA), as well as a computer-based structure-activity-relationship model (TOPKAT, Health Designs, Inc.). Compounds were selected using specific criteria for previously determined in vivo irritation potential, pH and solubility. Each company selected 1-6 test compounds from among synthetic intermediates isolated during the manufacture of pharmaceutical and chemical products. To assure technical consistency and evaluation, all tests were conducted at a single location (Merck Sharp and Dohme Laboratories in France for the BCOP test and Microbiological Associates, Inc. for the remaining tests) using coded samples. The results were pooled and analyzed relative to physical properties and in vivo activity. Among the assays evakuated, the BCOP test showed the most promise in predicting irritation class of the test compounds. The CAM-VA test and SAR analysis using TOPKAT may have application in predicting non-irritant, subject to some limitation. Results indicate that while it may not be possible to use any single alternative test, a battery of complementary tests may be used to classify the eye irritation potential of compounds. Alternative tests may be useful in setting priorities for and reducing the number of in vivo irritation tests conducted.

G5

CHARACTERIZATION AND EVALUATION OF AN ORDERED MACROMOLECULAR MATRIX TO BE USED TO PREDICT *IN VIVO* OCULAR IRRITATION

V. C. Gordon, InVitro International, 16632 Milliken Avenue, Irvine, California 92714

Mechanisms of ocular toxicity can include macromolecular events such as membrane perturbation, protein dehydration, protein alteration, the EYTEX® and protein denaturation. A transparent, highly ordered macromolecular matrix, was developed which could be studied spectrophotometrically when exposed to chemical irritants. The macromolecular matrix consists primarily of an oligomeric protein with a molar mass of approximately 300,000/mol, characterized by SDS gel electrophoresis and ultracentrifugation. The protein is incorporated into a matrix which can produce a hardened gel network on heating. The spectrophotometric assay determines quantitatively alterations on an ordered macromolecular matrix which contribute to the turbidity. Turbidity can serve as a sensitive indicator of alterations in the state of hydration and conformation of an ordered macromolecular matrix. Optical density changes are standardized with calibrators and controls. A score and classification is obtained when undiluted test samples are studied which compares to the *in vivo* Draize scores and classifications. Parallel responses between quantitated changes in the ordered macromolecular matrix and *in vivo* Draize scores for surfactants, solvents, salts, preservatives, and acids and bases were demonstrated. Evaluations of alterations in the order, spatial conformation, and hydration of this matrix can be used to screen test samples for their potential for ocular irritation.

G6

Title: **Application of the Computer Automated Structure Evaluation for Toxicology (CaseTox) methodology to the *in vitro* assessment of the eye irritation potential of chemicals, chemical mixtures and polymers.**

Gilles Klopman*, Dmitri Ptchelintsev*, Manton Frierson**, Stephen Pennisi^, Kevin Renskers^, Michael Dickenson^.

The Computer Automated Structure Evaluation for Toxicology (CaseTox) program has been applied to the semi-quantitative analysis of the eye-irritating ability of 186 organic chemicals. The results indicate that the following structural units are linked to the eye irritating effects: carboxylic and sulfonic groups in anionic sufactants, phenolic moieties in non-ionic surfactants, amino groups, halogenated and unsaturated structures, anhydride, and epoxide functionalities. Ester groups have been recongnized as having a low irritation potential. The CaseTox model based on these structural descriptors was successfully used for an *a priori* prediction of the eye irritating propensity of 1.) 21 individual chemicals, 2.) chemical mixtures such as, coconut oil, hydrogenated castor oil, rice bran and eucalyptus oils, potassium alginate, 3.) polymers including polyvinyl alcohols, polyvinyl butyral, polyvinyl pyrrolidone, corn starch and nylon. It was found that the structure of the repeat units, and not that of the monomers, can be used to predict the eye irritating properties of the corresponding polymers. Effects of the terminal groups are negligible.

The CaseTox eye irritation model can be used for 1.) *in vitro* presreening in eye irritation testing and 2.) design and modification of chemicals when low eye irritation potential is important.

*   Case Western Reserve University, Cleveland, OH 44106
** Biofor, Ltd., Waverly, PA 18471
^   Avon Products, Inc., Suffern, NY 10901

G7

USE OF FOUR *IN VITRO* ASSAYS TO EVALUATE THE OCULAR IRRITATION POTENTIAL OF HAIR CARE PRODUCTS. Lesile K. Lake*, Thomas J. Stephens, Ph.D.†, and E. Tiffany Spence†, *S.C. Johnson & Son, Inc., Racine WI and †Thomas J. Stephens & Associates, Inc., Carrollton, TX.

Eight hair care formulations were tested in a battery of four *in vitro* assays. The endpoints evaluated were: 1) cytotoxicity (MTT conversion) and 2) inflammation potential (PGE_2 release) from a reconstituted human dermal model, 3) vascular reactions in CAMVA, and 4) reduction of light emission in the Microtox™ Luminescent Bacteria Test. The purpose of the program was to evaluate whether these assays could correctly predict the ocular irritation potential of these surfactant systems. The test materials consisted of an antidandruff shampoo, two baby shampoos, one regular shampoo, and four shampoo/conditioner combinations. Analyses with Draize ocular data using Cooper's Criteria showed that all four assays were effective in classifying test materials as irritants or non-irritants.

G8

AN IN VITRO METHOD TO FORMULATE LOW ADVERSE EFFECTS SHAMPOOS.
Marina Marinovich, Barbara Viviani and Corrado Lodovico Galli
Research Center on Cosmetic Toxicology, University of Milan, Via Balzaretti 9, 20133 Milan, Italy

Shampoos and their ingredients, surfactants, were studied both *in vivo* (Draize eye test) and *in vitro*, using a murine epidermal cell line (HEL 30). The lactate dehydrogenase (LDH) leakage in cell medium, the inhibition of protein synthesis and the reduction of cell protein content were evaluated as markers of cytotoxicity. The cells were exposed for two hours to the material under treatment dissolved in the medium at concentrations of 0.05 to 0.5% (shampoos) or 1 to 1000 ug/ml (surfactants).

LDH leakage and the protein synthesis inhibition are the most sensitive parameters and the effective doses 50 (EC_{60} and IC_{60}) in producing the maximal effect have been used to rank both the shampoos and the surfactants from the most to the least cytotoxic.

A rank correlation has been observed between the *in vitro* toxicity and the eye irritation demonstrated for the same surfactants in the Draize test of $r=0.657$ when the LDH leakage was used and $r=0.524$ for the inhibition of the protein synthesis. This value drastically improved ($r=0.928$ LDH/Draize; $r=1$ protein synthesis inhibitio/Draize) when the anionic surfactants were not considered.

For what concerns the shampoos, the potency order in affecting the protein synthesis has been compared respectively to the surfactants total content ($r=0.768$) to those of non ionic ($r=0.809$) or amphoteric ($r=-0.724$) and to the Draize test ($r=0.607$). In the *in vivo/in vitro* comparison the parameter relative to the LDH leakage appears definitely preferable ($r=0.857$). The results obtained suggest the toxic (irritant) potential of raw materials and final product is predictable through an *in vitro* test; furthermore this model allows the quantitative evaluation of the effect and the influence of the single components on the final toxicity of a mixture.

Acknowledgements: this study was partially supported by a National Research Council project "Chimica Fine e Secondaria II"

G9

The Trans-Epithelial Permeability Assay As An In Vitro Assay For Predicting Ocular Irritation of Surfactant Formulations. K. M. Martin and C. W. Stott. JOHNSON & JOHNSON Consumer Products, Inc., Skillman, N.J. 08558

The trans-epithelial permeability assay has been evaluated as a model to predict the ocular irritation potential of surfactant based formulations. The corneal epithelium forms a relatively impermeable barrier to aqueous solutions. Monolayers of Mandin-Darby canine kidney cells on microporous filters, due to the presence of tight junctions, simulate the surface of the cornea. Changes in the permeability to sodium fluorescein following a 15min. exposure to dilutions of the formulations were used to calculate EC_{50}s for 28 products. These were compared with corneal reactions from prior rabbit eye test results and gave a correlation coefficient of 0.77. By the selection of an EC_{50} of 2% as the cutoff, products could be classified as slight to moderate (negative) or moderate to severe (positive). Based on this, the assay had a sensitivity of 0.87, a specificity of 1.00, a positive predictive value of 1.00 and a negative predictive value of 0.87.

G10
A TOXICITY EVALUATION BY THE MICROTOX® ASSAY OF TWENTY SURFACTANT-CONTAINING PRODUCTS AND THEIR CONSTITUENT SURFACTANTS AND PRESERVATIVES.
Karen A. Miller[1], Richard W. Stahl[1], Frank S. Marchesani[1], John W. Harbell[1], Kathleen A. Wallace[1], Francis H. Kruszewski[2], Kevin J. Renskers[2] and Rodger D. Curren[1]. [1]Microbiological Associates, Inc, Bethesda, Maryland; [2]Avon Products Inc., Suffern, New York.

The Microtox® Assay (Microbics Corporation, Carlsbad, CA) estimates toxicity by measuring changes in the light output of luminescent bacteria after exposure to a potentially toxic material. This assay has been previously reported to be predictive of ocular irritation for some surfactant-containing materials. We used the Microtox® assay to assess the toxicity of 20 cosmetic products (provided by Avon) which contained 4 - 40% surfactants. The individual constituent surfactants (29) and preservatives (9) were also tested.

Exposures and light measurements were made according to standard published procedures. Dilutions of the test materials were made in a high salt buffer (the bacteria are marine organisms) and incubated with the bacteria in a temperature controlled photometer. Measurements of light output were made immediately before the exposure and 5 minutes later. A ratio of light intensity pre- and post-exposure was plotted against the concentration of test material, and the EC_{50} - the amount of test material required to reduce light output by 50% - was calculated. We then compared Draize scores (24 Hr; Avon historical data) to the EC_{50} for each test material. In general, the Microtox assay was able to correctly predict the toxicity of the surfactant-containing products at either end of the Draize score scale, i.e. very mild or very irritating materials. It was not very predictive for those products with ocular irritation scores between 5 and 20. Slightly better estimations were found using the individual surfactants. The preservatives were the least well predicted with both over estimations and under estimations of irritancy. In some cases the irritation potential of the surfactant-containing products could be estimated by observing the toxicities of the individual component surfactants.

G11
CYTOTOXICITY OF BENZALKONIUM CHLORIDE (BAK) IS DEPENDENT ON THE ALKYL CHAIN LENGTH OF THE HOMOLOGS

Roger M. Oda, Ava Hayashi, Shawn Hickok and Steve Matsumoto
Allergan Inc., Irvine CA

Benzalkonium chloride (BAK) is a preservative that is commonly used in ophthalmic formulations. Commercial preparations are composed of a mixture of alkylbenzyldimethylammonium chlorides with alkyl chains ranging from eight to eighteen carbons in length. Pure homologs are available with even chain lengths of C_{12} to C_{18}. We used the CHO clonal assay to establish a possible relationship between the chain length and the cytotoxicity. This in-vitro assay measures irreversible changes in the growth or reproduction of chinese hamster ovary cells. The four homologs exhibited significant differences in their dose response curves. C_{12} was found to be least cytotoxic of the compounds tested. C_{18} and C_{14} were found to elicit an intermediate response. C_{16} was the most cytotoxic of the four chain lengths tested. Rank order comparisons of the homologs from least to most cytotoxic shows that:

$$C_{12} < C_{18} < C_{14} < C_{16}$$

The mean IC_{50} values for these four compounds were determined to be 5.78, 1.47, 1.25 and 0.89 ppm respectively. The results of these experiments clearly demonstrate that the cytotoxicity of the homolog is dependent on the length of the alkyl chain. Increasing or decreasing the length of the alkyl chain from sixteen carbons resulted in a corresponding decrease in the cytotoxicity. Comparisons of the single chain length compounds to two commercial BAK preparations suggests that the effect of the individual homologs is additive.

G12

DEVELOPMENT OF AN *IN VITRO* ASSAY FOR OCULAR IRRITANCY ASSESSMENTS OF AQUEOUS INCOMPATIBLE SUBSTANCES. Rosemarie Osborne, Mary A. Perkins, Deirdre A. Roberts and Leon H. Bruner. The Procter & Gamble Company, Human & Environmental Safety Division, Miami Valley Laboratories, Cincinnati, Ohio 45239-8707.

In order to address the need to reduce or replace the use of rabbits for prediction of human eye irritancy potential, we developed a new method utilizing a tissue equivalent approach. Currently available submerged cultures have limitations due to the aqueous buffered medium used for test material dilution. We have previously shown that these models are limited in their ability to predict irritancy potential for aqueous incompatible materials, certain product formulations, and acids/bases. To overcome these limitations, we developed a unique protocol utilizing Advanced Tissue Sciences Skin^2 cultures for topical application of neat (undiluted) test materials as an alternative model for eye irritancy testing. Skin^2 cultures are similar histologically to cornea. Methods were developed for topical application and removal of neat test materials for acute damage evaluations. Materials tested in this model included a wide array of product formulation types, including liquids, gels, creams, foams, pastes, solids, powders and granulars. Altered cell viability (MTT assay) was measured, representing a common pathway of corneal response to diverse chemicals and surfactant containing products. Results indicate that, with this protocol, eye irritancy potential in this *in vitro* model correlates well with the *in vivo* irritancy of the materials tested. We believe that this tissue equivalent *in vitro* assay will be a valuable method for predicting the ocular irritancy of solids, powders and other aqueous incompatible substances.

G13

The Chicken Enucleated-Eye-Test (CEET) as an alternative to the Draize Eye Test
M.K. Prinsen, H.B.W.M. Koëter, TNO Toxicology and Nutrition Institute, P.O. Box 360, 3700 AJ Zeist, the Netherlands, fax + 31 3404 57224.
In the past, the enucleated eye test method (EET) has been recognized as a valuable alternative to the Draize test, because it represents a test system nearest to the *in vivo* test and showed the best correlation with the *in vivo* test in a comparative study sponsored by the CEC[1]. In this *ex vivo* bioassay, three parameters are measured to detect possible adverse eye effects, namely corneal swelling, corneal opacity, and fluorescein retention. The measurement of corneal swelling in this assay guarantees an objective and discriminative parameter, this in contrast with the conventional rabbit test, which uses subjective, gross observations only. In combination with the measurement of corneal opacity and fluorescein retention, a reliable evaluation of the eye irritation potential of test materials is achieved. However, despite all these advantages, the main argument against its acceptance has always been that laboratory animals were still necessary as eye-donors. Therefore, in the present study, the use of various species of slaughter animals as possible eye-donor for the EET was examined. On the basis of this study, the **chicken** appeared to be the most practicable: no special provisions are necessary for collecting and transporting the eyes, and obtaining sufficient numbers of eyes with corneas suitable for testing did never pose any problem. Processing of chicken eyes with the standard apparatus used for this kind of testing could be done without major modifications. Twenty-one reference compounds, ranging from non-irritant to severe irritant, and previously tested in an CEC-validation study on alternative test methods for eye irritation testing[1] were examined in the CEET. When compared to the *in vivo* EC-classification, the CEET correctly classified all 21 compounds. Therefore, it was concluded that this *ex vivo* test system is highly accurate in the assessment of eye irritation potential of test materials without the use of live animals. Since in the latest update of the relevant OECD and EC guidelines the use of alternative *ex vivo/in vitro* test systems for prescreening and positive identification of eye irritants is recommended, the use of the CEET can make a valuable contribution to this intention. In order to allow this test also for the identification of non-irritants in case of a negative result in the CEET, it is recommended to additionally use a single animal test (OECD guideline no. 405) to confirm non-irritancy of test materials. By this approach, animal suffering and animal use is reduced to a minimum, and a vast amount of *in vivo* and *ex vivo* data on non-irritant materials will become available, allowing further international validation of this alternative test system.

[1] Commission of the European Communities (1991), Collaborative study on the evaluation of alternative methods to the eye irritation test. EC Document XI/632/91, V/E/1/131/91.

G14

Title: **The Computer Automated Structure Evaluation for Toxicology (CaseTox) methodology as an *in vitro* assessment of the eye irritation potential.**

Dmitri Ptchelintsev*, Manton Frierson**, Stephen Pennisi^, Kevin Renskers^, Michael Dickens^, Gilles Klopman*

The Computer Automated Structure Evaluation for Toxicology (CaseTox) program has been applied to the semi-quantitative analysis of the eye irritation potential of 186 organic chemicals. The results indicate that the following structural units are linked to the eye irritation potential: carboxylic and sulfonic acid groups in anionic sufactants, phenolic moieties in non-ionic surfactants, amino groups, halogenated and unsaturated structures, anhydrides, and epoxide functionalities. Ester groups have been recognized as having a low irritation potential. The CaseTox model based on these structural descriptors was successfully used for an *a priori* prediction of the eye irritation potential of 1.) 21 individual chemicals, 2.) chemical mixtures such as coconut oil, hydrogenated castor oil, rice bran and eucalyptus oils, potassium alginate, and 3.) polymers, including polyvinyl alcohols, polyvinyl butyral, polyvinyl pyrrolidone, corn starch and nylon. It was found that the structure of the repeating units together, and not that of the individual monomers, can be used to predict the eye irritation potential of the corresponding polymers. It appears as if the repeating units of polymers dilute out the irritation potential of terminal groups normally expected to contribute significant irritation potential to chemicals of lower molecular weight.

The CaseTox eye irritation model can be used for 1.) *in vitro* presreening for eye irritation potential, and 2.) design and modification of chemicals when low eye irritation potential is important.

*   Case Western Reserve University, Cleveland, OH 44106
** Biofor Ltd., Waverly, PA 18471
^   Avon Products Inc., Suffern, NY 10901

G15

The use of a Three-Dimensional Skin Model for Predicting Ocular Irritancy.

Barry Reece and Michael Rozen. Mary Kay Cosmetics, Inc. Dallas, Tx. 75247.

Fifteen surfactants, representing a broad range of ocular irritancy potentials, were evaluated for effects upon viability using a fibroblast dermal equivalency model. Coded samples were exposed to the dermal model for one hour followed by washing. Cellular viability was determined using the thiazolyl blue mitochondrial conversion assay (MTT). The concentration of sample that inhibited 50% (EC50) of the dye conversion relative to control was calculated and compared to the in vivo data. Samples yielding Draize scores greater than 15 were classified as positive irritants; using this criteria the MTT assay performed as follows: sensitivity = 83%, specificity = 88%.

G16
RESULTS OF THE GERMAN VALIDATION PROJECT OF ALTERNATIVES TO THE DRAIZE EYE TEST
H. Spielmann, M. Liebsch, I. Gerner, S. Kalweit, T. Wirnsberger
ZEBET (Zentralstelle zur Erfassung und Bewerttung von Eraatz-und Erganzungsmethoden zum Tierversuch) Bundesgesundheltsamt, Pf. 330013, D-1000 Berlin 33

Since 1988 ZEBET has coordinated a national German interlaboratory study on the validation of two alternative methods to the Draize rabbit's eye test, the neutral red/kenacid blue (NR/KB) cytotoxicity assay and the hen's egg chorioallantoic membrane (HET-CAM) test.

During the first two years the two methods were established in twelve laboratories to ensure intra-and interlaboratory reproducibility. Testing 32 chemicals from a variety of chemical classes indicated a better correlation between data from the HET/CAM test and both human and Draize test data than between cytotoxicity and the *in vivo* data.

During the final experimental stage of "data base development' (Balls et al., ATLA 18, 313-337, 1990) 165 chemicals were tested in both test systems to provide information whether and to what extent the *in vitro* tests might be able to replace the Draize rabbit's eye test. The test chemicals selected are representing a broad spectrum of both chemical classes and *in vivo* eye irritating properties.

The evaluation of a total of 200 chemicals tested during the validation study indicates a sufficient positive predictive value of the HET-CAM test and a poor correlation between cytotoxicity and *in vivo* data.

It will be discussed with industry and government agencies to which extent the validated *in vitro* methods can replace the mandatory Draize test in international guidelines of the CEC and OECD.

G17
In Vitro Cell Culture Investigation of Fish Eye Lens Cataract.
Christopher D. Williams, Robert J. Huggett, and Mohamed Faisal
Virginia Institute of Marine Science, College of William and Mary
Gloucester Point, VA., 23062

Cataract is the major cause of blindness in vertebrates, including fish. In this respect, the positive association of cataract development in fish with sediment levels of polycyclic aromatic hydrocarbons (PAH) has been reported. The lack of an *in vitro* cellular system has limited research into the mechanism responsible for cataractogenesis. Work by this laboratory has successfully established the first *in vitro* culture system for fish eye lens cells. Eye cells derived from the marine teleost spot (*Leiostomus xanthurus*) have been maintained for 22 months and successfully subcultured through 15 passages. Cultures showed a sequence of events at the cellular level which indicated crystalline synthesis similar to that described for murine animals. The synthesis of crystalline is indicative of cellular differentiation of epithelial cells to fiber cells. Investigations into the synthesis of macromolecules indicated that lens cells derived from cataractous fish showed a ten-fold increase in DNA as compared to control cells while non-cataractous fish, exposed to the same chemical environment as that of the cataract fish, displayed a seven-fold increase. In contrast, direct exposure of eye cells to the PAH benzo[a]pyrene-7,8-dihydrodiol showed inhibition, 0-67%, in the synthesis of DNA, RNA, and protein examined over a 15 day trial period. This indicates the presence of other factors that influence fish eye cells. Our studies indicate that the *in vitro* culture of fish eye lens cells is a promising non-mammalian model for research in the field of ocular toxicology.

H. Validation

H1
THE USE OF NORMAL HUMAN KERATINOCYTES AND THE NEUTRAL RED UPTAKE BIOASSAY TO ASSESS THE FIRST 30 MEIC COMPOUNDS.
R.D. Curren[*], K.A. Wallace[*], J. Janus[**], and J.W. Harbell[*]. [*]Microbiological Associates, Inc., 9900 Blackwell Rd., Rockville, MD 20850, U.S.A.; [**] Clonetics Corporation, 9620 Chesapeake Drive, San Diego, CA 92123, U.S.A.

A cytotoxicity assay (Neutral Red Uptake [NRU]) utilizing normal human keratinocytes (NHEK) obtained from the Clonetics Corporation, San Diego, CA, U.S.A., has been reported to give results which correlate well with a small data set of human lethal blood concentrations (LBC) and human acute oral lethal doses (OLD). This conclusion was based on results from the first ten compounds of the Multicentre Evaluation of In Vitro Cytotoxicity (MEIC) panel. We have now tested the next twenty chemicals in this panel and find that a good correlation between the in vivo and in vitro data still holds. The assay was conducted by exposing keratinocytes in exponential growth to test materials for 48 hours before measuring viability by neutral red uptake. NRU_{50} values (the amount of test material which reduces the neutral red uptake to 50% of the control cultures) for MEIC compounds 11 - 30 ranged over four orders of magnitude, from 0.23 μM (thallium sulfate) to ~3,800 μM (sodium chloride). Correlations with both LBC and OLD were good for the 20 new materials as well as all 30 materials combined. In general, the outliers were caused by the in vitro test overpredicting the toxicity of the materials. For example, 1,1,1-trichloroethane, thallium sulfate, malathion and 2,4-dichlorophenoxyacetic acid were more toxic in NHEK than in humans, while lithium sulphate and the short chained alcohols were slightly more toxic in humans than predicted in vitro.

H2

PRELIMINARY RESULTS OF THE MEIC PROGRAMME - A SUMMARY

Björn Ekwall* and Erik Walum**

*   Dept. Toxicology, University of Uppsala, Box 594, S-751 24 Uppsala, Sweden
** Dept. Neurochemistry & Neurotoxicology, University of Stockholm, S-10691, Stockholm, Sweden

The Multicenter Evaluation of In Vitro Cytotoxicity (MEIC) is an international project to evaluate the relevance and reliability of toxicity and toxicokinetic in vitro tests (1). It started in 1989 and will be finalized in 1994. Interested laboratories are still invited to test 50 chemicals in their respective in vitro systems. Results will be evaluated for prediction of various types of general toxicity, such as acute and chronic, target organ, skin, and eye toxicity, with use of human data. Presently, 80 laboratories have joined, representing over 200 methods. The first 10 chemicals have been tested in 100 systems.

The latter results have been used as a training set in preliminary evaluation, to demonstrate evaluation methods. First, a majority of 14 cytotoxicity tests predicted human lethal blood concentrations and doses better than rodent LD50 data (1). Second, in vitro IC10 (10% inhib. conc.) of the same tests predicted sublethal, moderately toxic human blood concentrations well (2). Third, all 100 in vitro data sets have been compared. The majority of assays tested toxicity to mammalian cells, with 24-72 h exposure and various toxicity criteria (MTT, LDH, NR, Protein etc.). Most of these tests gave similar results, independent of the toxic endpoint. This must be due to a close integration of basal cell functions - after 24h various types of primary chemical toxicity is spread to all organelles. Tests on organ specific cells/functions were more sensitive than the basal cytotoxicity tests for some chemicals, which could predict human target organ toxicity.

MEIC members have already published 16 independent papers on MEIC-connected research, some of them presenting own evaluation (listed in ref. 3).

References: 1. B. Ekwall et al., ATLA 17 (1989), 83-100. 2. E. Walum et al., MEIC Newsletter 2/3 (1990), 1-4. 3. MEIC Newsletter 3/4 (1992).

H3

IVT Databank Project Results: PC software for managing *in vitro* toxicity testing data. Green, M.R., Technical Database Services, Inc. (TDS) and Frazier, J.M., Johns Hopkins Center for Alternatives to Animal Testing (CAAT).

The In Vitro Toxicity Testing (IVT) Databank is a project initiated by TDS in consultation with CAAT. Our goal is to establish a central repository of verified data from which toxicologists in industry, testing labs, academia and government can draw detailed information on *in vitro* toxicity testing procedures. The IVT Databank was developed to provide detailed testing methods and related test results - *in vitro* and *in vivo* - for a large number of pure chemicals and formulations. We intend to keep the IVT Databank current by encouraging toxicologists who are active in the field to contribute data which cannot be found in the published literature. The practical tasks of entering and tracking data, and managing a complex and dynamic database involving many respondents can be daunting. To help meet this challenge, TDS developed the IVT Data Collection Instrument (IVT/DCI), a database management system for the PC, which can be used by respondents, CAAT, data verifiers and project staff. Now, we have released a new version of the IVT/DCI which can help toxicologists manage large inhouse databases of *in vitro* research findings for their laboratories.

H4

THE PROBLEM OF COLLINEARITY AND THE VALIDATION OF *IN VITRO* TESTS.
Robert L. Lipnick. U.S. Environmental Protection Agency, Office of Pollution Prevention and Toxics (TS-796), Washington, DC 20460.

At the turn of the century, H.H. Meyer and coworkers[1] at the University of Marburg were led to the discovery of the correlation between partition coefficient and anesthetic potency by the failure of certain chemicals to obey Richet's Rule (potency is inversely proportional to water solubility). Beginning in the 1930s, N.V. Lazarev,[2] at the Leningrad Institute of Industrial Hygiene and Worker Safety, investigated the high degree of intercorrelation of various physicochemical properties with both one another and with toxicity for simple nonreactive nonelectrolyte organic compounds acting by a narcosis mechanism. Within a large and diverse set of test chemicals, Lazarev found that the best correlations were obtained using partition coefficient. The problem of *collinearity* encountered by Meyer and Lazarev as well as numerous other scientists studying biological activity needs to be critically addressed in the development of schemes for the validation of *in vitro* tests. The ability to define the mechanistic foundation of an *in vitro* test and its mechanistic relationship to the *in vivo* biological system for which it would serve as a surrogate would increase its utility for predictive purposes by systematically defining the validity domain of chemical and physicochemical property space. Illustrations will be provided of how modern methods used in the area of QSAR can be applied to the rational selection of candidate test chemicals for the validation of *in vitro* tests.

[1]R.L. Lipnick, *Trends Pharmacol. Sci.* (1989) 10, 265-269; [2]*Ibid*, (1992) 13, 56-60.